ADVANCES IN

Ophthalmology and Optometry

Editor-in-Chief
Myron Yanoff, MD

Chair Emeritus, Ophthalmology, Professor, Departments of Ophthalmology and Pathology, College of Medicine, Drexel University, Philadelphia, Pennsylvania

ELSEVIER

PHILADELPHIA LONDON TORONTO MONTREAL SYDNEY TOKYO

ADVANCES IN
Ophthalmology and Optometry

VOLUMES 1 to 2 (OUT OF PRINT)

VOLUME 3

Director, Continuity Publishing: Taylor Ball
Editor: Lauren Boyle
Developmental Editor: Meredith Madeira

Printed in the United States of America.

Editorial Office:
Elsevier
1600 John F. Kennedy Blvd,
Suite 1800
Philadelphia, PA 19103-2899

International Standard Serial Number: 2452-1760
International Standard Book Number: 13: 978-0-323-71199-9

ADVANCES IN
Ophthalmology and Optometry

JOSEPH M. ORTIZ, MD, FRCOphth – Glaucoma
Consultant in Ophthalmology, Sacred Heart Hospital, Allentown, Pennsylvania; Consultant in Ophthalmology, Abington Memorial Hospital, Abington, Pennsylvania; Formerly Assistant Professor of Ophthalmology, Hahnemann University Hospital, Drexel University School of Medicine, Philadelphia, Pennsylvania

LEONARD J. PRESS, OD, FAAO, FCOVD – Optometry
Optometric Director, The Vision & Learning Center, Fair Lawn, New Jersey; Adjunct Professor, Southern College of Optometry, Memphis, Tennessee

APARNA RAMASUBRAMANIAN, MD – Pediatric Ophthalmology
Pediatric Ophthalmology/Oncology, Department of Ophthalmology and Visual Sciences & Graham Brown Cancer Center, University of Louisville, Louisville, Kentucky

CONTRIBUTORS

SARINA AMIN, MD, Vitreoretinal Surgery Fellow, Department of Ophthalmology, USC Roski Eye Institute, Keck School of Medicine of USC, Los Angeles, California, USA

PETER J. BELIN, MD, Chief, Resident, Department of Ophthalmology, Donald and Barbara Zucker School of Medicine at Hofstra/Northwell, Great Neck, New York, USA

JESSE L. BERRY, MD, Associate Professor, Department of Ophthalmology, USC Roski Eye Institute, Keck School of Medicine of USC, Associate Director of Ocular Oncology, The Vision Center, Children's Hospital Los Angeles, Los Angeles, California, USA

KRITI BHAGAT, OD, FAAO, Adjunct Assistant Professor of Optometric Medicine, Former Director, Ocular Surface Disease Clinic, The Eye Institute of the Pennsylvania College of Optometry at Salus University, Philadelphia, Pennsylvania, USA

POOJA BHAT, MD, Assistant Professor, Department of Ophthalmology, Illinois Eye and Ear Infirmary, The University of Illinois at Chicago, Chicago, Illinois, USA

ETTY BITTON, OD, MSc, FAAO, FBCLA, Associate Professor of Optometry, Director, Dry Eye Clinic, École d'Optométrie, Université de Montréal, Montreal, Quebec, Canada

DONALD L. BUDENZ, MD, MPH, Professor and Chair, Department of Ophthalmology, The University of North Carolina at Chapel Hill, Chapel Hill, North Carolina, USA

BRETT CAMPBELL, MD, PGY-2 Resident, Department of Ophthalmology, College of Medicine, Drexel University, Philadelphia, Pennsylvania, USA

CARA E. CAPITENA YOUNG, MD, Assistant Professor, Department of Ophthalmology, University of Colorado Hospital, Aurora, Colorado, USA

JUDY L. CHEN, MD, Department of Ophthalmology, Illinois Eye and Ear Infirmary, The University of Illinois at Chicago, Chicago, Illinois, USA

JEFFREY COOPER, MS, OD, FAAO, Professor Emeritus, SUNY College of Optometry, New York, New York, USA

STUART G. COUPLAND, PhD, Department of Ophthalmology, University of Ottawa Eye Institute, Ottawa Hospital Research Institute, The Ottawa Hospital, Ottawa, Ontario, Canada

DAVID A. CRANDALL, MD, Glaucoma Fellowship Director, Department of Ophthalmology, Henry Ford Health System, Detroit, Michigan, USA; John Moran Eye Center, University of Utah, Salt Lake City, Utah, USA

ALIREZA GHAFFARIEH, MD, Clinical Pathology Fellow, Department of Pathology, Keck School of Medicine of USC, University of Southern California (USC), Los Angeles, California, USA

BENJAMIN KAMBIZ GHIAM, MD, Oakland University, William Beaumont School of Medicine, Rochester, Michigan, USA

ROBIN N. GINSBURG, MD, Department of Ophthalmology, Icahn School of Medicine at Mount Sinai, Department of Ophthalmology, New York Eye and Ear Infirmary of Mount Sinai, New York, New York, USA

JONATHAN P. GREENBERG, MBBCh, Department of Ophthalmology, Northwell Health, New York, New York, USA

DAVID L. GUYTON, MD, The Johns Hopkins University, The Johns Hopkins Hospital, Baltimore, Maryland, USA

MADELEINE HASBROOK, MD, Department of Ophthalmology, Henry Ford Health System, Detroit, Michigan, USA

ISABELLA IRRCHER, PhD, MSc, Assistant Professor, Department of Ophthalmology, Kingston Health Sciences Centre-HDH Site, Queen's University, Kingston, Ontario, Canada

MALIK Y. KAHOOK, MD, Professor, Department of Ophthalmology, University of Colorado Hospital, Aurora, Colorado, USA

EVAN KALIN-HAJDU, MD, Assistant Professor, Department of Ophthalmology, Affiliated to Université de Montréal, Montréal, Québec, Canada

RUSTUM KARANJIA, MD, PhD, FRCSC, DABO, Department of Ophthalmology, David Geffen School of Medicine at UCLA, Doheny Eye Institute, Los Angeles, California, USA; Department of Ophthalmology, University of Ottawa Eye Institute, Ottawa Hospital Research Institute, The Ottawa Hospital, Ottawa, Ontario, Canada

AHMED M. KASSEM, MD, Attending Physician, Pediatric Ophthalmology, Sanford Health, Sanford South University Medical Center, Fargo, North Dakota, USA

IRFAN KHAN, MD, Assistant Professor, Department of Ophthalmology, University of Virginia, Charlottesville, Virginia, USA

YASSER KHAN, MD, Associate Clinical Professor, Oculoplastics, Orbital and Ophthalmic Surgery, McMaster University, Hamilton, Ontario, Canada; Carrot Eye Clinic, Brampton, Ontario, Canada

BRUCE H. KOFFLER, MD, Department of Ophthalmology, Associate Clinical Professor, University of Kentucky, Lexington, Kentucky, USA

RONNI M. LIEBERMAN, MD, Assistant Professor, Director, Department of Ophthalmology, Icahn School of Medicine at Mount Sinai, New York, New York, USA

MICHAEL J. LIPSON, OD, FAAO, FSLS, Department of Ophthalmology and Visual Science, Associate Professor, University of Michigan, Ann Arbor, Michigan, USA

ANN-MARIE LOBO-CHAN, MD, Assistant Professor, Department of Ophthalmology, Illinois Eye and Ear Infirmary, The University of Illinois at Chicago, Chicago, Illinois, USA

SARA NÚÑEZ MÁRQUEZ, MD, Fellow, Oculoplastics, Orbital and Ophthalmic Surgery, McMaster University, Hamilton, Ontario, Canada

ANNA J. MATHEW, MD, Assistant Professor, Department of Pathology, Keck School of Medicine of USC, University of Southern California (USC), Keck Hospital of USC, Los Angeles, California, USA

OSAMA MUFTI, MD, Kentucky Lions Eye Center, University of Louisville, Louisville, Kentucky, USA

JEAN-CLAUDE MWANZA, MD, MPH, PhD, Associate Professor, Department of Ophthalmology, The University of North Carolina at Chapel Hill, Chapel Hill, North Carolina, USA

AMY C. NAU, OD, FAAO, Korb & Associates, Boston, Massachusetts, USA

SAGAR PATEL, MD, Vitreoretinal Surgery Fellow, Department of Ophthalmology, USC Roski Eye Institute, Keck School of Medicine of USC, Los Angeles, California, USA

KRISHI PEDDADA, MD, PGY-3 Resident, Department of Ophthalmology, College of Medicine, Drexel University, Philadelphia, Pennsylvania, USA

TIMOTHY J. PEIRIS, MD, Department of Ophthalmology, Northwell Health, New York, New York, USA

BRIANA PLY, MD, PGY-2 Resident, Department of Ophthalmology, College of Medicine, Drexel University, Philadelphia, Pennsylvania, USA

ASHLEY POLSKI, BS, Department of Ophthalmology, USC Roski Eye Institute, Keck School of Medicine of USC, Los Angeles, California, USA

APARNA RAMASUBRAMANIAN, MD, Assistant Professor, Kentucky Lions Eye Center, University of Louisville, Louisville, Kentucky, USA

SHERIEF RAOUF, MD, PGY-2 Resident, Department of Ophthalmology, Donald and Barbara Zucker School of Medicine at Hofstra/Northwell, Great Neck, New York, USA

ASHVINI REDDY, MD, Associate Professor of Ophthalmology, Retina Division, Dean McGee Eye Institute, Oklahoma City, Oklahoma, USA

RICHARD RIVERS, MD, PhD, MBA, Hopkins Epic Anesthesia Physician Champion and Physician Builder, Associate Professor of Anesthesiology and Critical Care Medicine, Associate Professor of Ophthalmology, The Johns Hopkins University, Baltimore, Maryland, USA

MARIA SIBUG SABER, MD, Assistant Professor of Clinical Pathology and Ophthalmology, Associate Director of Ocular Pathology, Department of Pathology, USC Roski Eye Institute, Keck School of Medicine of USC, University of Southern California (USC), Keck Hospital of USC, Los Angeles, California, USA

LEONARD K. SEIBOLD, MD, Associate Professor, Department of Ophthalmology, University of Colorado Hospital, Aurora, Colorado, USA

JOEL A. SILBERT, OD, FAAO, Professor of Optometric Medicine, Cornea & Specialty Contact Lens Service, The Eye Institute of the Pennsylvania College of Optometry at Salus University, Philadelphia, Pennsylvania, USA

ETHAN K. SOBOL, MD, Department of Ophthalmology, Icahn School of Medicine at Mount Sinai, New York, New York, USA

JEFFREY R. SOOHOO, MD, Associate Professor, Department of Ophthalmology, University of Colorado Hospital, Aurora, Colorado, USA

RAN STEIN, MD, Attending, Division of Oculoplastics, Department of Ophthalmology, Shamir Medical Center, Affiliated to Tel-Aviv University, Tel-Aviv, Israel

MARTIN WILLIAM TEN HOVE, MEng, MD, FRCSC, Department Head and Associate Professor, Department of Ophthalmology, Kingston Health Sciences Centre-HDH Site, Queen's University, Kingston, Ontario, Canada

AN VO, MD, Faculty, Department of Ophthalmology, College of Medicine, Drexel University, Philadelphia, Pennsylvania, USA

CARL S. WILKINS, MD, Department of Ophthalmology, Icahn School of Medicine at Mount Sinai, New York, New York, USA

KELLY WILLIAMSON, MD, Assistant Professor of Ophthalmology, Drexel University College of Medicine, Philadelphia, Pennsylvania, USA

EDWARD J. WLADIS, MD, FACS, Professor and Chairman, Lions Eye Institute, Department of Ophthalmology, Ophthalmic Plastic Surgery, Albany Medical College, Albany, New York, USA

CONTENTS

VOLUME 4 • 2019

Microinvasive Glaucoma Surgeries and When to Use Them

Cara E. Capitena Young, Leonard K. Seibold, Jeffrey R. SooHoo, and Malik Y. Kahook

Video content accompanies this article at http://www.advancesinophthalmology.com.

Section VII: Neuro-ophthalmology

Electrophysiology in Neuro-Ophthalmology

Rustum Karanjia and Stuart G. Coupland

Advances in Teleophthalmology: Is It Ready for Neuro-Ophthalmology?

Isabella Irrcher and Martin William ten Hove

Section VIII: Cornea and External Diseases

Section IX: Oculoplastics

Section X: Uveitis

Advances in Ophthalmology and Optometry 4 (2019) xxiii

ADVANCES IN OPHTHALMOLOGY AND OPTOMETRY

Preface

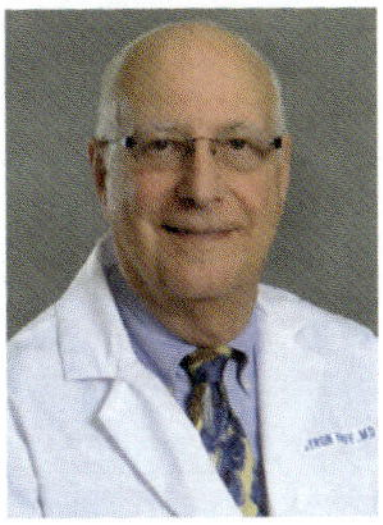

Myron Yanoff, MD
Editor

In Volume 4 of *Advances in Ophthalmology and Optometry* we continue to explore the new ideas, new treatments, new ways of doing things to give us a fresh frame of reference to sort through the crush of data and to make sense in a real way of how to proceed. We again have asked experts in each of the pertinent fields to sift through current literature to give us insights on the latest developments such as: adjustable suture strabismus surgery in children; advances in diagnosis and management of dry-eye disease; sterile intraocular inflammation after intravitreal injection–diagnosis and management; biopsy techniques in ocular oncology; perioperative management of uveitic cataracts; light-adjustable intraocular lens; the flanged, intrascleral, intraocular-lens fixation with double-needle technique; orthokeratology for myopia control in children; and much more.

We do hope that you enjoy reading this volume and share our enthusiasm for what the authors have accomplished in giving us their wisdom and perceptions.

Myron Yanoff, MD
Departments of Ophthalmology and Pathology
Drexel University College of Medicine
219 North Broad Street, 3rd Floor
Philadelphia, PA 19107, USA

E-mail address: my26@drexel.edu

https://doi.org/10.1016/j.yaoo.2019.05.004
2452-1760/19/

Section I: Optometry

Advances in Ophthalmology and Optometry 4 (2019) 1–12

ADVANCES IN OPHTHALMOLOGY AND OPTOMETRY

Medical Application of Contact Lens Technology

Amy C. Nau, OD

Korb & Associates, 400 Commonwealth Avenue, Suite 2, Boston, MA 02215, USA

Keywords

• Contact lens technology • Myopia control • Ocular surface protection
• Scleral lens • Ortho-Keratology

Key points

The worldwide increase in the incidence of myopia has spurred advancements in contact lens approaches to myopia reduction.

Amniotic membrane lenses are being used to treat advanced ocular surface disease, and improvements in tissue reproducibility are being developed.

Scleral contact lenses are now mainstream and are being used to correct complex refractive errors and corneal irregularity, and are increasingly used as therapy for ocular surface rehabilitation.

Although historically contact lenses have provided primarily cosmetic benefits to patients, now they are able to provide therapeutic benefits to restore ocular surface health, prevent more invasive surgical procedures, and help control myopia. Contact lens manufacturers have worked in tandem with the eyecare community to push their technologies to accommodate these contemporary needs. It is stimulating to be immersed in this expanded use of contact lenses, which now are seen as much as a way to treat and prevent ocular disease as they are a way to increase cosmesis. Related to this is the need to be well-versed in the identification and management of anterior segment disorders. If patients are relying on their contact lenses for medical treatment, there must be an understanding of the complex interplay between a contact lens, the eye, and the lid, and the ability to recognize and treat problems that may arise from their use.

Disclosures: A.C. Nau has received payment for speaking from Johnson & Johnson, Avedro, and Review of Optometry.

E-mail address: anau@korbassociates.com

https://doi.org/10.1016/j.yaoo.2019.04.001
2452-1760/19/

The goal of this article is to provide an overview of how modern contact lens technologies can be exploited in the context of myopia control and management of ocular surface diseases in ways that have heretofore been impossible.

MYOPIA CONTROL

Pathologic myopia, which usually begins to manifest during childhood, represents an endemic vision-threatening problem in many industrialized countries. The goal of myopia control is to blunt rapid ametropization, which can lead to high amounts of myopia (generally considered to be >6 diopters [D]). Candidates for therapy include children who are showing rapid progression, many of whom also have a genetic predisposition. There have historically been inconsistent definitions of what constitutes pathologic or degenerative myopia, and it is important to distinguish it from high myopia. The former includes elongation of axial length and the presence of posterior staphyloma. The ensuing changes to the shape of the globe carry risk of acquired pathologic conditions such as glaucoma, macular atrophy, choroidal neovascularization, retinal detachment, macular hole formation, and cataract. It is now indisputable that myopia progression can be slowed to at least some degree with certain patients [1]. Studies show that the antimuscarinic agents, such as pirenzepine or atropine eye drops, tend to be very effective [2]; however, not all patients want to approach myopia control in this way. Single-vision rigid gas permeable (GP) lenses [3] and single-vision soft contact lenses [4] are not effective means of myopia control. Two types of contact lenses exist that have been proven to provide some degree of myopia control: center distance bifocals and overnight orthokeratology (ortho-k) lenses.

Bifocal contact lenses

Bifocal contact lenses come in aspheric, center near, and center distance options, and in soft, hybrid, corneal GP, and scleral lenses modalities. Myopia control using contact lenses is based on the idea that once axial elongation occurs, the periphery of the retina is no longer in focus, with images peripheral to the macula falling behind the retina. This peripheral hyperopic error acts as a stimulus to further eye growth even if the macular area is fully corrected [5]. Eventually, practitioners deduced that exploiting optical correction in contact lenses to create ametropic errors in the retinal periphery might affect the stimulus to continued axial elongation. This was shown to occur in chicks [6] and later with marmosets [7]. A meta-analysis in 2017 concluded that concentric ring and multifocal soft contact lenses could reduce myopia progression between 30% and 50% over a 2-year period, and that concentric ring bifocal soft lenses seem to have greater effect than peripheral add multifocal soft lenses [8]. Some practitioners try any type of multifocal soft lens for myopia control, thinking that just reducing accommodation will produce an effect. However, center near contact lens designs will fail to introduce the necessary peripheral retinal hyperopic defocus. Generally, when fitting contacts for myopia control, higher add powers will generate larger effects. Fortunately, visual acuity seems not to suffer much with high add designs [9].

A newer development in the multifocal lens category is the introduction of customized optic zones that are based on pupil size. Although smaller optic zones generally are preferable, young people have larger pupils and, therefore, designs generated for presbyopes (who have smaller pupils) might cause glare, especially under mesopic or scotopic conditions. Some companies will allow for customizable center distance optic zones, which can be adjusted depending on pupil size.

In the soft lens category, few center distance multifocal options exist for patients with astigmatism. If the astigmatism is primarily corneal, then a corneal GP, center distance bifocal lens could be considered. In addition to the benefits of sharp vision, ease of handling, and reduced incidence of infection, they often are cost-effective. Topography-guided systems allow for optimal alignment fitting with astigmatic corneas, provided a good scan is obtained. GP lenses offer ultimate customization for bifocal designs with essentially unlimited parameters, allowing practitioners to design lenses as they wish. An especially good attribute is that the bifocal add power can be made quite high, so that if a patient's myopia is not responding with a certain add power, then a higher add power can be ordered, which is not always possible with commodity soft lenses. However, if the patient is participating in contact sports or is often outside in dirty environments, GP lenses can be less desirable. That said, when designed properly, GP lenses should be comfortable, and if a patient has not previously been exposed to soft lenses, adaptation is rarely an issue.

A nice alternative to more traditional GP contacts are hybrid lenses that can similarly neutralize relatively large amounts of astigmatism. Synergeyes™ (Carlsbad, CA, USA) has recently expanded their parameters so that a distance center bifocal lens is available. Their distance center hybrid features Center Distance FlexOptics, which provides for adjustable center distance optics, depending on photopic pupil size, and add powers range from +0.75 to +5.00 D. Moreover, hybrid lenses tend to center very well, which can be an issue with a corneal-based GP. Compared with GP lenses, hybrid lenses may be more tolerable and may be better suited for dusty or dirty conditions, such as a soccer field, and are less likely to become dislodged or come out of the eye. Of course, hybrid lenses are a great option even for patients without astigmatism as an alternative to corneal GP lenses or a soft distance center bifocal.

Full scleral and miniscleral lenses are becoming very popular for presbyopes, given their stability, ability to correct astigmatism, essentially unlimited add powers and customizable optic zones, which are especially helpful for controlling centration. Many practitioners are more comfortable with miniscleral designs because they can be less intimidating and are easier to handle. However, larger lenses offer several advantages, including spreading the load-bearing weight of the lens over a larger surface area, increased vault capabilities, and avoiding conjunctival vascular impingement. Generally, larger diameter lenses are more comfortable and, for patients with ocular surface issues, larger lenses confer greater potential for rehabilitation and protection.

Scleral lenses theoretically are an excellent option for myopia control because the optics are completely stable, which promotes correct placement of the optic zone. However, use of scleral lenses in children is not common outside of pathologic indications, and scleral lenses for myopia reduction have not been well-studied. It should be noted that none of the available multifocal contact lens designs are approved by the US Food and Drug Administration (FDA) for myopia control, so patients and parents must be informed that this is an off-label usage.

Orthokeratology

The first ortho-k lenses in the 1960s were unpredictable and were made from polymethyl methacrylate (PMMA) material [10]. The 1980s saw the initial development of reverse zone lens designs. Further developments coincided with advanced manufacturing with computer-assisted lathing, improvements in corneal topography, and the introduction of highly oxygen-permeable polymers. These factors culminated in lenses that could produce more predictable refractive results, and ortho-k achieved FDA approval for the correction of myopia in 1994. That same year in Asia, clinicians began to postulate that ortho-k might be an approach to control myopia progression [11]. It was not until 2002 that the FDA approved ortho-k lenses that could be worn overnight. Currently, there are several laboratories that make proprietary lenses, which are often referred to as retainer devices.

A properly fit ortho-k lens has to be centered perfectly with tear exchange present but with minimal movement. The treatment zone has to be flat enough to be effective at instigating epithelial migration while avoiding formation of central islands; however, if the central curve is too flat, the lens will irritate the cornea and/or be uncomfortable. Decentration of the lens might cause irregular astigmatism that will blur vision. Currently, ametropias of +2.00 to −6.00 D with less than 1.75 D of corneal cylinder are potential candidates for ortho-k. Patients with high amounts of astigmatism are not considered good candidates for spherical ortho-k lenses because decentration may be an issue, which would cause irregular astigmatism [12]. New toric designs are now available for patients with moderate myopia and low astigmatism, which expands the number of patients who can be treated [13]. Although in some studies visual acuity between toric and nontoric designs was similar, posttreatment topography with toric designs demonstrated smoother corneal profiles. This may not affect high-resolution visual acuity but could help reduce higher order aberrations, which have been shown to increase after corneal reshaping with lenses [14]. Topography-guided ortho-k lenses are an excellent choice for truly customizing low amounts of astigmatic correction and can help achieve stable centration. Although these systems represent powerful tools for optimizing lens fits, success is predicated on acquiring good topography scans, which sometimes can be challenging in children.

Overnight ortho-k for correction of ametropia works by causing a redistribution of corneal epithelial cells from the center to the periphery in a controlled manner that is dictated by the shape of the reverse geometry lens design. This has been postulated for some time and has been confirmed by a recent study using anterior segment optical coherence tomography (OCT) [15]. This same study validates prior literature regarding the linear relationship between degree of correction and the amount of central epithelial thinning (an inverse relationship with treatment zone diameter), and a lack of effect of mid peripheral stromal thickening on refractive change.

Ortho-k is an option for patients who work in dusty or dirty environments during the day or who are exposed to recreational or occupational water sources. It is an option for patients who cannot tolerate other forms of lenses, if the patient's eyes are not too dry. Patients with environmental allergies or with poor blinking habits also are potential candidates. Like all contact lenses, reported complications include glare, infection, and irregular astigmatism. Another consideration is the transition period in and out of these lenses, during which time corneal topography and refraction are unstable. Starting in the 1990s, investigations began to be published that explored in earnest the usefulness of ortho-k lenses for myopia control. Several studies, which are effectively summarized in a recent article by Cooper and Tkatchenko [1], have shown that ortho-k lenses can slow myopia progression by about 45% and, therefore, should also be considered as an option for reducing myopia progression. This is a popular method for control in Asia but less so in Western countries. The mechanism by which ortho-k lenses control myopia is through control of peripheral defocus, similar to the center distance bifocals discussed previously. Lens-induced peripheral migration of the epithelial cells creates an oblate corneal profile, thereby effectively reducing central myopic defocus and simultaneously allowing for peripheral placement of the image on the retinal plane; if the oblate cornea can be sufficiently remodeled, myopic defocus might even be achieved.

Myopia control summary

Using contact lenses for control of myopia is typically restricted to pediatric populations. When determining which type of lens for myopia control is right for a given patient, several factors must to be considered. A child's motivation to use contact lenses is the most important determinant; a child who is hesitant will likely not use the lenses and, therefore, will not be successful with myopia control. Second, the child has to be sufficiently responsible to handle lens care and use independently. If a child cannot use lenses when not in the presence of a parent or caregiver, use atropine drops. Participation in sports is another factor. If a patient is involved in water sports and cannot see well enough in the water to not be corrected, then ortho-k lenses are a good option. If a patient plays contact sports without eye protection, then rigid lenses should probably be avoided. When prescribing contact lenses for children, careful follow-up is needed and working parents with sometimes overscheduled children must accept the extra visits required compared with atropine drops for myopia control. Having spare lenses on hand also is recommended (especially for ortho-k) and represents an additional expense.

An important new issue to consider is the multitude of reports that prove that meibomian gland dysfunction (MGD) occurs in children [16,17]. Contact lenses have been shown to impair blinking, which will also potentially cause MGD [18]. Therefore, meibography and assessment of meibomian gland status should be conducted at baseline and thereafter annually. If MGD begins, then a change in lens type (ortho-k) or a switch to atropine drops should be considered. Early education about prophylactic lid care and blinking is imperative for all young people.

OCULAR SURFACE PROTECTION

Amniotic membranes

Amniotic membrane (AM) lenses are a newer category, used exclusively for ocular surface restoration and rehabilitation. Initially used for burn and wound care, starting as early as 1910 [19], their use has greatly expanded. These biologic devices are now used when there are nonhealing corneal or conjunctival defects, or ocular surface inflammation that is recalcitrant to other therapies and surgery [20]. The AM is easily harvested, easily stored for use when needed, and is not immunogenic. The tissue has been shown in multiple studies to have healing properties, antimicrobial and antiinflammatory effects, and may reduce pain [21]. However, AMs are far from a miracle cure for all conditions, and their results not only vary but recurrence of pathologic conditions such as neurotrophic keratitis and dry eye can occur [22]. Reviewing the available literature shows few randomized, investigator-masked studies with good control groups [23], and many more studies represent case series. These are valuable; however, the zeal for these devices could be premature without more rigorous investigation. Refractory pathologic conditions are not always remedied by these devices; however, for acute exacerbations, there is certainly an emerging place for them in clinical practice.

There are anecdotal reports that AM lenses have not been effective. What is important to remember when using biologics is that the health and integrity of donor tissue may vary. Although membrane donors are screened for infectious diseases, there are some infections for which screening protocols have not been developed, such as prion diseases. A detailed social and medical history is important to try to eliminate ineligible donors. However, the system is imperfect and lifestyle events or a biologic idiosyncrasy that could affect the healing properties of the membrane exist. It is for this reason that the use of porcine membranes is being investigated. Animals raised on medical farms in highly controlled environments might produce a more consistent product; however, the myriad of issues surrounding this practice have not yet been legislated.

Human AM is the innermost part of amnion that is made up of 3 layers: the single-layered epithelium, a thick basement membrane, and an avascular stroma [24]. The membranes are obtained from planned cesarean sections from donors who have been screened for transmissible diseases. There are different methods for processing AM: cryopreservation or dehydration. The cryopreservation process involves washing the placenta, then separating the AM from the chorion. The membrane is cut, then placed in glycerol or dimethyl sulfoxide preservation media at -80°C to allow slow freezing without ice formation. This method retains extracellular matrix components, which promote healing and antiinflammatory effects. The membrane must be maintained in a frozen state (-80°C) and be thawed immediately before use. Prokera by BioTissue (Miami, FL, USA) is a cryopreserved AM corneal bandage, suspended within a circular ring for direct placement of the stromal side on the surface of the affected eye. If patients find the insert uncomfortable, a tape tarsorrhaphy can be used.

Dehydration of the AM is another processing technique in which vacuum application removes all moisture, thereby reducing enzymatic activity and inhibiting growth of pathogens. The patented PURION™ (MiMedx, Marietta, GA, USA) process results in a durable graft that has a shelf life of up to 5 years. Studies show that biological activity is maintained [25]. Examples of dehydrated membranes include AmbioDisc (Katena, Denville, NJ, USA), BioDOptix (Integra Life Sciences, Plainsboro, NJ, USA), and Aril (Seed Biotech, Dallas, TX, USA). Dehydrated AM bandage lenses are stored at room temperature but must be rehydrated before use and covered with a bandage soft contact lens once on the eye. Similar to the cryopreserved version, the stromal side of the membrane is placed in contact with the ocular surface. Although it is not yet routine to use AMs, their use is becoming more widespread. Interested practitioners must get proper training on their indications and insertion or removal techniques, which vary by manufacturer. Otherwise, identify a local eye care provider to whom you can refer patients.

Scleral lenses

Use of contact lenses for the correction of irregular astigmatism is well-established. Rico-Del-Viejo and colleagues [26] provide an excellent 20-year review of GP, hybrid, piggyback, and scleral lenses in the management of keratoconus. GP lenses are extremely versatile, and their designs are sometimes extremely advanced with quadrant-specific edge designs and topography-guided freeform lens capabilities. They remain the most common form of correction for irregular astigmatism; however, the number of doctors prescribing scleral lenses has increased substantially in the past few years [27]. The primary indication for scleral lens use is corneal irregularity. Unlike corneal GP lenses, scleral lenses tend to be more comfortable. Many patients with keratoconus are being refit into scleral lenses, particularly because of their comfort and ability to provide clearer vision due to their stability, even when the topography is highly abnormal [28].

This has been an exciting development in the contact lens field, for it has enabled eye care practitioners who are interested to become more involved in managing sometimes severe ocular surface pathologic conditions alone or in cooperation with corneal specialists. Scleral lenses have been shown to improve the ocular surface for almost every pathologic condition for which they have been tried, including exposure keratitis, infections, neurotrophic keratitis, refractive surgery induced ectasia, graft-versus-host disease, Stevens Johnson Syndrome, recurrent erosions, dry eye, and other complex ocular surface diseases [29,30]. This is accomplished by creating a fluid reservoir, which bathes the cornea and conjunctiva, and also probably by decreasing the constant mechanical trauma caused by interactions with the eyelids. Scleral lenses also have been used as a drug delivery vehicle [31]. Scleral lens success has now piqued the interest of the entire eyecare community, which has encouraged referrals to those who specialize in such lenses. In some patients, the use of scleral lenses has avoided the need for more invasive surgical procedures, causing many to choose between the bowl and the knife. A recent retrospective case series in Belgium demonstrated a nearly 50% reduction in the need for keratoplasty in 75 eyes with severe keratoconus with the use of scleral lenses [32].

Contact lens manufacturers have responded to the increased interest in scleral lenses by generating better lens architectures, which are easier to fit and more customizable. Older lenses were essentially spherical; however, the sclera becomes less regular with increasing distance from the limbus [33]. The Boston Foundation for Sight, established by Perry Rosenthal MD, who developed the Prosthetic Replacement of Ocular Surface Ecosystem (PROSE) lens, recently released the BostonSight lens (Boston Sight, Needham, MA, USA), which has a quadrant-specific haptic eccentricity design based on scleral anatomy derived from databases of previous fits. Topography-guided systems also are now leveraging their existing software programs to be able to create freeform haptic designs. The newest entry into this field is the EyePrint impression-based lens (EyePrint Prosthetics, Denver, CO, USA), which, because of computer software–driven design capabilities, is a quantum leap better than the historical scleral molds. The impression, once taken, is scanned and then can be manipulated to provide custom vaults and haptics so that lens adherence is not an issue. This particular lens also enables incorporation of limited amounts of vertical prism for patients with binocular imbalances. As long as a good impression is achieved, the lens fits in a single visit, making it convenient for patients who require a lens on an expedited basis. Scleral profiles can now be evaluated with several methods, including Eaglet Eye Surface Profiler (Eaglet-eye, Houten, The Netherlands), and anterior segment OCT. These emerging technologies are in-office devices for creating custom maps outside the limbus and have been introduced for scleral lens fitting. However, their use is not yet widespread, and many practitioners rely entirely on slit lamp evaluation of the lens features. Seasoned contact lens fitters are more likely to use toric haptics because the fit generally is worth the extra effort and cost needed to incorporate these parameters [34]. One remarkable consequence of the optics of scleral lenses is that it is now possible to incorporate multifocal designs into medical contact lenses, even for irregular surfaces. This can be quite successful (unless there is corneal scarring) and is a huge benefit for presbyopic patients with pathologic conditions.

Increasingly, scleral and miniscleral lenses are being used for refractive indications. In the absence of a pathologic condition, the fits are more straightforward and can be especially successful with presbyopic patients who have astigmatism. Scleral lenses also can be a way to allow patients whose dry eye is precluding comfortable lens use to remain in lenses, although patients who are fit with scleral lenses for correction of ametropia did not realize any improvement in signs or symptoms of ocular surface disease [35]. Bifocal scleral lenses now come in aspheric, center near, and center distance options, with a wide variety of options for add powers. Although the Scleral Lens in Ophthalmic Practice Evaluation

(SCOPE) research group showed that the complications of scleral lenses were low, they definitely can cause problems such as epithelial bogging [36], conjunctival prolapse, and post lens fogging [37]. Compression of conjunctival vasculature has been shown with anterior segment OCT [38], and the ultimate consequences for this are unknown. As anterior segment OCT-angiography becomes more available, checking for conjunctival blood flow integrity may become part of the standard fitting procedure. Another concern revolves around whether scleral lenses can increase intraocular pressure (IOP) [39]. This study was done on healthy subjects wearing scleral lenses for only a short time. It is known that corneal swelling can influence IOP measurements, especially in eyes with pathologic conditions [40]; therefore, the author suggests that, given the uncertainty surrounding IOP and scleral lens use, baseline pachymetry and IOP should be a routine part of scleral lens fitting. These parameters should be followed at regular intervals until the risks are better understood. Also, caution should be exercised when using scleral lenses for the correction of ametropia because iatrogenic complications can occur. There certainly are conditions for which scleral lenses should be used cautiously, including Fuchs dystrophy, patients who will insist on overnight use, pseudophakic bullous keratopathy, corneal grafts with low endothelial counts, or other conditions causing endothelial dysfunction, severe corneal neovascularization, uncontrolled epithelial bogging, excessive conjunctival chalasis, and possibly glaucoma. Given that the vast number of patients who wear scleral lenses have an underlying pathologic condition, it is imperative that these patients are closely monitored and refit as soon as complications related to lens use occur.

No accepted consensus exists on scleral lens fitting guidelines. Survey results of prescription and management practices among attendees at the 2017 Global Specialty Lens Symposium demonstrated that practitioners who have been fitting scleral lenses for more than 5 years tend to schedule follow-up visits to assess conjunctival compression, conjunctival staining, and corneal staining after contact lens removal, whereas less experienced providers exhibited more variability. In addition, new prescribers consider base curve, whereas experienced providers use sagittal depth for initial lens selection [40]. With scleral lenses, we do not know what we do not know. Therefore, until design philosophies have been standardized, practitioners must be prepared to refit if needed, and patients must be willing to accept the cost of new lenses if necessary.

Insurance companies are not keeping up with the trend toward use of contact lenses for medical management. Carriers will sometimes cover part of the cost of AMs; however, this varies highly by state and by insurance company. Despite increasing evidence of their benefit in wound care, many companies still consider the procedure experimental. Therefore, it is important to discuss all potential costs with patients beforehand and have them sign an advanced beneficiary notice form. Coverage for corneal GP and scleral lenses is becoming more common but only for limited indications, usually keratoconus. In general, insurance companies are less likely to authorize coverage for other types of ocular surface diseases, such as severe dry eye or neurotrophic keratitis. Methods for billing for medical contact lenses are beyond the scope of this article; however, operationally, the practitioner must determine how to proceed in such cases, which should be spelled out to the patient before the initiation of any new fit.

In the not too distant future, patients will have access to intelligent contact lenses having both medical and entertainment applications. Google, Sony, Novartis, Alcon, and multiple startup companies are heavily invested in contact lenses as a means to integrate technology and biology. Lenses that overcome presbyopia, enable night vision, record video, create the perception of virtual objects within real environments, release drugs, and monitor glucose and IOP are just some of the ideas being pursued. Smart lenses are being powered by everything from tiny solar receptors to using the motion of natural blinking. Some of these devices will likely interface with smartphones and, in some cases, will pair with auditory devices to eliminate the physical phone altogether. Beyond the obvious technological difficulties of incorporating electronics into a medium that is not only moist but requires biocompatibility, physiologic barriers exist that will need to be overcome. For example, patients with diabetes and glaucoma have a higher incidence of dry eye and thus may not be able to tolerate a lens worn on an all-day basis. Additionally, lenses incorporating electronics could be bulkier, causing hypoxic stress or comfort issues. There also will be legislative issues surrounding whether fittings from a licensed practitioner will be required or if entertainment-based lenses will be available direct to the consumer without a prescription.

SUMMARY

With an increased capacity to treat and manage ocular surface disease and myopia with contact lenses, there comes an ensuing opportunity for closer cooperation between anterior segment and medical contact lens specialists. Ultimately, input from each discipline will enhance patient outcomes and potentially reduce health care expenditures. The future is indeed bright for the contact lens industry.

References

[1] Cooper J, Tkatchenko A. A review of current concepts of the etiology and treatment of myopia. Eye Contact Lens 2018;44(4):231–47.

[2] Walline JJ. Myopia control: a review. Eye Contact Lens 2016;42(1):3–8.

[3] Walline JJ, Jones LA, Mutto DO, et al. A randomized trial of the effects of rigid contact lenses on myopia progression. Arch Ophthalmol 2004;122:1760–6.

[4] Walline JJ, Jones LA, Sinnott L, et al. A randomized trial of the effect of soft contact lenses on myopia progression in children. Invest Ophthalmol Vis Sci 2008;49:4702–6.

[5] Smith EL III, Hung LF, Huang J. Relative peripheral hyperopic defocus alters central refractive development in infant monkeys. Vision Res 2009;49:2386–92.

[6] Liu Y, Wildsoet C. The effective add inherent in 2-zone negative lenses inhibits eye growth in myopic young chicks. Invest Ophthalmol Vis Sci 2012;53(8):5085–93.

[7] Troilo D, Judge SJ. Ocular development and visual deprivation myopia in the common marmoset (Callithrix Jacchus). Vis Res 1993;33(10):1311–24.

[8] Benaventa-Perez A, Nour A, Troilo D. Axial eye growth and refractive error development can be modified by exposing the peripheral retinal to relative myopic or hyperopic defocus. Invest Ophthalmol Vis Sci 2014;55(10):6765–73.

[9] Li SM, Kant MT, Wu SS, et al. Studies using concentric ring bifocal and peripheral add multifocal contact lenses to slow myopia progression in school aged children: a meta-analysis. Ophthalmic Physiol Opt 2017;37(1):51–9.
[10] Coon LJ. Orthokeratology: part I historical perspective. J Am Optom Assoc 1982;53(3): 187–95.
[11] Heng LS, Khoo CY. Can contact lenses control the progression of myopia? Singapore Med J 1994;35(4):367–70.
[12] Cheung SW, Cho P, Chan B. Astigmatic changes in orthokeratology. Optom Vis Sci 2009;86(12):1352–8.
[13] Lyu B, Hwang KY, Kim SY, et al. Effectiveness of toric orthokeratology in the treatment of patients with combined myopia and astigmatism. Korean J Ophthalmol 2016;30(6):434–42.
[14] Hiraoka T, Matsumoto Y, Okamoto F, et al. Corneal higher order aberrations induced by overnight orthokeratology. Am J Ophthalmol 2005;139(3):429–36.
[15] Kim W, Kim BJ, Ryu IK, et al. Corneal epithelial and stromal thickness changes in myopic orthokeratology and their relationship with refractive change. PLoS One 2018;13(9): e0203652.
[16] Gupta PK, Stevens MN, Kashyap N, et al. Prevalence of meibomian gland atrophy in a pediatric population. Cornea 2018;37(4):426–30.
[17] Mizoguchi T, Arita R, Fukuoka S, et al. Morphology and function of meibomian glands and other tear film parameters in junior high school students. Cornea 2017;36(8):L922–6.
[18] McMonnies CW. Incomplete blinking: exposure keratopathy, lid wiper epitheliopathy and dry eye, refractive surgery and dry contact lenses. Cont Lens Anterior Eye 2007;30(1): 37–51.
[19] Davis JW. (1910) Skin transplantation with a review of 550 cases at the Johns Hopkins Hospital. Johns Hopkins Med J. 15: 307. Cited in: Dua H. Amniotic membrane transplantation. Br J Ophthalmol 1999;83(6):748–52.
[20] Cheng AMD, Tighe S, Sheha H, et al. Adjunctive role of self-retained cryopreserved amniotic membrane in treating immune related dry eye disease. Int Ophthalmol 2018;38(5): 2219–22.
[21] Dua H. Amniotic membrane transplantation. Br J Ophthalmol 1999;83(6):748–52.
[22] Suri K, Kosker M, Raber IM, et al. Sutureless amniotic membrane ProKera for ocular surface disorders: short term results. Eye Contact Lens 2013;39(5):341–7.
[23] McDonald MB, Sheha H, Tighe S, et al. Treatment outcomes in the Dry Eye Amniotic Membrane (DREAM) study. Clin Ophthalmol 2018;12:677–81.
[24] Niknejad H, Peirovi H, Jorjani M, et al. Properties of the amniotic membrane for potential in tissue engineering. Eur Cell Mater 2008;15:88–99.
[25] Lei J, Priddy L, Lim J, et al. Dehydrated human amnion/chorion membrane allograft therapy for orthopedic tissue repair. Tech Orthop 2017;32(3):149–57.
[26] Rico-Del-Viejo L, Garcia-Montero M, Hernandez Verdejo JL, et al. Nonsurgical procedures for keratoconus management. J Ophthalmol 2017;2017:9707650.
[27] Nau CB, Harthan J, Shorter E, et al. Demographic Characteristics and prescribing patterns of scleral lens fitters: the SCOPE study. Eye Contact Lens 2018;44(Suppl 1):S265–72.
[28] Harthan J, Nau CB, Barr J, et al. Scleral Lens prescription and management practices: The SCOPE study. Eye Contact Lens 2018;44(Suppl 1):S228–32.
[29] Shorter E, Harthan J, Nau CB, et al. Scleral lenses in the management of corneal irregularity and ocular surface disease. Eye Contact Lens 2018;44(6):372–8.
[30] Schornack MM. Scleral lenses: a literature review. Eye Contact Lens 2015;41(1):3–11.
[31] Yin J, Jacobs DS. Long-term outcome of using Prosthetic Replacement of Ocular Surface Ecosystem (PROSE) as a drug delivery system for bevacizumab in the treatment of corneal neovascularization. Ocul Surf 2018; https://doi.org/10.1016/j.jtos.2018.11.008.
[32] Koppen C, Kreps EO, Anthonissen L, et al. Scleral lenses reduce the need for corneal transplants in severe keratoconus. Am J Ophthalmol 2018;185:43–7.

[33] Fadel D. The influence of limbal and scleral shape on scleral lens design. Cont Lens Anterior Eye 2018;41(4):321–8.
[34] Harthan J, Shorter E, Nau C, et al. Scleral lens fitting and assessment strategies. Contact Lens Anterior Eye 2019;42(1):9–14.
[35] Schornack M, Nau C, Nau A, et al. Visual and physiological outcomes of scleral lens wear. Cont Lens Anterior Eye 2019;42(1):3–8.
[36] Isozaki VL, Chiu GB. Transient corneal epithelial bullae associated with large diameter scleral lens wear: a case series. Cont Lens Anterior Eye 2018;41(5):463–8.
[37] Walker MK, Bergmanson JP, Miller WL, et al. Complications and fitting challenges associated with scleral contact lenses: a review. Cont Lens Anterior Eye 2016;39(2):88–96.
[38] Gimenez-Sanchis I, Palacios-Carmen B, Garcia-Garrigos A, et al. Anterior segment optical coherence tomography angiography to evaluate the peripheral fitting of scleral contact lenses. Clin Optom (Auckl) 2018;10:103–8.
[39] Michaud L, Samaha D, Giasson CJ. Intraocular pressure variation associated with the wear of scleral lenses of different diameters. Cont Lens Anterior Eye 2019;42(1):104–10.
[40] Doughty MJ, Zaman ML. Human corneal thickness and its impact on intraocular pressure measures: a review and meta-analysis approach. Surv Ophthalmol 2000;44(5):367–408.

Advances in Ophthalmology and Optometry 4 (2019) 13–38

ADVANCES IN OPHTHALMOLOGY AND OPTOMETRY

Advances in Diagnosis and Management of Dry Eye Disease

Joel A. Silbert, OD, FAAO[a,*], Etty Bitton, OD, MSc, FBCLA[b], Kriti Bhagat, OD[c]

[a]Cornea & Specialty Contact Lens Service, The Eye Institute of the Pennsylvania College of Optometry at Salus University, 1200 West Godfrey Avenue, Philadelphia, PA 19141, USA; [b]Dry Eye Clinic, École d'Optométrie, Université de Montréal, 3744 Jean Brilliant St., Montreal, Quebec H3T 1P1, Canada; [c]Ocular Surface Disease Clinic, The Eye Institute of the Pennsylvania College of Optometry at Salus University, 1200 West Godfrey Avenue, Philadelphia, PA 19141, USA

Keywords

• Dry eye disease (DED) • Meibomian gland dysfunction (MGD)
• Tear Film and Ocular Surface Society (TFOS) • Dry Eye Workshop II (DEWS II)
• Hyperosmolarity • Homeostasis • Tear film instability

Key points

- Dry eye disease (DED) is a disease entity, although a multifactorial one.
- It is now thought that the tear film is a 2-phase structure, comprising an outer lipid layer overlying a single mucoaqueous phase, with the entire tear film being involved in preventing or limiting evaporation.
- The causes of DED stem from either aqueous deficiency conditions, classified as aqueous-deficient dry eye , or evaporative conditions, classified as evaporative dry eye (EDE), and exist as a continuum. Elements of each must be considered in the clinical diagnosis and management of DED.
- Meibomian gland dysfunction constitutes the major cause of EDE.
- Common to most types of DED is the development of hyperosmolarity, which leads to tear film instability, inflammatory changes to the ocular surface, and ultimately loss of homeostasis.

INTRODUCTION

Open almost any ophthalmic journal and you will likely find one or more articles discussing some aspect of dry eye. The literature on dry eye is vast,

Disclosures: Dr E. Bitton has received research funding from Alcon Canada, Allergan Canada, I-med Pharma Inc., Shire, and Valeant. Drs J.A. Silbert and K. Bhagat have nothing to disclose.

*Corresponding author. *E-mail address:* joel@salus.edu

https://doi.org/10.1016/j.yaoo.2019.04.002

growing exponentially, and confusing at the same time. In order to bring order and good evidence-based science to this almost limitless field of data, the Tear Film and Ocular Surface Society (TFOS) Dry Eye Workshop (DEWS II) in 2017 published the most comprehensive meta-analysis of this expansive literature, updating the prior TFOS DEWS report from 2007. Published in *The Ocular Surface* (Elsevier), the TFOS DEWS II report used 150 experts in 23 countries who reviewed and analyzed the many articles published in the ensuing decade. It updated the definitions as well as the classification of dry eye; considered the causes, epidemiology, mechanisms, pathophysiology, and diagnostic testing; and ultimately created a consensus opinion among experts to assist practicing clinicians in formulating sound treatment plans for dry eye disease (DED). The TFOS DEWS II report recognized that DED is, by its new definition, a disease, although a multifactorial one.

DEFINITION AND CLASSIFICATION

The new definition of DED by TFOS DEWS II is as follows:

> Dry eye is a multifactorial disease of the ocular surface characterized by a loss of homeostasis of the tear film, and accompanied by ocular symptoms, in which tear film instability and hyperosmolarity, ocular surface inflammation and damage, and neurosensory abnormalities play etiological roles [1].

The TFOS DEWS II classification of ocular surface disease is useful in that it presents clinicians with a patient-based schema that first addresses the presence or absence of symptoms. It then addresses whether such symptoms (or lack thereof) correspond with clinical signs. Thus, there are 4 subtypes (Fig. 1):

- Asymptomatic patients without signs (no dry eye)
- Asymptomatic patients with signs (such patients may be at risk for developing symptoms from ocular procedures [eg, refractive surgery] or from the use of topical or systemic medications)
- Symptomatic patients with signs (eg, typical dry eye or other ocular surface conditions)
- Symptomatic patients without signs (eg, patients who may have a preclinical dry eye, or who may have neuropathic pain) [1].

THE PRECORNEAL TEAR FILM

The best way to understand current thinking about the tear film is to focus on the TFOS DEWS II *Tear Film* report. Historically, the tear film has been thought to be a 3-layered structure consisting of an outermost lipid, a thicker middle aqueous, and an inner mucin layer, which interacts with the glycocalyx, which interdigitates with the corneal epithelial microvilli. The report updates a large body of new research to suggest that the tear film is a 2-phase structure, composed of an outer lipid layer overlying a single mucoaqueous phase, with the entire tear film being involved in preventing or limiting evaporation [2].

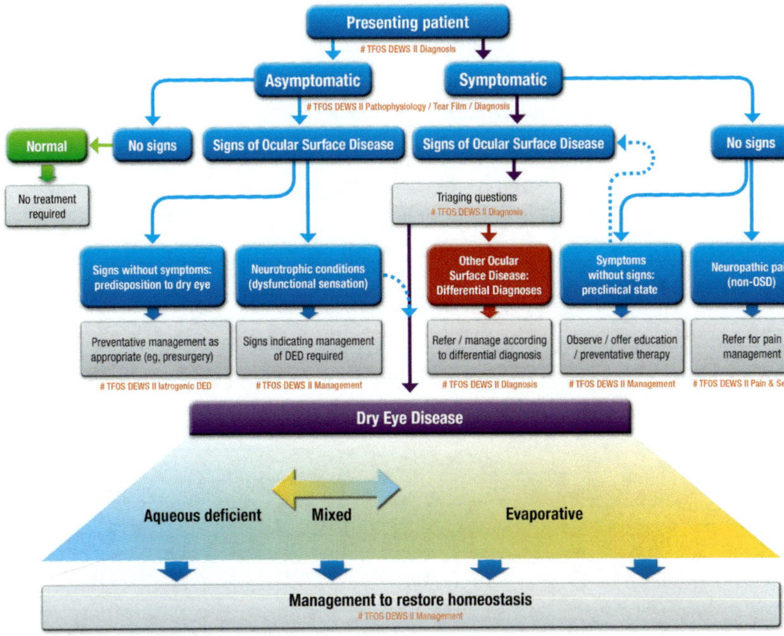

Fig. 1. Classification of DED. The upper portion of the figure represents a clinical decision algorithm, beginning with the assessment of symptoms, and followed by review for signs of ocular surface disease. The lower portion represents the etiologic classification of DED, highlighting aqueous-deficient dry eye (ADDE) and evaporative dry eye (EDE), which may for some patients, be mixed. OSD, ocular surface disease. (*From* Craig JP, Nichols KK, Akpek EK et al. TFOS DEWS II definition and classification report. Ocul Surf 2017;15(3), 276–283, with permission.)

The lipid layer contains both nonpolar and polar lipids whose role is to stabilize the entire tear film via reduction in surface tension. It has long been thought that the lipid layer prevents tear evaporation. The TFOS DEWS II report suggests that, although this is possible, it is not a certainty because of variability in the role of polar and tear lipid profiles among various studies [3]. More research is still needed to better the understanding of this layer.

The mucoaqueous phase is composed of more than 1500 different proteins and peptide chains, including at least 4 major mucins, the purpose of which is to increase hydration. Reduced mucin production, such as the frequently seen reduction in expression of mucin 5AC, is implicated in ocular surface disease. However, more research is needed to help identify specific proteins or changes in protein levels to specifically identify with DED (Fig. 2).

PATHOPHYSIOLOGY OF DRY EYE DISEASE

The TFOS DEWS II report on pathophysiology describes 2 main subtypes of DED: aqueous-deficient dry eye (ADDE) and evaporative dry eye (EDE)[4].

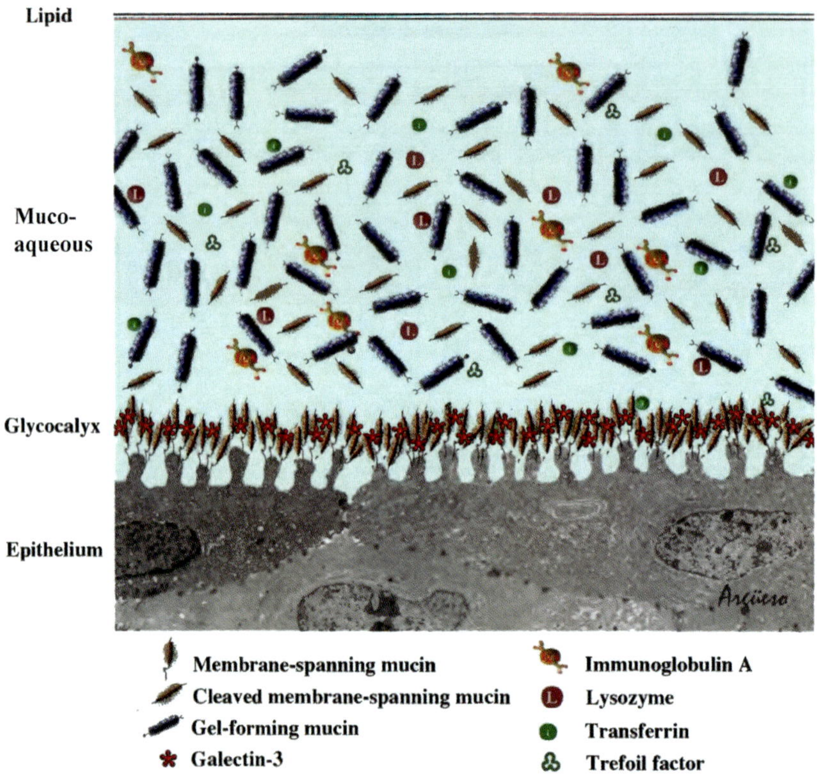

Fig. 2. The tear film structure showing the mucins and galectin of the glycocalyx, soluble mucins and proteins in the mucoaqueous layer, and the surface lipid layer. (*From* Willcox MDP, Argueso P, Georgiev GA, et al. TFOS DEWS II tear film report. Ocul Surf 2017;15(3), 366–403, with permission.)

ADDE describes eyes in which insufficient tears are secreted by the lacrimal glands, but in which there is a normal evaporative rate, which in turn creates hyperosmolarity. This condition can be caused by:

- Obstruction of the lacrimal gland
- Sjögren syndrome with autoimmune cellular infiltration of the lacrimal gland
- Systemic drugs (eg, ophthalmic β-blockers, antihistamines, diuretics, antispasmodics, and some psychotropic medications) [5]

Patients with ADDE may develop instability of the tear film from hyperosmolarity, corneal or conjunctival staining, and ocular discomfort or gritty sensation.

EDE describes eyes with sufficient tear secretion but with excessive evaporation, which also produces hyperosmolarity. EDE is commonly seen with meibomian gland dysfunction (MGD), the most common form of DED, caused by tear film lipid layer deficiency [5].

TFOS DEWSII emphasizes the retention of both of these dry eye designations

> ...to describe the initiating basis of a dry eye, but it should be recognized that with progression any form of DED may take on additional evaporative features.

It should be noted that patients can have mixed dry eye, in which DED occurs along the spectrum between ADDE and EDE.

Regardless of initiating type, with hyperosmolarity comes instability of the tear film, and, as a result, a vicious circle of ocular surface inflammation, exacerbating DED desiccation stress (Fig. 3).

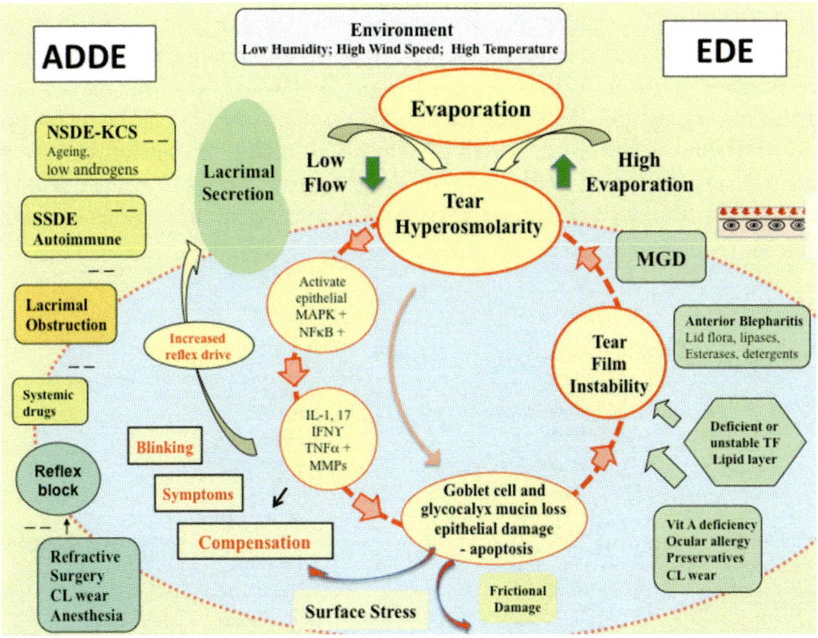

Fig. 3. The vicious circle of DED. The core mechanism of DED is tear hyperosmolarity, the hallmark of the disease. It damages the ocular surface both directly and by initiating inflammation. In ADDE, tear hyperosmolarity results when lacrimal secretion is reduced, in conditions of normal evaporation from the eye. In EDE, tear hyperosmolarity is created by excessive evaporation from the exposed tear film in the presence of a normally functioning lacrimal gland. Hyperosmolarity sets up a cascade of events leading to inflammatory mediator release, which likely causes goblet cell and epithelial cell loss (punctate epithelial staining of DED) and damage to the epithelial glycocalyx, with tear film instability leading to tear film break-up. This process, in turn, worsens the hyperosmolarity, thus completing the vicious circle of events that lead to ocular surface damage and self-perpetuation of the disease. Although hyperosmolarity is often the initiating point for DED, any dry eye cause may have other entry points in the vicious circle. IFN, interferon; IL, interleukin; MAPK, mitogen-activated protein kinase; MMPs, matrix metalloproteinases; NF-κB; nuclear factor kappa-B; TF, tear film; TNF, tumor necrosis factor; Vit A, vitamin A. (*From* Bron AJ, dePaiva CS, Chauhan SK et al. TFOS DEWS II Pathophysiology report. Ocul Surf 2017;15(3), 438–510, with permission.)

As can be seen in Fig. 3, besides low tear production and evaporation, many other factors can be present that may worsen the vicious circle, including contact lens wear, refractive surgery, concurrent anterior and posterior blepharitis, lid abnormalities, ocular allergy, and topical and systemic medications.

MEIBOMIAN GLAND DYSFUNCTION

Korb and Henriquez [6,7] introduced the term MGD in 1980, to identify the most common cause of EDE. Although beginning as an impairment to delivery of meibum to the lid margin, the clinical course leads to a pathologic and potentially irreversible disease state [8]. Noncicatricial MGD occurs in acne rosacea, atopic dermatitis, seborrheic dermatitis, and psoriasis, all of which develop hyperkeratinization of the terminal gland ducts, leading to duct obstruction and glandular atrophy. In addition, inflammatory mediators are released into the tears and onto the ocular surface, causing subsequent epithelial damage [5]. With cicatricial MGD, seen in pemphigoid, trachoma, and erythema multiforme, scarring leads to dragging of meibomian ducts and orifices, impairing delivery of meibum to the tear film, which in turn causes tear film instability and increased evaporation, and leads to EDE (Fig. 4).

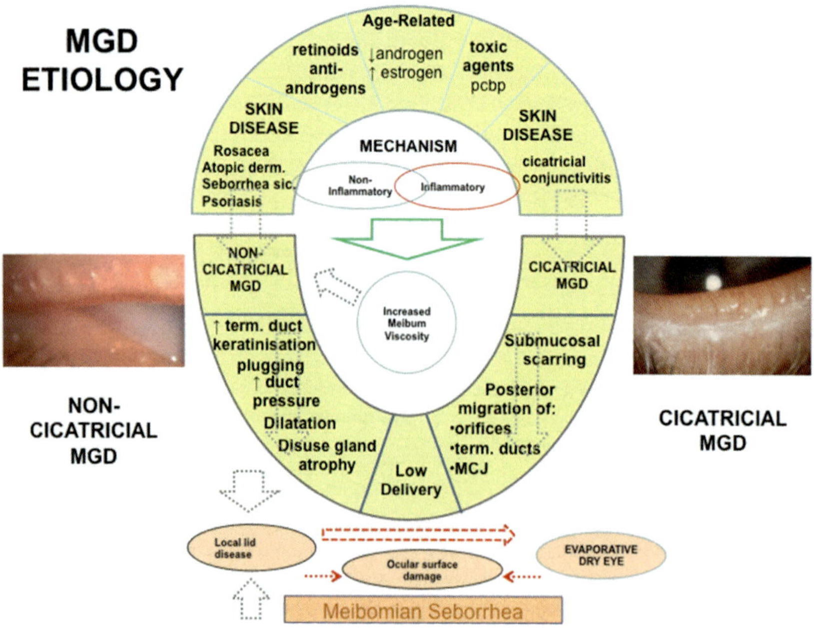

Fig. 4. The cause and mechanism of MGD, which constitutes the major cause of EDE. It accounts for the low delivery of meibum to the ocular surface, in both cicatricial as well as noncicatricial MGD. MCJ, mucocutaneous junction; term, terminal. (*From* Bron AJ, dePaiva CS, Chauhan SK et al. TFOS DEWS II Pathophysiology report. The Ocular Surface. 2017;15(3), 438-510, with permission.)

PREVALENCE AND THE EFFECTS OF SEX, GENDER, AND HORMONES

The TFOS DEWS II report on sex, gender, and hormones confirms that these issues play an important role in DED differences between women and men [9]. Although sex and gender are intertwined, sex refers to reproductive organs and functions, according to chromosomal status, whereas gender refers to a person's representation of self as male or female. The literature supports that female sex is a risk factor for DED as well as DED-related autoimmune diseases such as Sjögren syndrome [10]. In the United States alone, women are 70% more likely to be diagnosed with DED than men [11,12], and they experience a greater impact of this disease on vision quality and on activities requiring sustained visual attention. Evidence of sex differences also exists in anterior segment structures and lacrimal-associated adnexa. The sex-related difference in DED prevalence is attributed in large part to the effects of sex steroids (eg, androgens, estrogens), hypothalamic-pituitary hormones, glucocorticoids, insulin, insulinlike growth factor 1 and thyroid hormones, and the sex chromosome complement [9].

Gender-based differences exist as well in terms of access to care, care-seeking behavior depending on whether the person is in a developed or nondeveloped country, and health outcomes that differ around the world. Both gender and biological sex affect patients' risk for DED, disease presentation, level of pain, immune response, and the degree to which they seek care [9].

DIAGNOSTIC TECHNIQUES FOR DRY EYE DISEASE

The TFOS DEWS II report has provided a framework for a more systematic approach to diagnostic testing for DED than was previously used.

Dry eye questionnaires

The TFOS DEWS II definition of DED incorporates an evaluation of symptoms. Consequently, diagnostic testing should begin with symptom assessment using a validated DED questionnaire. Many available questionnaires exist specific to DED, such as the McMonnies questionnaire [13–17], the Ocular Surface Disease Index (OSDI) [18,19], Dry Eye Questionnaire (DEQ-5) [20], Standard Patient Evaluation of Eye Dryness (SPEED) [21,22], and Impact of Dry Eye on Everyday Life (IDEEL) [23–25], some of which may be more suitable for research. TFOS DEWS II proposes the use of 2 validated tools easily integrated into a clinical setting, namely the OSDI and the DEQ-5.

The OSDI (Allergan, Inc., Irvine, CA) is a self-administered 12-question symptom assessment, divided into 3 main sections:

- Frequency of symptoms (eg, dryness, blurry vision, grittiness)
- Effects on daily tasks (eg, reading, computer use, driving at night)
- Aggravation by environmental factors (eg, wind, air conditioning) over the past week

Each response has a numerical value and there is a subtotal for each section. The total is then multiplied by 25 and divided by the number of questions answered (some may not apply, such as air conditioning in the winter months) to arrive at the final OSDI score. The OSDI score can range from 0 to 100 and offers a symptom severity as follows: less than 12 (normal), 13 to 22 (mild), 23 to 32 (moderate), and greater than 33 (severe). The sensitivity (80%) and specificity (79%) of the OSDI is high to discriminate patients with DED from those without DED [18].

The DEQ-5 is a self-administered questionnaire related to the frequency and intensity of symptoms within the prior month. A numerical value is associated with each response and the sum serves as the total score. A cutoff score of greater than or equal to 6 discriminates asymptomatic from symptomatic DED with a high degree of sensitivity (90%) and specificity (81%) [20]. A cutoff score of greater than or equal to 12 offers a good discrimination between patients with and without Sjögren (sensitivity 82%, specificity 54%). This second parameter provides an advantage of the DEQ-5 compared with the OSDI. Both questionnaires are easily accessible online and can be integrated at low to no cost within a practice setting. Questionnaires can be sent electronically to the patient before an appointment or can be completed while in the waiting room. Evaluating symptoms with a validated questionnaire is not only an important characteristic to measure during an initial DED work-up but also can be used to measure treatment outcomes.

- OSDI questionnaire that can be easily administered in-office before the examination: https://static1.squarespace.com/static/51ba5346e4b09459e2a8c0aa/t/55e5e844e4b0b7789bdf80f2/1441130564021/osdi.pdf
- Dry Eye OSDI downloadable smartphone app useable by office staff, as well as by patients who can self-monitor during treatment: https://www.allerganoptometry.com/_/docs/DryEye/APC11CB14-OSDI-App-Instructions.pdf
- DEQ-5 questionnaire: https://www.reviewofoptometry.com/CMSDocuments/2017/09/ro0917_mededicusi.pdf

Assessment of tear breakup stability

Following a symptom assessment, the evaluation of homeostatic markers is needed to assess characteristics of the tear film and ocular surface. Numerous tear tests have been reported and summarized in the literature [26–30]. This article focuses on 3 markers, namely tear film stability, tear film osmolarity, and ocular surface staining, which are presented as part of the TFOS DEWS II diagnostic algorithm [31].

The tear breakup time (TBUT) has a long clinical history as a measure of tear film stability [32]. Once sodium fluorescein has been instilled in the eye and distributed evenly with a few blinks, the patient is asked to refrain from blinking. The time (in seconds) between the last blink and the first appearance of a break in the fluorescein-stained tear film is known as the F-TBUT and recorded. Typically, an F-TBUT of greater than 10 seconds is considered the norm. Despite its popularity as one of the most used clinical tests for DED, several factors can affect it, including inconsistent methodology [33]. One way of reducing this variability is to wet a standard fluorescein strip with sterile saline, shake off the excess (to control the volume), and to tap the lower tarsal (not bulbar) conjunctival surface with a small volume [34,35]. It is recommended to take 2 consecutive measurements to calculate an average [27]. To control the volume even further, smaller 1-mm fluorescein strips are available [36–38]. Optimal viewing of the F-TBUT is between 1 and 3 minutes following instillation [39].

It is important not to use a topical anesthetic or combination anesthetic-fluorescein, because this would further disrupt the tear film and give an artificially reduced value. Some clinicians have argued that the addition of fluorescein is invasive to the tear film and can negatively affect the TBUT. Consequently, several noninvasive breakup time (NIBUT) methods have been elucidated, providing longer tear film stability times [40–47]. These instruments require mires that can be reflected off the corneal surface to view any distortions following the blink (Fig. 5). The TFOS DEWS II report recommends, when possible, to use a NIBUT technique rather than the F-TBUT and that a value of less than 10 seconds is considered a positive finding.

Assessment of tear film hyperosmolarity

Tear film hyperosmolarity is considered to be a core mechanism of ocular inflammation [1,4,48–52]. Tear osmometers, such as the TearLab Osmolarity System (TearLab Corporation, Escondido, CA), measure the concentration of ions in only a 50-nL sample of tears [53]. The test should be performed on the lower temporal tear meniscus (Fig. 6), preferably before any manipulation of the eye or lid. The instrument is user-friendly and can easily be integrated in clinical practice with little training other than appropriate positioning on the

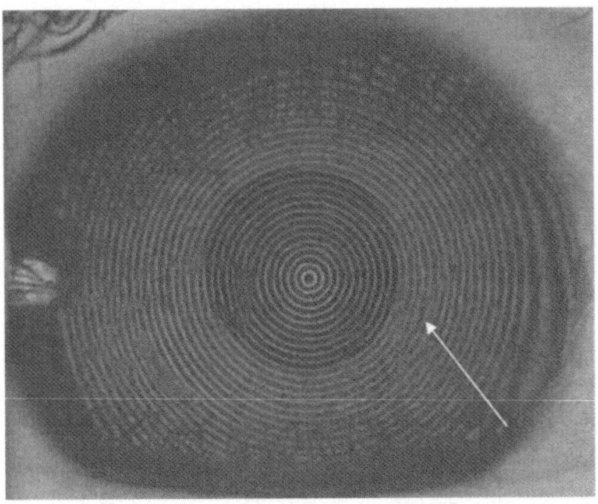

Fig. 5. NIBUT measured in seconds between a blink and the first observable distortion of corneal topographic mires (Medmont topographer). Arrow denotes mire distortion. (*Courtesy of* Etty Bitton, OD., Université de Montréal, Montreal, Quebec, Canada)

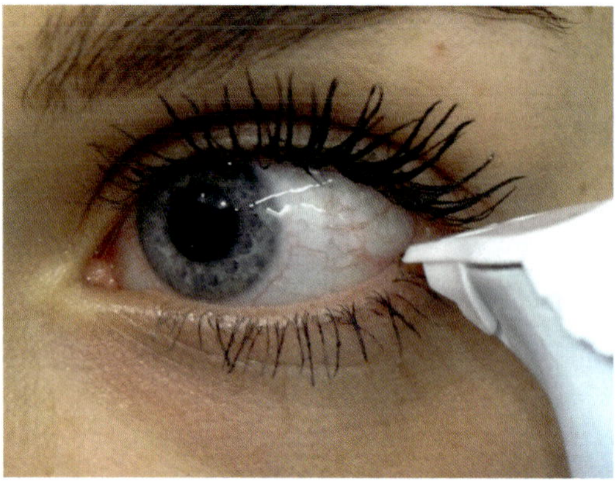

Fig. 6. Tear osmolarity measured at the lower temporal tear meniscus using the TearLab instrument. (*Courtesy of* Etty Bitton, O.D., Université de Montréal, Montreal, Quebec, Canada)

lower lid margin. A value of greater than or equal to 308 mOsm/L in either eye has been widely accepted as a cutoff for mild to moderate DED [52], and an intereye asymmetry of greater than 8 mOsm/L is expected, especially with increasing severity [54]. Despite the reported variability of instrumentation [55–57], osmolarity remains one of the most sensitive objective tests correlated to DED diagnosis and severity [54,58,59].

Assessment of ocular surface staining

Ophthalmic vital dyes, such as sodium fluorescein, rose bengal, and lissamine green, have a long-standing history in clinical practice to assess the integrity of the ocular surface [28,29,60]. Several grading scales and schemes have been proposed to establish the severity of both conjunctival and corneal staining. These schemes include the van Bijsterfeld system [26], the National Eye Institute/Industry Workshop system [49], the Oxford system [34], the Brien Holden Vision Institute grading scale [61–63], and the Ocular Staining Score proposed by the Sjögren International Collaborative Clinical Alliance [64]. Objective photometric methods have been evoked with emerging imaging technologies [65,66]. Although numerous grading scales are available, eye-care practitioners are often remiss in documenting the severity of the staining observed [67].

- Sodium fluorescein highlights areas of compromised ocular surface integrity, such as loss of cell tight junctions or defective glycocalyx [68,69]. To maximize fluorescence, a cobalt blue filter housed in most slit lamps is needed and the addition of a yellow barrier filter enhances the contrast [39,70]. Corneal staining, even among normal non–contact lens wearers, is mainly found in the inferior quadrant [71,72].
- Rose bengal stains mucus, cells unprotected by mucin or glycocalyx, and devitalized (desiccated) cells. This red dye is most useful in assessing conjunctival cells in DED [73,74].

Lissamine green 1% has largely replaced rose bengal in current clinical practice because of its enhanced patient comfort and decreased toxicity to epithelial cells [75,76] Lissamine green is particularly useful [77,78] in staining the upper lid margin in contact lens wearers with dry eye symptoms, when a lid-wiper epitheliopathy is present [79] (Fig. 7).

To simplify a positive staining diagnosis, the TFOS DEWSII algorithm has proposed cutoffs that are greater than 5 corneal spots, greater than 9 conjunctival spots, or lid margin staining (≥2 mm in length and ≥25% width) [31].

Assessment of dry eye disease subtypes (aqueous vs evaporative dry eye disease)

According to the TFOS DEWS II diagnostic algorithm [31], DED is classified as having both symptoms (OSDI>13 or DEQ-5>6) and at least 1 positive sign (TBUT/osmolarity/ocular staining). A differential of other ocular surface diseases (eg, blepharitis, conjunctivochalasis, corneal dystrophies, contact lens discomfort) with similar clinical presentations needs to be ruled out before a definitive DED diagnosis. Once DED is considered, additional testing is needed to determine the subtype. To do this an evaluation of the tear meniscus height (TMH) is performed to establish whether an aqueous deficiency exists. To determine whether there is an evaporative component, typically caused by MGD, an assessment of the gland secretions is needed.

The TMH, measured in millimeters, can be evaluated directly at the slit lamp using the graduated scale on the slit beam (for most slit lamps, the smallest measurement is 0.2 mm). More recent imaging technologies, such as the Keratograph 5M (Oculus, Inc., Arlington, WA) can capture an image of the meniscus, which can subsequently be measured [80–82] This measurement is quick and simple to integrate in a DED assessment to determine whether there is an aqueous deficiency component. To establish severity, a TMH of 0.2 mm is considered mild, 0.1 mm moderate, and 0 is severe [31].

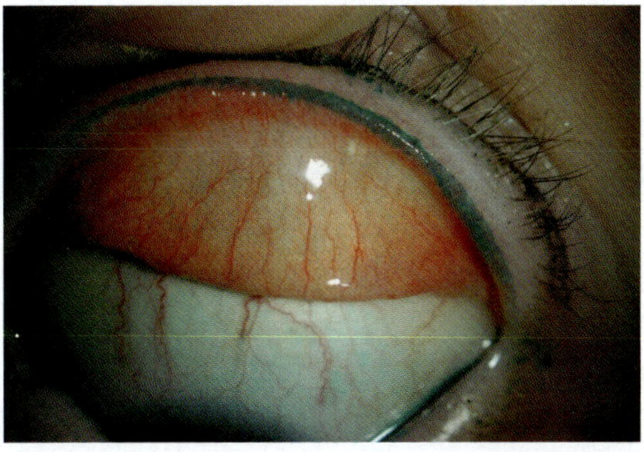

Fig. 7. Upper lid margin staining or lid-wiper epitheliopathy as observed with lissamine green under white diffuse illumination, seen in contact lens dry eye. (*Courtesy of* Etty Bitton, OD., Université de Montréal, Montreal, Quebec, Canada).

Assessment of gland secretions

To establish the severity of evaporative DED, such as MGD, expression of the glands is needed, preferably with a calibrated tool such as the Meibomian Gland Evaluator (MGE) (TearScience, Johnson & Johnson Inc.), although other lid expressers exist in the market [83–86]. The MGE is a 6 × 1.5 cm handheld instrument with a retractable end that, when pressed gently against the edge of the lid margin, provides a calibrated pressure of 0.8 to 1.2 g/mm^2, equivalent to that of a deliberate blink. It covers approximately the width of 5 meibomian glands and a subjective value of 3 is given for each gland that secretes clear liquid, 2 if cloudy, 1 if the gland is inspissated, and 0 if there are no secretions, for a total possible score of 15. This test is performed for 5 glands in each of 3 zones of the lower lid margin, namely temporally, centrally, and nasally. A total meibomian gland evaluation score of 0 means there are no functional glands, whereas a total of 45 means that all 15 glands assessed produce clear liquid secretions.

A video demonstration is available online for this diagnostic technology (https://vimeo.com/243680939).

Other tests

In assessing DED, it is recommended to choose a testing order that goes from least to most invasive so as not to affect subsequent tests. A suggested order of testing is shown in Table 1. Additional testing, such as lipid layer thickness (LLT) or testing for inflammatory markers, such as matrix metalloproteinase-9 (MMP-9), may affect the order of testing.

Interferometric fringe patterns from the reflective properties of the tear film allow the LLT to be measured, more recently using an automated noninvasive instrument such as the LipiView II Interferometer (TearScience, Johnson & Johnson Inc.). Reduced values of LLT (<60 nm) seem to be well correlated with increasing DED symptoms [87]. The instrument has a good validity when 75 nm is used as a cutoff for MGD (sensitivity 65.8%; specificity 63.4%) and can engage the practitioner to discuss how anatomic changes of the glands can directly affect function (ie, lipid secretion) [88].

Table 1
Suggested order of testing for DED

Least invasive ↑	Symptoms (OSDI/DEQ-5)
	Tear osmolarity
	TMH (Keratograph)
	NIBUT
	Anterior segment assessment (biomicroscopy)
	Ocular surface staining
	F-TBUT
	Meibomian gland expression
↓ Most invasive	MMP-9

Abbreviation: MMP, matrix metalloproteinase.

MMP-9 is a nonspecific inflammatory biomarker found in low concentration in the normal eye, but increases (>40 ng/mL) with ocular surface inflammation, such as DED. InflammaDry (Quidel Corp., San Diego, CA) is an in-office test that measures MMP-9 levels within 10 minutes of tear collection from the lower palpebral conjunctiva, with a high degree of validity (sensitivity 85%; specificity 94%) [89,90]. Because this test is more invasive, it should be performed later in the series of testing.

ADVANCES IN MANAGEMENT OF DRY EYE DISEASE

With better understanding of the physiologic mechanisms of ADDE, EDE, and combined forms of DED, in tandem with enhanced diagnostic testing protocols, clinicians are now in a better position to design more tailored treatment algorithms for their patients with dry eye. Current evidence-based and consensus-based recommendations outlined in the latest TFOS DEWS II report [91] are discussed next. Treatment algorithms can be summarized by the underlying cause: tear insufficiency, lid abnormalities, inflammation, decreased dacryoreservoirs, dietary insufficiencies, and/or environmental causes.

Tear insufficiency treatments

Over-the-counter ocular lubricants have been used as a first-line therapy for DED for many years. Traditionally, artificial tear substitutes (ATSs) were given to provide temporary relief, despite how they target the specific layer of the tear film. Several ATS products have been designed to be hypo-osmolar, to counter the hyperosmolarity of the dry eye [92]. Newer artificial tear formulations include supplements that target tear film osmolarity by including osmoprotectants. Studies show that osmoprotectants can protect corneal epithelial cells, decrease inflammatory cytokine response, and increase conjunctival goblet cell density [93]. Trehalose is a disaccharide that is incorporated in newer artificial tears to prevent cells from death by desiccation [94]. Antioxidants are being incorporated in artificial tears to decrease the presence of oxygen free radicals found in the tear film of patients with DED. For example, Visomitin is an ophthalmic solution, currently available in Russia, containing an antioxidant, SkQ1, designed to penetrate the mitochondria and neutralize excessive free radicals found in DED [95]. Phase III trials of Visomitin have begun in the United States (https://www.mitotechpharma.com/news/mitotech-completes-first-patient-visit-in-vista-1-phase-3-clinical-study-of-skq1-for-dry-eye-disease).

The normal tear film has been shown to be rich in electrolytes. Electrolyte-enhanced artificial tears have been shown to increase conjunctival goblet cell density and promote corneal wound healing [96,97]. With expanding knowledge about the vital role of the lipid layer of the tear film, various types of lipids, phospholipids, fatty acids, and triglycerides have been incorporated in ATSs to create a stable lipid layer but there is as yet no definite algorithm of which lipid can be specifically recommended for a corresponding lipid-deficient tear film.

Biologic tear substitutes, previously reserved for patients with severe dry eye, are a growing option for patients with DED. Autologous serum eye drops are preservative free and manufactured from the patient's own blood serum, which contains fibronectin, vitamins, and growth factors that encourage epithelial wound healing [98]. Autologous serum has been shown to inhibit the release of inflammatory cytokines and increase goblet cells and mucin expression [99]. Despite these benefits, autologous serum is not widely used because of cost, quality control, product storage issues, and risk of infection. Other biologic options include adult allogeneic serum (serum from a donor), umbilical cord serum, and platelet preparations, but these also share similar disadvantages, leading to underuse of this promising therapy [91].

In addition to tear supplementation, tear conservation via punctal plugs has long been popular for blocking drainage (temporarily or permanently) of endogenously produced tears. Conservation options include collagen plugs, silicone plugs, cyanoacrylate adhesives, and/or surgical occlusion of the puncta.

Tear stimulation using pharmacologic agents, through the use of aqueous and mucin secretagogues as well as stimulation of lipids, has had limited clinical application and success [91]. The recent introduction of the TrueTear neurostimulation device (Allergan, Inc., Dublin, Ireland) has sparked renewed interest, without the need to use pharmaceutical agents. The device is an intranasal tear neurostimulator that allows patients to self-deliver pulses to create a nasolacrimal reflex creating additional, albeit temporary, tear production (Fig. 8).

Treatments for dry eye disease–associated lid abnormalities

Lid abnormalities, including anterior blepharitis, MGD, and lid-globe incongruity, can lead to various types of DED. Patient management for blepharitis and MGD are based on severity of signs and symptoms, degree of inflammation, and cause. Proper lid hygiene recommendations, including lid scrubs using mild lid cleansers and warm compresses, have been the mainstay of treatment of patients with mild to moderate blepharitis and MGD. A careful examination of the lid margins and lashes reveals whether the patient has squamous, seborrheic, or ulcerative blepharitis, or cylindrical dandruff from *Demodex* infestation, all of which can cause dryness symptoms or exacerbate a preexisting dry eye. New advances for demodicosis treatment include the use of tea tree oil, a natural, essential oil that has antimicrobial, antiinflammatory, antifungal, and antiparasitic properties (the last of which is toxic to *Demodex*) [100,101].

Microblepharoexfoliation is used to remove bacterial biofilm, scurf, and debris from the lid margins [102]. BlephEx (Scope Ophthalmics, London) is one such instrument, consisting of a spinning microsponge, soaked in a lid cleanser, which glides over the lash line. In-office treatments are often performed monthly (Fig. 9).

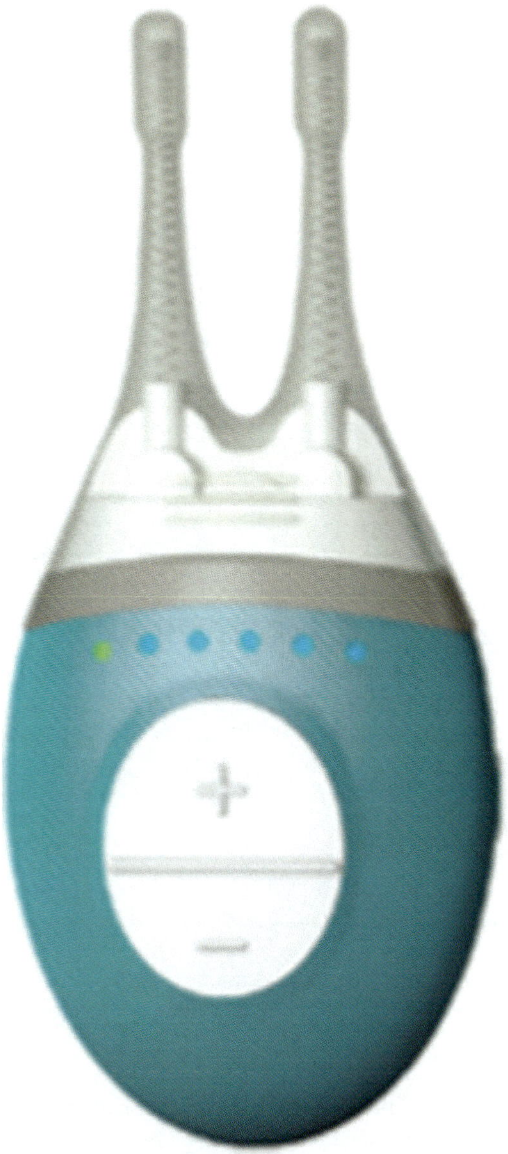

Fig. 8. TrueTear neurostimulator device (Used with permission from Allergan Plc, Dublin, Ireland)

Other blepharoexfoliative instruments recently entering the market include:

- NuLids system (NuSight Medical; Rancho Santa Fe, CA), prescribed in the office and designed for daily home use by patients with chronic meibomian gland congestion (Fig. 10).
- LidPro (Mibo Medical Group; Dallas, TX) (Fig. 11).

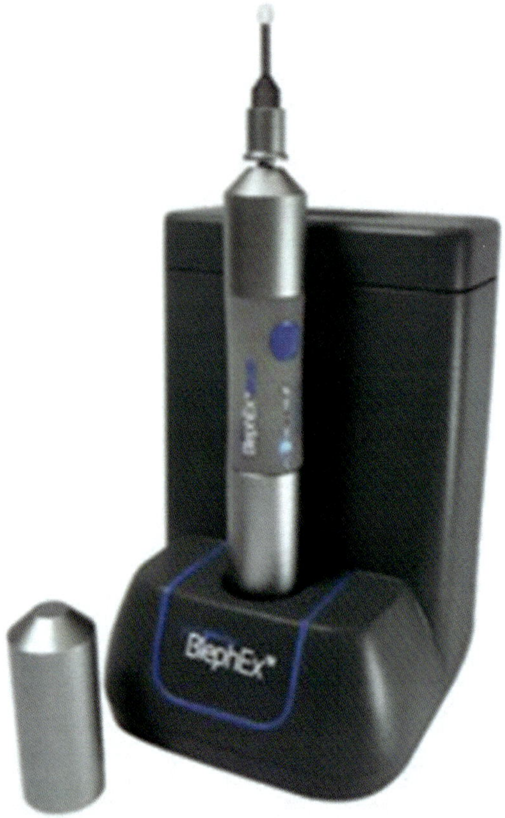

Fig. 9. BlephEx device for removing lid margin debris and scurf. (Used with permission from Scope Ophthalmics, London.)

Although clinicians often recommend the application of warm heat to the lids for MGD and other lid conditions, poor patient compliance in the use of a washcloth, which does not retain the desired heat for long enough periods, is problematic.

Newer eyelid warming products include microbeaded masks that can hold heat much longer. These reusable moist heat devices consist of an eye mask that is heated in the patient's microwave and is used for prolonged heating of obstructed meibomian glands to facilitate meibum and lipids to the tear film [103].

An in-office procedure, the MiBo ThermoFlo device (Mibo Medical Group, Dallas, TX) delivers consistent emissive heat to the meibomian glandular apparatus. Inspissated lipid secretions are softened and mobilized through gentle ocular massage (Fig. 12).

Treatment modalities for MGD involve not just applying heat for obstructed glands but also applying physical expression of glands. Manual expression of

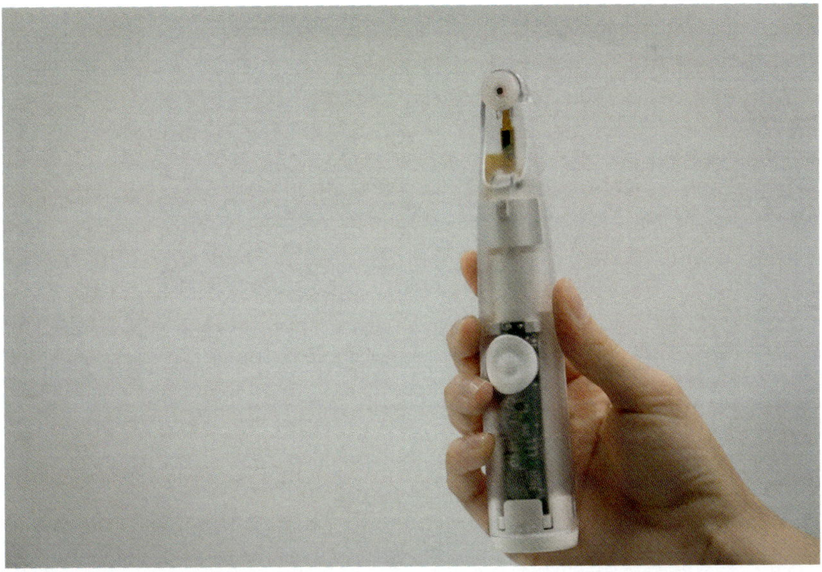

Fig. 10. NuLids device. (Used with permission from NuSight Medical; Rancho Santa Fe, CA)

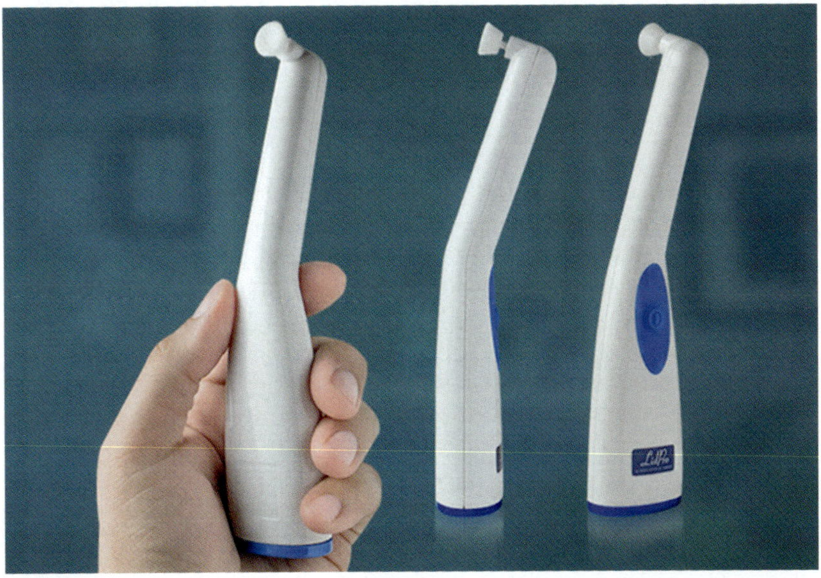

Fig. 11. LidPro lid margin blepharoexfoliative device. (Used with permission from Mibo Medical Group; Dallas, TX)

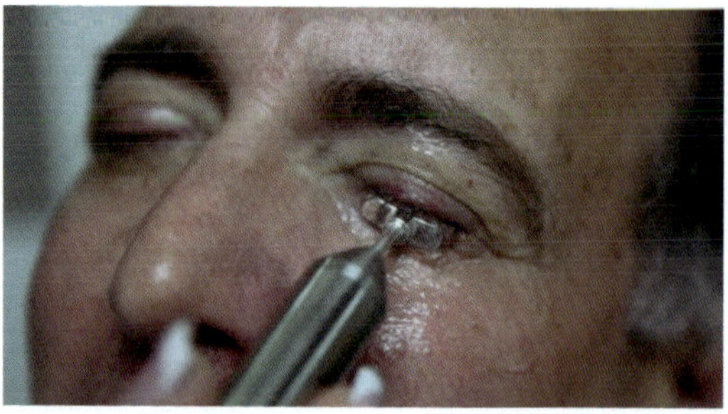

Fig. 12. MiBo ThermoFlo (Mibo Medical Group; Dallas, TX) treatment with a single-pad thermal applicator. A dual pad is also available for simultaneous treatment of upper and lower lids. (*Courtesy of* James S. Lewis, MD.)

glands has been the traditional therapy, which takes much chair time and is uncomfortable for the patient. The LipiFlow system (TearScience Inc., Johnson & Johnson Vision) is a new treatment option for patients with MGD that allows one 12-minute application of heat and gentle pressure to remove meibomian gland obstructions (Fig. 13). This process is done by applying a single-use activator to the eyelid, designed to protect the cornea while sliding under and over the eyelid to provide targeted therapy to the meibomian glands. This treatment has been successfully compared with a 3-month, twice-a-day warm compress lid hygiene, and lid massage at-home therapy [104]. It is able to increase the

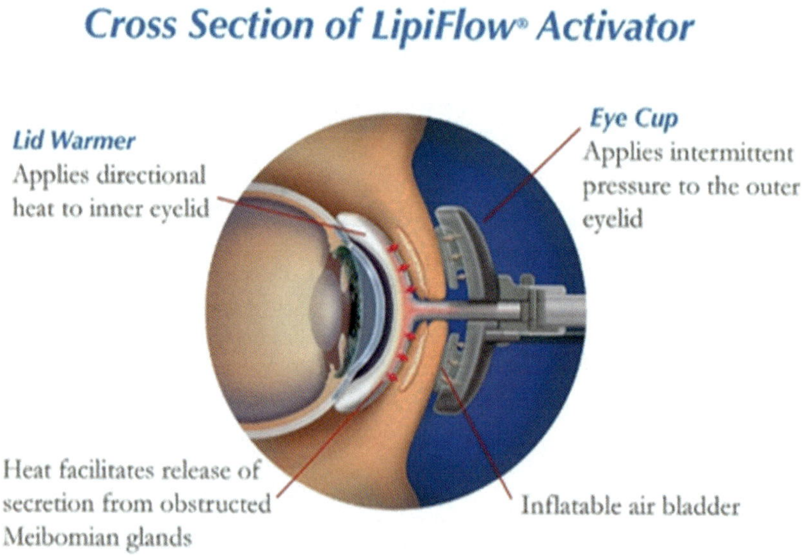

Fig. 13. LipiFlow system. (Used with permission from TearScience Inc., Johnson & Johnson Vision)

inner lid surface temperatures to the reported 40°C minimum therapeutic threshold for melting obstructed meibum [105].

Intense pulsed light therapy has been used extensively in dermatology to treat chronic skin conditions, especially acne rosacea, and is an emerging technology for patients with EDE disease [101]. Monthly treatments with 500-nm to 1200-nm light pulses have been found to improve meibum quality in MGD. The few existing studies show clinical safety as well as improvements in lid margin vascularity and edema, TBUT, meibum viscosity, and OSDI score [106]. However, it is not yet clear which type of patients would benefit the most from this adjunctive therapy [107].

Treatment of inflammation

Topical corticosteroids are an effective treatment of inflammatory DED by inhibiting the activation and degranulation of inflammatory cells [108]. Despite newer preservative-free formulations becoming available, long-term maintenance with topical steroid therapy is not advised because of complications of steroid-response glaucoma and early cataract formation. When topical steroids are indicated in severe DED, the use of a so-called soft-steroid such as loteprednol etabonate is helpful because of its reduced complication profile [109].

Cyclosporine is an immunosuppressive drug that is used to decrease inflammation by binding to the cytosolic protein cyclophilin and blocking T-helper 2 lymphocyte proliferation, resulting in inhibiting the interleukin (IL)-2 activation and decreasing the total T cells on the ocular surface.

Newer topical solutions include lifitegrast, a small molecule integrin antagonist that binds to lymphocyte function–associated antigen-1, blocking intercellular adhesion molecule 1, resulting in inhibition of T-cell migration, cytokine release, and further T-cell activation [110]. Other antiinflammatory approaches include recombinant human nerve growth factor, tumor necrosis factor, interleukin receptor antagonist, and neuropeptides, but these therapies are still undergoing clinical trials and have not been FDA approved for DED [91].

Treatment of decreased dacryoreservoirs

In severe cases of decreased tear production or a lack of natural tear coating of the ocular surface, surgical approaches are warranted. Techniques such as tarsorrhaphy, conjunctival resection, and blepharoplasty have been well established. Amniotic membrane application is beneficial on a temporary or permanent basis for ocular surface disease. It derives from the innermost layer of fetal membranes from growing embryos and has antiinflammatory, antiscarring, and antiangiogenic activity [111]. The use of amniotic membranes has greatly increased because of improved availability, ease of use, and effectiveness in treating ocular surface disease signs and symptoms. A temporary amniotic membrane patch is used to promote healing, decrease inflammation, and decrease chances of scarring. A permanent graft is used as a scaffold for epithelial cornea and conjunctival healing and/or to replace ulcerated tissue. See Boxes 1 and 2.

Box 1: Indications for amniotic membrane use as a temporary treatment

Persistent epithelial defect without ulceration

Acute Stevens-Johnsons syndrome

Acute chemical burns

High-risk corneal transplantation

After superficial keratectomy

TREATMENT OF DIETARY DEFICIENCIES

Diet and nutritional support can promote healing and maintenance of the ocular surface. Essential fatty acids are an important part of a healthy dietary intake. Omega-3 fatty acids have long been thought by clinicians to play an essential role in treating patients with ocular surface disease, decreasing inflammation by inhibiting the production of IL-1, IL-2, and tumor necrosis factor alpha, and preventing T-cell activation [112]. T-cell activation is a key part of the inflammatory cascade in inflammatory DED, and inhibition of this step would be expected to decrease inflammatory markers on the ocular surface. Clinical trials have shown that a therapeutic dosage of omega-3 fatty acids (1000 mg of eicosapentaenoic acid/500 mg of docosahexaenoic acid) can improve TBUT and Schirmer scores [113].

However, much of what clinicians believed regarding the benefits of omega-3 fatty acid supplementation for DED and MGD has been challenged by the recent DREAM (Dry Eye Assessment and Management) study [114], which showed no benefits compared with placebo (pills containing small amounts of olive oil, amounts currently found in most North American diets) [115]. In this large, randomized, multicenter clinical trial over 12 months, using daily oral supplementation with 3000 mg of n-3 fatty acids for treatment of moderate

Box 2: Indications for amniotic membrane use as a permanent graft

Persistent epithelial defects with ulceration

Scar or tumor removal

Band keratopathy

Bullous keratopathy

Partial limbal stem cell deficiency

Symblepharon excision and fornix reconstruction

Conjunctival tumor excision

Pterygium excision

Conjunctivochalasis

Leaking filtering blebs

to severe DED, signs and symptoms improved both among patients receiving the supplement and those receiving the placebo, with no significant difference between groups. Furthermore, there was no significant difference between the two groups in 4 key signs of DED: conjunctival staining score, corneal staining score, TBUT, and Schirmer test [114].

Modifying environmental factors

Environmental factors can affect tear film stability and exacerbate dry eyes; for example, computers and video displays, contact lens use, cosmetics, medications, and climate. Depending on the severity of DED, clinicians should counsel their patients on modification of these factors when feasible. Suggestions can be as simple as informing patients to increase blink rate during digital device use, or increasing humidification. Eliminating smoking to decrease local environmental pollutants can also be of value [91]. Contact lens wearers with moderate to severe levels of DED are advised to decrease wear time, change to daily replacement modality, eliminate or change care systems (oxidative systems preferred), change lens materials, switch to a scleral contact lens, increase ocular surface lubrication, and/or eliminate contact lens wear.

SUMMARY

As the TFOS DEWS II treatment and therapy report suggests, many options exist for DED treatment and management. Optimal management requires a precise diagnosis and clinical plan that is specific to each patient. Using the recommendations from the TFOS DEWS II reports and reviewing them with patients may help increase DED awareness and compliance with medical treatments. At the same time, additional constructs may expand the conceptualization of DED [116,117]. As DED awareness increases, newer research and advancements are on the horizon and ever changing.

References

[1] Craig JP, Nichols KK, Akpek EK, et al. TFOS DEWS II Definition and Classification report. Ocul Surf 2017;15(3):276–83.

[2] Doane MG. Abnormalities of the structure of the superficial lipid layer on the in vivo dry-eye. In: Sullivan DA, editor. Lacrimal gland, tear film, and dry eye syndromes. Advances in Experimental Medicine and Biology, vol 350. Boston (MA): Springer; 1994. p. 489–93.

[3] Willcox MDP, Argueso P, Georgiev G, et al. TFOS DEWS II tear film report. Ocul Surf 2017;15(3):366–403.

[4] Bron AJ, DePaiva CS, Chauhan SK, et al. TFOS DEWS II pathophysiology report. Ocul Surf 2017;15(3):438–510.

[5] Craig JP, Nelson JD, Azar DT, et al. TFOS DEWS II report executive summary. Ocul Surf 2017;15(4):802–12.

[6] Korb DR, Henriquez AS. Meibomian gland dysfunction and contact lens intolerance. J Am Optom Assoc 1980;51:243–51.

[7] Henriquez AS, Korb DR. Meibomian glands and contact lens wear. Br J Ophthalmol 1981;65:108–11.

[8] Blackie CA, Korb DR, Knop E, et al. Nonobvious obstructive meibomian gland dysfunction. Cornea 2010;29:1333e45.

[9] Sullivan DA, Rocha EM, Aragona P, et al. TFOS DEWSII sex, gender, and hormones report. Ocul Surf 2017;15(3):284–333.

[10] Brandt JE, Priori R, Valesini G, et al. Sex differences in Sjogren's syndrome: a comprehensive review of immune mechanisms. Biol Sex Differ 2015;6:19.
[11] Schaumberg DA, Dana R, Buring JE, et al. Prevalence of dry eye disease among US men: estimates from the Physicians' Health Studies. Arch Ophthalmol 2009;127:763–8.
[12] Moss SE, Klein R, Klein BE. Prevalence of and risk factors for dry eye syndrome. Arch Ophthalmol 2000;118:1264–8.
[13] McMonnies CW. Key questions in a dry eye history. J Am Optom Assoc 1986;57(7): 512–7.
[14] McMonnies C, Ho A. Patient history in screening for dry eye conditions. J Am Optom Assoc 1987;58(4):296–301.
[15] McMonnies C. Responses to a dry eye questionnaire from a normal population. J Am Optom Assoc 1987;58:588–9.
[16] McMonnies C, Ho A, Wakefield D. Optimum dry eye classification using questionnaire responses. In: Sullivan DA, Dartt DA, Meneray MA, editors. Lacrimal Gland, Tear Film, and Dry Eye Syndromes 2. Advances in Experimental Medicine and biology, vol 438. Boston (MA): Springer; 1998. p. 835–8.
[17] Nichols KK, Nichols JJ, Mitchell GL. The reliability and validity of McMonnies dry eye index. Cornea 2004;23(4):365–71.
[18] Schiffman RM, Christianson MD, Jacobsen G, et al. Reliability and validity of the ocular surface disease index. Arch Ophthalmol 2000;118(5):615–21.
[19] Ozcura F, Helvaci MR. Ocular surface disease index for the diagnosis of dry eye syndrome. Ocul Immunol Inflamm 2007;15:389–93.
[20] Chalmers RL, Begley CG, Caffery B. Validation of the 5-item dry eye questionnaire (DEQ-5): discrimination across self-assessed severity and aqueous tear deficient dry eye diagnoses. Cont Lens Anterior Eye 2010;33(2):55–60.
[21] Asiedu K. Rasch analysis of the standard patient evaluation of eye dryness questionnaire. Eye Contact Lens 2017;43(6):394–8.
[22] Asiedu K, Kyei S, Mensah SN, et al. Ocular surface disease index (OSDI) versus the Standard Patient Evaluation of Eye Dryness (SPEED): a study of a nonclinical sample. Cornea 2016;35(2):175–80.
[23] Rajagopalan K, Abetz L, Mertzanis P, et al. Comparing the discriminative validity of two generic and one disease-specific health-related quality of life measures in a sample of patients with dry eye. Value Health 2005;8:68–74.
[24] Abetz L, Rajagopalan K, Mertzanis P, et al. (Impact of Dry Eye on Everyday Life (IDEEL) Study Group). Development and validation of the impact of dry eye on everyday life (IDEEL) questionnaire, a patient-reported outcomes (PRO) measure for the assessment of the burden of dry eye on patients. Health Qual Life Outcomes 2011;9:111.
[25] Fairchild CJ, Chalmers RL, Begley CG. Clinically important difference in dry eye: change in IDEEL- symptom bother. Optom Vis Sci 2008;85(8):699–707.
[26] Van Bijsterveld OP. Diagnostic tests in the sicca syndrome. Arch Ophthalmol 1969;82: 10–4.
[27] Nichols KK, Mitchell GL, Zadnik K. The repeatability of clinical measurements of dry eye. Cornea 2004;23(3):272–85.
[28] Norn M. Vital staining of the cornea and conjunctiva. Acta Ophthalmol (Copenh) 1973;51:483–91.
[29] Kim J. The use of vital dyes in corneal disease. Curr Opin Ophthalmol 2000;11:241–7.
[30] Methodologies to diagnose and monitor dry eye disease: report of the Diagnostic Methodology Subcommittee of the International Dry Eye WorkShop (2007). Ocul Surf 2007;5(2): 108–52.
[31] Wolffsohn JS, Arita R, Chalmers R, et al. TFOS DEWS II Diagnostic Methodology report. Ocul Surf 2017;15(3):539–74.
[32] Cho P, Brown B. Review of the tear break-up time and a closer look at the tear break-up time of Hong Kong Chinese. Optom Vis Sci 1993;70(1):30–8.

[33] Lemp MA, Hamill JR. Factors affecting tear film breakup in normal eyes. Arch Ophthalmol 1973;89(2):103–5.
[34] Bron AJ, Evans VE, Smith JA. Grading of corneal and conjunctival staining in the context of other dry eye tests. Cornea 2003;22(7):640–50.
[35] Abdul-Fattah AM, Bhargava HN, Korb DR, et al. Quantitative in vitro comparison of fluorescein Delivery to the eye via impregnated paper strip and volumetric techniques. Optom Vis Sci 2002;79:435–8.
[36] Korb DR, Greiner JV, Herman J. Comparison of fluorescein break-up time measurement Reproducibility using standard fluorescein strips versus the Dry Eye Test (DET) method. Cornea 2001;20(8):811–5.
[37] Pult H, Riede-Pult BH. A new modified fluorescein strip: its repeatability and usefulness in tear film break-up time analysis. Cont Lens Anterior Eye 2012;35(1):35–8.
[38] Mooi JK, Wang MTM, Lim J, et al. Minimizing instilled volume reduces the impact of fluorescein on clinical measurements of tear film stability. Cont Lens Anterior Eye 2017;40(3):170–4.
[39] Peterson RC, Wolffsohn JS, Fowler CW. Optimization of anterior eye fluorescein viewing. Am J Ophthalmol 2006;142:572–5.
[40] Mengher LS, Bron AJ, Tonge SR, et al. Effect of Fluorescein instillation on the pre-corneal tear film stability. Curr Eye Res 1985;4(1):9–12.
[41] Mengher LS, Bron AJ, Tonge SR, et al. A non-invasive instrument for clinical assessment of the pre-corneal tear film stability. Curr Eye Res 1985;4(1):1–7.
[42] Mengher LS, Pandher KS, Bron AJ. Non-invasive tear film break-up time : sensitivity and specificity. Acta Ophthalmol 1986;64:441–4.
[43] Cho P, Douthwaite W. The relation between invasive and noninvasive tear break-up time. Optom Vis Sci 1995;72:17–22.
[44] Guillon JP. Use of the Tearscope Plus and attachments in the routine examination of the marginal dry eye contact lens patient. Adv Exp Med Biol 1998;438:859–67.
[45] Cho P, Ho KY, Huang YC, et al. Comparison of noninvasive tear break-up time measurements from black and white background instruments. Optom Vis Sci 2004;81(6):436–41.
[46] Hong J, Sun X, Wei A, et al. Assessment of tear film stability in dry eye with a newly developed keratograph. Cornea 2013;32(5):716–21.
[47] Bhandari V, Reddy JK, Relekar K, et al. Non-invasive assessment of tear film stability with a novel corneal topographer in Indian subjects. Int Ophthalmol 2016;36(6):781–90.
[48] Farris RL. Tear osmolarity—a new gold standard? Adv Exp Med Biol 1994;350:495–503.
[49] Lemp MA. Report of the national eye institute/industry workshop on clinical trials in dry eyes. CLAO J 1995;21:221–32.
[50] Gilbard JP, Rossi SR. Changes in tear ion concentrations in dry-eye disorders. Adv Exp Med Biol 1994;350:529–33.
[51] Tomlinson A, Khanal S, Ramaesh K, et al. Tear film osmolarity: determination of a referent for dry eye diagnosis. Invest Ophthalmol Vis Sci 2006;47(10):4309–15.
[52] Lemp MA, Bron AJ, Baudouin C, et al. Tear osmolarity in the diagnosis and management of dry eye disease. Am J Ophthalmol 2011;111:792–8.
[53] Benelli U, Nardi M, Posarelli C, et al. Tear osmolarity measurement using the TearLab Osmolarity System in the assessment of dry eye treatment effectiveness. Cont Lens Anterior Eye 2010;33(2):61–7.
[54] Sullivan BD, Whitmer D, Nichols KK, et al. Tear film osmolarity: determination of a referent for dry eye diagnosis. Invest Ophthalmol Vis Sci 2010;47:4309–15.
[55] Bunya VY, Fuerst NM, Pistilli M, et al. Variability of tear osmolarity in patients with dry eye. JAMA Ophthalmol 2015;133:662–7.
[56] Szczesna-Iskander DH. Measurement variability of the TearLab osmolarity system. Cont Lens Anterior Eye 2016;39(5):353–8.

[57] Baenninger PB, Voogeli S, Buchmann LM, et al. Variability of tear osmolarity measurements with a point-of-care system in healthy subjects-systematic review. Cornea 2018;37(7):938–45.
[58] Versura P, Profazio V, Campos EC. Performance of tear osmolarity compared to previous diagnostic tests for dry eye diseases. Curr Eye Res 2010;35(7):553–64.
[59] Potvin R, Makari S, Rapuano CJ. Tear film osmolarity and dry eye disease: a review of the literature. Clin Ophthalmol 2015;9:2039–47.
[60] Guillon M, Maissa C. Bulbar conjunctival staining in contact lens wearers and non-lens wearers and its association with symptomatology. Cont Lens Anterior Eye 2005;28: 67–73.
[61] Terry R, Sweeney D, Wong R, et al. Variability of clinical investigators in contact lens research. Optom Vis Sci 1995;72(suppl 12):16.
[62] Carnt N, Willcox M, Evans V, et al. Corneal staining: the IER matrix study. Contact Lens Spectrum 2007;22(9):38–43.
[63] Efron N. Clinical application of grading scales for contact lens complications. Optician 1997;213(5604):26–35.
[64] Whitcher JP, Shiboski CH, Shiboski SC, et al. A simplified quantitative method for assessing keratoconjunctivitis sicca from the Sjogren's Syndrome International Registry. Am J Ophthalmol 2010;149:405–15.
[65] Pritchard N, Young G, Coleman S, et al. Subjective and objective measures of corneal staining related to multipurpose care systems. Cont Lens Anterior Eye 2003;26:3–9.
[66] Sorbara L, Simpson T, Duench S, et al. Comparison of an objective method of measuring bulbar redness to the use of traditional grading scales. Cont Lens Anterior Eye 2007;30(1): 53–9.
[67] Efron N, Pritchard N, Brandon K, et al. How optometrists record corneal staining. Clin Exp Optom 2011;94(1):82–6.
[68] Feenstra RP, Tseng SC. Comparison of fluorescein and rose bengal staining. Ophthalmology 1992;99:605–17.
[69] Bron AJ, Argueso P, Irkec M, et al. Clinical staining of the ocular surface: mechanisms and interpretations. Prog Retin Eye Res 2015;44:36–61.
[70] Cox I, Fonn D. Interference filters to eliminate the surface reflex and improve contrast during fluorescein photography. International Contact Lens Clinic 1991;18:178–81.
[71] Schwallie JD, McKenney CD, Long WD, et al. Corneal staining patterns in normal non-contact lens wearers. Optom Vis Sci 1997;74(2):92–8.
[72] Dundas M, Walker A, Woods RL. Clinical grading of corneal staining of non-contact lens wearers. Ophthalmic Physiol Opt 2001;21(1):30–5.
[73] Khan-Lim D, Berry M. Still confused about rose bengal. Curr Eye Res 2004;29:311–7.
[74] Argueso P, Tisdale A, Spur-Michaud S, et al. Mucin characteristics of human corneal-limbal epithelial cells that exclude the rose bengal anionic dye. Invest Ophthalmol Vis Sci 2006;47:113–9.
[75] Manning FJ, Wehrly SR, Foulks GN. Patient tolerance and ocular surface staining characteristics of lissamine green versus rose bengal. Ophthalmology 1995;102(12):1953–7.
[76] Kim J, Foulks GN. Evaluation of the effect of lissamine green and rose Bengal on human corneal epithelial cells. Cornea 1999;18:328–32.
[77] Varikooty J, Keir N, Jones L. Optimization of assessment and grading for Lid Wiper Epitheliopathy. Presented at the Annual Meeting of the American Academy of Optometry, Phoenix (AZ), October 24-27, 2012. e-abstract #120241.
[78] Efron N, Brennan NA, Morgan PB, et al. Lid wiper epitheliopathy. Prog Retin Eye Res 2016;53:140–74.
[79] Korb DR, Greiner JV, Herman JP, et al. Lid-wiper epitheliopathy and dry eye symptoms in contact lens wearers. CLAO J 2002;28(4):211–6.

[80] Baek J, Doh SH, Chung SK. Comparison of tear meniscus height measurements obtained with the Keratograph and Fourier domain optical coherence tomography in dry eye. Cornea 2015;34(10):1209–13.
[81] Tian L, Qu JH, Zhang XY, et al. Repeatability and reproducibility of noninvasive Keratograph 5M measurements in patients with dry eye disease. J Ophthalmol 2016;2016: 8013621.
[82] Lee KW, Kim JY, Chin HS, et al. Assessment of the tear meniscus by strip meniscometry and Keratograph in patients with dry eye disease according to the presence of Meibomian gland dysfunction. Cornea 2017;36(2):189–95.
[83] Korb DR, Blackie CA. Meibomian gland therapeutic expression: quantifying the applied pressure and the limitation of resulting pain. Eye Contact Lens 2011;37(5):298–301.
[84] Opitz DL, Harthan JS, Formstein SR, et al. Diagnosis and management of meibomian gland dysfunction: optometrists' perspective. Clin Optom 2015;5:59–69.
[85] Kunnen CM, Borwn SH, Lazon de la Jara P, et al. Influence of meibomian gland expression methods on human lipid analysis results. Ocul Surf 2016;14(1):49–55.
[86] Aketa N, Shinzawa M, Kawashima M, et al. Efficacy of plate expression of meibum on tear function and ocular surface findings in Meibomian gland disease. Eye Contact Lens 2018; https://doi.org/10.1097/ICL.0000000000000535. Accessed on November 21, 2018.
[87] Blackie CA, Solomon JD, Scaffidi RC, et al. The relationship between dry eye symptoms and lipid layer thickness. Cornea 2009;28:789–94.
[88] Finis D, Pischel N, Schrader S, et al. Evaluation of lipid layer thickness measurement of the tear film as a diagnostic tool for meibomian gland dysfunction. Cornea 2013;32: 1549–53.
[89] Chotikavanich S, de Paiva CS, de Quan Li, et al. Production and activity of matrix metalloproteinase-9 on the ocular surface increase in dysfunctional tear syndrome. Invest Ophthalmol Vis Sci 2009;50(7):3203–9.
[90] Sambursky R, Davitt WF 3rd, Latkany R, et al. Sensitivity and specificity of a point-of-care matrix metalloproteinase 9 immunoassay for diagnosing inflammation related to dry eye. JAMA Ophthalmol 2013;131(1):24–8.
[91] Jones L, Downie LE, Korb D, et al. TFOS DEWS II management and therapy report. Ocul Surf 2017;15(3):575–628.
[92] Bitton E, Perugino C, Charette S. Comparison of ocular lubricant osmolalities. Optom Vis Sci 2017;94:694–9.
[93] Chen W, Zhang X, Li J, et al. Efficacy of osmoprotectants on prevention and treatment of murine dry eye. Invest Ophthalmol Vis Sci 2013;54(9):6287–97.
[94] Matsuo T. Trehalose protects corneal epithelial cells from death by drying. Br J Ophthalmol 2001;85(5):610–2.
[95] Brzheskiy VV, Efimova EL, Vorontsova TN, et al. Results of a multicenter, randomized, double- masked, placebo-controlled clinical study of the efficacy and safety of Visomitin eye drops in patients with dry eye syndrome. Adv Ther 2015;32(12):1266–79.
[96] Ho WT, Chiang TH, Chang SW, et al. Enhanced corneal wound healing with hyaluronic acid and high-potassium artificial tears. Clin Exp Optom 2013;96(6):536–41.
[97] Gilbard JP, Rossi SR. An electrolyte-based solution that increases corneal glycogen and conjunctival goblet-cell density in a rabbit model for keratoconjunctivitis sicca. Ophthalmology 1992;99(4):600–4.
[98] Freire V, Andollo N, Etxebarria J, et al. Corneal wound healing promoted by 3 blood derivatives: an in vitro and in vivo comparative study. Cornea 2014;33(6):614–20.
[99] Esquenazi S, He J, Bazan HE, et al. Use of autologous serum in corneal epithelial defects post- lamellar surgery. Cornea 2005;24(8):992–7.
[100] Carson CF, Hammer KA, Riley TV. Melaleuca alternifolia (Tea Tree) oil: a review of antimicrobial and other medicinal properties. Clin Microbiol Rev 2006;19(1):50–60.

[101] Gao YY, Di Pascuale MA, Li W, et al. In vitro and in vivo killing of ocular Demodex by tea tree oil. Br J Ophthalmol 2005;89(11):1468–73.

[102] Rynerson JM, Perry HD. DEBS - a unification theory for dry eye and blepharitis. Clin Ophthalmol 2016;10:2455–67.

[103] Goto E, Monden Y, Takano Y, et al. Treatment of non-inflamed obstructive meibomian gland dysfunction by an infrared warm compression device. Br J Ophthalmol 2002;86(12):1403–7.

[104] Finis D, Konig C, Hayajneh J, et al. Six-month effects of a thermodynamic treatment for MGD and implications of meibomian gland atrophy. Cornea 2014;33(12):1265–70.

[105] Kenrick CJ, Alloo SS. The limitation of applying heat to the external lid surface: a case of recalcitrant meibomian gland dysfunction. Case Rep Ophthalmol 2017;8(1):7–12.

[106] Gupta PK, Vora GK, Matossian C, et al. Outcomes of intense pulsed light therapy for treatment of evaporative dry eye disease. Can J Ophthalmol 2016;51(4):249–53.

[107] Toyos R, McGill W, Briscoe D. Intense pulsed light treatment for dry eye disease due to meibomian gland dysfunction: a 3-year retrospective study. Photomed Laser Surg 2015;33(1):41–6.

[108] Holland EJ, Mannis MJ, Lee WB. Ocular surface disease: cornea, conjunctiva and tear film. Amsterdam: Elsevier Inc.; 2013.

[109] Belvisi MG, Hele DJ. Soft steroids: a new approach to the treatment of inflammatory airways diseases. Pulm Pharmacol Ther 2003;16(6):321–5.

[110] Zhong M, Gadek TR, Bui M, et al. Discovery and development of potent LFA-1/ICAM-1 antagonist SAR 1118 as an ophthalmic solution for treating dry eye. ACS Med Chem Lett 2012;3(3):203–6.

[111] Tseng SCG, Espana EM, Kawakita T, et al. How does amniotic membrane work? Ocul Surf 2004;2(3):117–87.

[112] Purasiri P, Mckechnie A, Heys S, et al. Modulation in vitro of human natural cytotoxicity, lymphocyte proliferative response to mitogens and cytokine production by essential fatty acids. Immunology 1997;92(2):162–72.

[113] Liu A, Ji J. Omega-3 essential fatty acids therapy for dry eye syndrome: a meta-analysis of randomized controlled studies. Med Sci Monit 2014;20:1583–9.

[114] Maguire M, Asbell P, Pistilli M, et al, Dry Eye Assessment and Management (DREAM) Study Research Group. n-3 fatty acid supplementation for the treatment of dry eye disease. N Engl J Med 2018;378(18):1681–90.

[115] Caffery B. Dry eye therapy: keeping it simple. Rev Optom 2018;155(11):58–65.

[116] Press LJ. Editorial: the eye as a specialized joint adapted for sight. Vis Devel Rehab 2016;2(1):4–5.

[117] Karpecki PM. The dry eye misalignment. Rev Optom 2018;155(8):80–1.

Advances in Ophthalmology and Optometry 4 (2019) 39–64

ADVANCES IN OPHTHALMOLOGY AND OPTOMETRY

Etiology and Management of Myopia: A Clinical Guide

Jeffrey Cooper, MS, OD*

SUNY College of Optometry

Keywords

• Myopia control • Orthokeratology • Atropine • Myopia • Multifocal soft contact lenses • Progressive glasses • Axial length • Axial elongation

Key points

- Reviews the etiology of myopia
- Creates a relationship between the process of emmetropization and the development of myopia
- Integrates the etiology with treatment
- Reviews treatment using optical and pharmeucalogical methods
- Provides clinicians with clinical insight into how to manage myopia control treatment

INTRODUCTION

Myopia is a common ocular disorder previously viewed as a benign refractive condition. However, even at low levels, myopia is now associated with increased risk for numerous ocular diseases [1]. Researchers have acknowledged a myopia epidemic is occurring worldwide [2]. Although the exact cause of myopia remains elusive, it has both genetic and environmental components, making prevention and treatment both challenging and individualized [3]. Stopping the progression of myopia has the potential to positively affect quality of life and ocular health. The most common options for control include progressive addition lenses (PALs), topical atropine drops (hereafter referred to as atropine), orthokeratology lenses (ortho-k), and multifocal contact lenses. This article provides the most current information about myopia causes and

Disclosure: Dr J. Cooper is a consultant for VTI, Treehouse.

*539 Park Ave, New York, NY 10065. *E-mail address:* cooperjsc1@gmail.com

https://doi.org/10.1016/j.yaoo.2019.04.015

treatment strategies with the goal that ocular health may be preserved. This article is an update of previous reviews by this author [4–6].

PREVALENCE AND CAUSE OF MYOPIA

Myopia is the most common ocular disorder worldwide [7]. The prevalence of myopia in the United States increased dramatically from 25% to 44% between 1972 and 2004 [8–10]. In many urban communities in Asia, the prevalence is now greater than 80% [11,12]. The prevalence is much lower in underdeveloped areas in the world such as Sherpa in Nepal [13].

Myopia is associated with cataract, glaucoma, retinal detachment, and myopic maculopathy, which is similar to the risks associated with hypertension for stroke and myocardial infarction [1,14]. Myopia negatively affects self-perception, job/activity choices, and ocular health [15–17], and is the sixth leading cause of blindness in the world [18]. The incidence of retinal detachments per year is 0.015% in patients with less than 4.75 diopters (D) myopia and increases to 3.2% when myopia is greater than 6 D [19,20]. Myopic patients have a greater risk of developing macular choroidal neovascularization, specifically twice the risk when myopia is in the range of 1 to 2 D, and 9 times the risk when myopia exceeds 5 D; that is, 2× with 1 D to 2 D; and 9× for more than 5 D [21]. It is estimated that almost one-half of the world's population will be myopic by 2050 [22]. As the incidence increases, so does the magnitude. In a recent study, more that 10% of Asian high school students had high myopia increasing the risk for future retinal disease [23].

Human and animal studies conducted over the last 4 decades suggest that development of myopia is controlled by both environmental and genetic factors [24–27]. Human population studies have suggested that environmental factors, such as near work and reading, play an important factor in the development of myopia [28–34], although this is controversial [35]. Zylbermann and colleagues [36] analyzed the incidence of myopia in 2 groups: Orthodox Jewish students (among whom men, unlike women, spent most of the day reading) and secular Jewish students (both men and women spent equal but less time reading than the male students in the Orthodox Jewish schools). They reported that the Orthodox Jewish male students had a higher incidence and magnitude of myopia compared with the other groups of students. They concluded that reading was the factor that caused myopia.

In addition, there are several studies that show that myopia is more common in urban areas, among professionals, educated patients, computer users, university students, and people of high intelligence [37–45]. There is evidence that the intensity of reading may be more important than the time spent reading [46]. Myopia is also associated in individuals who perform sustained near tasks, such as microscopists [47]. Near vision tasks, such as reading, are associated with an increased lag of accommodation, which causes the plane of accommodation to be located behind the retina (hyperopic defocus) when the person performs near work tasks [48,49]. It has been postulated that the optical blur produced by the lag of accommodation may be a signal that drives excessive eye growth and causes myopia [29,48,50–53]. This theory is supported by animal studies that have reported that blur using diffusers or negative lenses results in excessive eye growth and myopia in species as diverse as fish, chickens, tree shrews, monkeys, guinea pigs, and mice [54–69].

Wiesel and Raviola [63,70] induced myopia by placing a translucent screen over a monkey's eye; however, when total occlusion was used instead, there was no alteration in the length of the eye. When animals had either positive or negative lenses placed in front of an eye for an extended time, axial length increased to accommodate the lens placed in front of the eye [71–74]. However, this change is reversible in some animals because they are able to recover when the visual stimuli is removed [75]. This change in axial length occurred even if the optic nerve was severed [76]. This alteration occurs in half the eye, if only half the eye was exposed to blur using a diffuser, or plus or minus lenses [77]. The eye responds to local blur with local changes even when the optic nerve is severed, which shows that the signaling cascade that regulates refractive eye development or axial length is within the eye and does not need feedback from the brain. Rada and colleagues [78] reported that the retina provides remodeling signals to the sclera by which the eye alters it shape to place an image on the retina (ie, emmetropization).

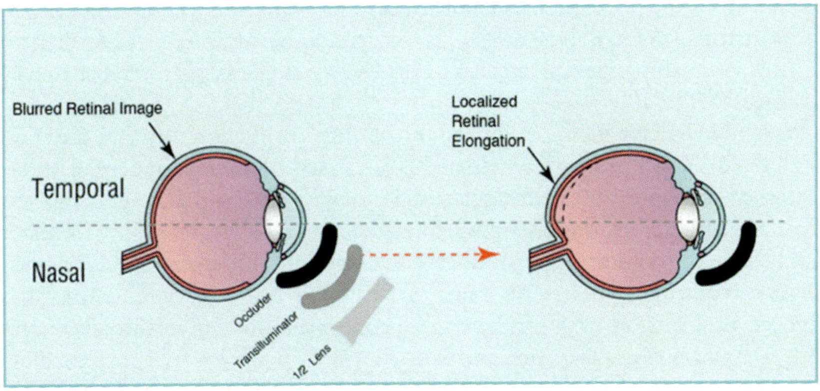

Fig. 1. If a minus lens, transilluminator, or occluder is placed over half of an animal's eye, the portion of the eye receiving a blurred image elongates, trying to eliminate the induced blur. This process of emmetropization is local to the retina and occurs even if the optic nerve is cut, but not if atropine is injected into the eye. (*From* Cooper J, Schulman E, Jamal N. Current status on the development and treatment of myopia. Optometry 2012;83:179–99; with permission.)

Smith and colleagues [79,80] have experimentally asked the most important question regarding refractive development: does the growth of the eye respond more to foveal blur, peripheral blur, or equally to both (Fig. 1)? Smith created a series of lenses in which the center was either plus or minus and the periphery was the opposite; for example, plus in the center with the periphery being minus. In both cases, the length of the eye changed in response to the peripheral lens power. For instance, if the central lens was plus and the peripheral part of the lens was minus, the eye elongated. Smith and colleagues [81] then ablated the macula in several monkeys. In this instance, the eyes still changed their axial length in response to the lens power, which only affected peripheral vision. These studies suggest that defocused information is summed across the entire surface of the retina and that the integrated signal regulates the growth of the eye [76,80,82]. Normal physiologic development of the eyeball results in increased axial elongation primarily along the Z axis, then growth in the X and Y coordinates. Thus, normal spherical spectacles and contact lenses correct the posterior pole and create a relative hyperopic focus of the peripheral retina. The peripheral defocused light becomes the stimulus for axial elongation [80]. Many clinicians and researchers have concluded that these animal studies have a direct relationship with the development of myopia and believe that treatment should be based on these models [2,4,80].

Myopia progresses the most between ages 8 and 15 years (white people X = 0.6 D/y and Asian people X = 0.7 D/y) and then begins to slow down [83–85]. Before the onset of myopia, hyperopic defocus develops in the periphery of the eye along the horizontal meridian [86]. This relative hyperopia is thought to be a growth signal. If this hyperopic defocus is altered optically to create myopic defocus by using plus power in the periphery, according to this theory, a stop signal is created. This theory is the basis for most optical treatments [79].

Myopia increases the most during the winter and the least during the summer [87,88]. It is unknown whether this is caused by increased school work, decreased sunlight, or decreased time outside. In previous generations, myopic progression was assumed to end at age 18 years [89]. However, that has changed since more students have entered graduate school followed by jobs requiring 8 hours or more of sustained near/computer work [45]. Myopic progression was studied in a cohort of postuniversity graduates with a mean age of 35 years and was found to progress in approximately 10% of the cohort who spent a lot of time in front of computers [90]. Those subjects who did not spend time in front of computers did not progress as much. Recently, Bullimore and colleagues [91] reported that 21% of contact wearers between the ages of 20 and 40 years progressed at least 1 D over a 5-year period of follow-up.

These human and animal studies strongly suggest that environmental factors play an important role in the development and progression of myopia; however, human population studies suggest that genetic factors account for as much as 70% of variance in refraction, and the other 30% is from the environment [92–96]. It is clear that the incidence of myopia increases when both parents have myopia [40,97], and this is the most important predictor of the development of myopia [98,99]. Support also comes from studies comparing monozygotic [100] and dizygotic twins [92,101,102]. In summary, refractive error is thought to be influenced by multiple interacting genes [92–94].

Multiple chromosomal loci, which are linked to human myopia, have been identified [25,103–129]. Myopia seems to be a heterogeneous disease, because the genetic loci and genetic variants associated with myopia in different families and ethnic groups may be distinct. Only a small fraction of chromosomal regions that control refractive eye development have been identified [25,27,103–128,130].

Thus, both environmental and genetics factors have been shown to contribute to myopia development [24–27]; Recent work by Tkatchenko and colleagues [3] has helped consolidate the dichotomy of views related to the cause of myopia; that is, genes versus environment. These investigators studied the interaction between age, time spent reading, and genetic variation at the *APLP2* gene locus. Children who spent a high amount of time reading (ie, >3 h/d reading) and who had the myopic version of the *APLP2* gene were 5 times more likely to develop myopia compared with those children who spent a low amount of time reading (ie, <3 h/d reading). In contrast, children who carried a normal version of *APLP2* did not develop myopia even if they were exposed to high levels of reading. Similar findings were found with mice. In a more recent study, Tkatchenko and colleagues [131] showed that the primate retina responds to defocus of different signs by activation or suppression of distinct genetic pathways.

MYOPIA TREATMENT

The incidence of retinal detachment and macular degeneration increases logarithmically at more than 2 D of myopia [1]. Thus, keeping myopia in the −1.00 D versus −3.00 D range may reduce the risk of macular degeneration by 4 times, and retinal detachment by 3 times. Brennan [132] reported that reducing progression by 50% would reduce the risk by almost 90%. Thus, myopia control has become an increasingly important issue with the dramatic increase in the incidence of myopia worldwide, thus patients should be presented with the current risks and benefits of the various treatment options available for myopia control.

The results of both animal and human studies suggest that reducing lag of accommodation, reducing both central and peripheral defocus, and/or blocking myopiagenic signaling in the eye might slow the progression of myopia. The currently considered treatment modalities for control of myopic progression include optical correction, such as bifocal spectacle lenses, PALs, undercorrection, orthokeratology (ortho-k), multifocal contact lenses, and increased exposure to outdoor activities, with the notable exception of atropine, which has been shown to block myopiagenic signaling, albeit with some uncomfortable side effects [4].

Spectacles

Bifocal spectacle lenses have been used extensively to control myopia progression. The lenses were prescribed based on the assumption that myopia was a response to prolonged accommodation [4,53,133,134]. Numerous retrospective studies showed that bifocals and PALs slow the progression of myopia [135–137]. On average, myopia was slowed by 40%. However, these studies had experimental design issues, such as being retrospective and unmasked. The Correction of Myopia Evaluation Trial (COMET) study tried to determine whether a +2.00 D PAL slowed the progression of myopia more than a single-vision full-correcting spectacle lens [138]. This National Institutes of Health/National Eye Institute prospective, multicenter clinical trial reported that, in the first year, PALs slowed the progression of myopia by 20%. However, after 4 years the net myopic reduction was 0.2 D, which was clinically insignificant but statistically significance. The progressive lenses were the most effective when both parents were myopic, there was a large lag of accommodation, and/or the children had esophoria at near [53,139].

Cheng and colleagues [140], in a nonmasked study, evaluated the use of high-fitting executive bifocal spectacle lenses with base-in prism versus single-vision lenses in a group of Canadian Asian people. The experimental lens slowed the progression of myopia by 40%. In 2011, Li and colleagues [141] performed a meta-analysis of 9 clinical trials evaluating PALs that ranged from +1.5 to +2.0 D and found that PALs slowed myopic progression by 0.25 D/y compared with single-vision lenses. The effect was greater in Asian children, who had a higher level of myopia at baseline and who progressed at a more rapid rate compared with white counterparts.

Various novel spectacle lenses have been designed to reduce peripheral hyperopic defocus [142]. None of the spectacle lenses reported had any significant effect in slowing the progression of myopia. Failure to achieve a significant result is thought to be related to the constant changing of eye position when viewing through the lenses.

Historically, many eye care professionals have undercorrected myopia in the belief that the myopic progression will slow down as a result of reduced accommodation. Two studies have shown that undercorrection actually results in minimal acceleration of myopia progression [143,144]. Thus, undercorrection is of questionable therapeutic value in slowing myopic progression.

Contact lenses

For years, it was thought that gas-permeable contact lenses slowed the progression of myopia. In 2 clinical trials, it was shown that neither conventional soft nor gas-permeable contact lenses alter the progression of myopia [145,146].

Reim and colleagues [147] in a retrospective study of 253 children (aged 6–18 years) measured the ability of ortho-k to slow the progression of myopia. They found that the rate of progression was slowed from 0.5 D/y to 0.13 D/y. Since then, there have been several prospective clinical trials that have shown that ortho-k slows the progression of myopia by 40% [148–156]. Two separate meta-analyses of ortho-k, each including more than 400 patients in 7 studies, found that myopic progression was slowed by approximately 45% using axial length measurements [157,158].

Swarbrick and colleagues [154] studied 26 myopic children (11–17 years of age) of east Asian ethnicity using an A-B reversal design. Each child was fitted with an overnight ortho-k lens in 1 eye and a conventional rigid gas-permeable (RGP) lens for daytime wear in the other eye. After 6 months, the lens-eye combinations were crossed over for another 6 months. After the first 6 months of lens wear, the average axial length of the RGP eye had increased by an average of 0.04 mm, whereas the ortho-k eye showed no change. After the second 6-month phase of lens wear, the ortho-k eye showed no change from baseline in axial length, whereas the conventional RGP eye showed a significant increase in mean axial length (ie, 0.09 mm). In summary, the conventional RGP lens–wearing eye showed progressive axial length growth (myopic progression) throughout the study, whereas the ortho-k eye did not.

There have been 2 ortho-k studies that have long-term data (5 years and 7 years) showing the myopia control effect of ortho-k [155,156]. Ortho-k provides patients with a so-called wow factor, and the elimination of daily wearing of contact lenses or glasses. This benefit is particularly important for more athletic children. Visual acuity is good, with most achieving 20/20 and more than 90% achieving 20/30 [159].

The true risk of infection for ortho-k is unknown [160]. Any risk of infection in a voluntary treatment program that involves children must be weighed against the potential benefit of the future reduction of ocular complications such as retinal detachment and macular degeneration. The best estimate of the risk of microbial keratitis (MK) from ortho-k is less than from extended wear of contact lenses. The overall rate for ortho-k is 7.7 per 10,000 years of wear [161]. This rate compares with 1.4 per 10,000 patient years of wear in nonwearers, 11.9 per 10,000 patient years of wear in silicone hydrogel daily wearers, and 20 per 10,000 patient years of wear in soft contact lens extended wear [162]. Ortholenses are worn for a maximum of 8 to 10 hours per day, whereas extended-wear contacts are worn for 24 hours, ortho-k lenses are more oxygen permeable than soft lenses, and the surface of ortho-k lenses is smoother or slipperier than soft lenses, so that a biofilm does not stick to the lens as easily. The incidence of MK is higher in children than in adults [163]. The rare cases from acanthamoeba or fusarium infection often result in permanent damage to the cornea, thus it is important to maintain proper hygiene and cleaning [164]. However, because ortho-k lenses are worn at night, there is greater opportunity for the parents to supervise wearing these lenses versus regular soft lenses.

The largest effect from ortho-k is achieved in children who have moderate myopia (between 1.25 and 4.0 D) and have larger pupils. It is more difficult to get good results with lower or higher myopia [156,165–167]; dropout rates are around 20% [150].

Cho and Cheung [168] evaluated the rebound effect when ortho-k lenses were discontinued by comparing the axial lengths in both an ortho-k group and spectacle group. Stopping ortho-k lens wear was associated with a more rapid increase in axial length compared with those wearing spectacles. When ortho-k was resumed, axial elongation slowed again. This study suggests that there is a rebound effect with ortho-k lenses.

Recently, there has been increased interest in the use of soft lenses to create similar effects to ortho-k [169–175]. To design an optically similar lens, a multifocal lens would need to be manufactured with a distance center that has a small optic zone. Walline and colleagues [174] fitted 40 children with soft multifocal contact lenses (Proclear Multifocal D; CooperVision, Fairport, NY) with a +2.00 D add power, which they compared with a historical age-matched control group of single-vision distance lens wearers. The adjusted mean increase of myopia at 2 years was −1.03 ± 0.06 D for the single-vision contact lens wearers and −0.51 ± 0.06 D for the soft multifocal contact lens wearers. The adjusted mean axial elongation was 0.41 ± 0.03 mm and 0.29 ± 0.03 mm for the single-vision and soft multifocal contact lens wearers respectively ($P < .0016$). They concluded that soft multifocal contact lens wear results in a 50% reduction in the progression of myopia and a 29% reduction in axial elongation over a 2-year treatment period. A major criticism of this study is that there was no true control, only a historical control. The results from the COMET study suggest that the greatest myopia-controlling effect occurs during the first year.

In a recent study, progressive myopic children, were placed in 1 of 3 groups: (1) soft radical gradient (SRRG) contact lenses, (2) orthokeratology, and (3) single-vision glasses [175]. The SRRG is an experimental soft contact lens with a distance center and high plus in the midperiphery. After 2 years, the mean myopia progression value for the SRRG was −0.56 D or 43%; for ortho-k, −0.32 D or 67%; and for single vision, −0.98 D. Measurement of axial length increase was less by 27% and 38% in the SRRG and ortho-k groups respectively, compared with the single-vision group. However, the SRRG lens is not currently commercially available. Aller and colleagues [176] used an Acuvue Bifocal (Johnson & Johnson, Jacksonville, FL) center distance bifocal soft contact lens in a group of myopic esophoric patients, and achieved almost a 70% reduction of myopia after 1 year. A meta-analysis, which included 587 subjects from 8 studies, found that concentric ring and distance centered multifocal designs slowed myopia progression by 30% to 38% and axial elongation by 31% to 51% over 24 months [177]. Turnbull and colleagues [178] performed a retrospective case series analysis of 110 myopic children and reported that multifocal soft lens and ortho-k slowed myopic progression equally. Cooper and colleagues [179] performed a retrospective case series analysis on 32 myopic children and reported that a center distance extended depth of focus soft multifocal contact lens design (NaturalVue by VTI) slowed myopic progression from X = −0.85 D before treatment to 0.04 D/y after, almost a 90% decrease in the progression of myopia. These findings support the concept that both ortho-k and multifocal lenses slow the progression of myopia by similar mechanisms, and the greater the plus over the largest retinal area, the greater the effect.

Pharmaceutical agents

Atropine 1%, which was first used by Wells around 1900 to slow the progression of myopia by "paralyzing" accommodation, has been shown in several retrospective studies to slow the progression of myopia by almost 80% [180–192]. The effect is by a nonaccommodative mechanism [72,82,193], because it inhibits axial length in animals that have no accommodative mechanism [194]; when the optic nerve has been cut, eliminating visual feedback necessary for accommodation [76]; or when regionally induced axial length changes occur from blur [73]. The exact mechanism by which atropine inhibits myopia progression is unknown; multiple studies have suggested that atropine has an effect altering the sclera [195–197]. Another proposed mechanism is that increased ultraviolet (UV) light (secondary to pupil dilatation) may increase collagen cross-linking within the sclera, thereby slowing scleral growth [198].

The most common complaints when using atropine are pupillary dilatation and temporary paralysis of accommodation; however, they can be reduced by the use of photochromic PAL glasses. There have also been some concerns of increased UV exposure and long-term retinal damage [199], which is reduced by the use of UV coatings on the lenses. Besides having a good safety profile with long-term clinical use [200], ERG results (which are a sensitive indicator for early retinal damage) are normal in patients using atropine in the long term [4,200–202]. In the 2-year Atropine in the Treatment of Myopia (ATOM) study (N = 400) there were no serious adverse effects. Reasons for withdrawal included allergic or hypersensitivity reactions, discomfort (4.5%), glare (1.5%), blurred near vision (1%), logistical difficulties (3.5%), and others (0.5%). Similar low adverse rates have been reported by other atropine studies. Although atropine 1% may have its strongest effect in year 1, several earlier studies have shown the long-term effectiveness of atropine [185,188,191]. Chiang and colleagues [203] evaluated the effect of atropine 1% used once a week for 1 month to 10 years. They reported a mean progression rate of 0.08 D/y in the compliant group and 0.23 D/y in the partially compliant group.

Chua and colleagues [204] (ATOM 1) studied the effect of atropine 1% in a group of 400 children (13.5% dropout rate) in which 1 group received atropine in 1 eye and the other group received a placebo. The mean progression in the control eye after 2 years was 0.6 D/y, whereas the atropine-treated eye progressed 0.14 D/y, which represents a 77% reduction in the progression of myopia. More importantly, the axial length measurements in the eyes that received atropine remained essentially unchanged (0.02 mm over 2 years). There were no serious adverse events, with atropine being generally well tolerated.

There have been several studies that evaluated the relationship of the concentration of atropine to the rate of progression of myopia. Shih and colleagues [205] evaluated the effect of different concentrations of atropine in children (6–13 years of age) who were prescribed 0.5%, 0.25%, or 0.1%

atropine, or 0.5% tropicamide (control group) in both eyes nightly. The mean progression of myopia was 0.04 ± 0.63 D/y in the atropine 0.5% group, 0.45 ± 0.55 D/y in the atropine 0.25% group, and 0.47 ± 0.91 D/y in the atropine 0.1% group, compared with 1.06 ± 0.61 D/y in the control group. At the end of the 2-year treatment period, 61% of children in the atropine 0.5% group, 49% in the atropine group 0.25%, and 42% in the atropine 0.1% group had no myopic progression. In another study, the concentration of atropine was varied from winter (0.5%) to summer (0.1%) based on the assumption that myopia progresses less during the summer. The children had less pupillary dilatation during the summer months when the sunlight and photophobia was the greatest [206]. This regimen slowed myopic progression by 77%. Fang and colleagues [207] evaluated the efficiency of atropine 0.025% to prevent the development of myopia in a group of children presenting with the signs of myopic progression. There was a 50% reduction in the number of children who converted from emmetropia to myopia. Cooper and colleagues [208] found that the highest concentration of atropine, which does not cause any symptoms related to pupil dilatation or decreased accommodation when atropine is used, is 0.02%.

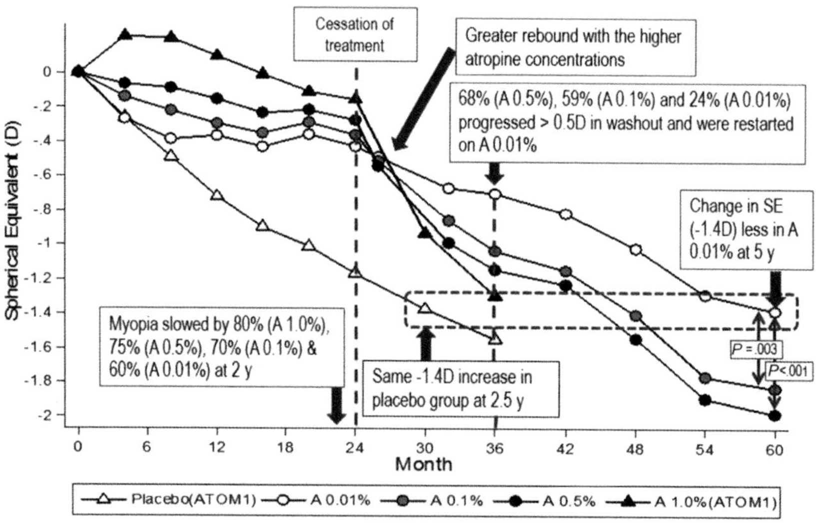

Fig. 2. Combined data from ATOM 1 and 2 in which patients used various concentrations over 3 phases of the study: experimental for the first 2 years; cessation of treatment, which occurred for the third year; and resumption of treatment of those patients who showed progression during the cessation period. The most effective treatment during the first phase was atropine 1%; however, during the cessation phase there was the most rebound with the higher dosages. During the resumption phase, atropine 0.01% was again effective in slowing the progression of myopia. SE, spherical equivalent. (*From* Chia A, Lu QS, Tan D. Five-year clinical trial on atropine for the treatment of myopia 2: myopia control with atropine 0.01% eyedrops. Ophthalmology 2016;123(2):391–399; with permission.)

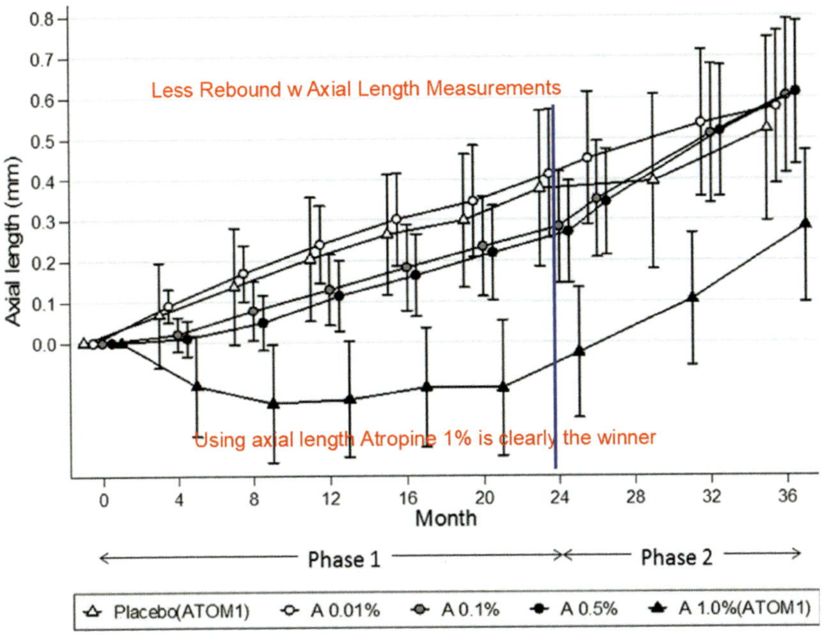

Fig. 3. It is clear that, when axial length is used, atropine 1% reduces the progression more than any other concentration. The higher the concentration, the more effective atropine is in slowing the progression of myopia. Atropine 0.01% and placebo are not clinically or statistically different. At 2 years, all atropine treatment is terminated for a year. There is greater progression than before treatment, but the progression is still less than if atropine of any concentration was used. (*Reprinted from* American Journal of Ophthalmology, Volume 157, Issue 2, Audrey Chia, Wei-Han Chua, Li Wen, Allan Fong, Yar Yen Goon, Donald Tan, Atropine for the treatment of childhood myopia: changes after stopping atropine 0.01%, 0.1% and 0.5%, 451–7, Copyright 2014, with permission from Elsevier.)

The ATOM 2 study [199] evaluated various concentrations of atropine (ie, 0.5%, 0.1%, and 0.01%). After 2 years, Chia and colleagues [209] reported that all 3 concentrations slowed the progression of myopia. The mean progression with each concentration (spherical equivalent) was 0.15 D/y (0.5% atropine), 0.19 D/y (0.1% atropine), and 0.25 D/y (0.01% atropine). (Fig. 2) On first glance, the ATOM 2 study suggests that myopic progression was slowed equally for all concentrations. However, this conclusion is not justified if axial length is used to measure myopic progression rather than refractive error. Fig. 3 shows the axial change measurements from the ATOM 1 and 2 studies combined at the end of 2 years. The ATOM 1 study showed a minimal 0.02-mm change in axial length over 2 years with the use atropine 1%, whereas ATOM 2 showed no statistical difference between the placebo and atropine 0.01% groups. This finding is important for 2 reasons. First, if the primary purpose of slowing myopia progression is to reduce axial elongation, which in turn decreases future retinal complications, then the lower concentrations are not nearly as effective as atropine 1%. Second, minimal difference between placebo and atropine 0.01% axial length changes versus significant refractive changes between placebo and atropine 0.01% should make clinicians question the true effect of atropine 0.01%.

After 2 years, all participants in the ATOM 2 study discontinued the use of atropine for 1 year. At the end of that year, 24% of the 0.01% group, 59% of the 0.1% group, and 68% of the 0.5% groups in the original ATOM 2 trial progressed more than 0.5 D of myopia and required retreatment with 0.01% atropine for an additional 2 years [210]. This rebound effect was much greater with cycloplegic refractions compared with axial length changes. The rebound effect observed in the ATOM studies can be partially explained by atropine having a greater cycloplegic effect than the 1% cyclopentolate used to measure refractive error, creating an impression that atropine slows the progression of myopia more than it really does in the first year, which creates a false impression of a rebound effect. Because atropine suppresses the signal for axial elongation, an abrupt stopping of higher dosages would result in faster elongation than discontinuation of lower concentrations. These findings suggest that atropine use should be tapered down rather than abruptly discontinued [211].

After stopping the use of atropine drops for 1 year, the patients were reassessed [212]. It was noted that the progression of myopia resumed in some patients and stopped in others. Those who progressed after phase 2 were restarted on 0.01% atropine and reassessed 2 years later (total of 5 years) [210]. Those who did not progress after the discontinuation phase generally did not progress during the next 2 years. The investigators falsely concluded that 0.01% atropine was more effective than the higher dosages in slowing the progression of myopia. The investigators' conclusion may be incorrectly supported by a recent meta-analysis that suggests that there is no clinical difference between the effectiveness of low and high concentrations of atropine to slow the progression of myopia [213]. This conclusion must be viewed cautiously in light of axial length measurements where there are significant dosage-related differences in the effect of atropine in slowing the progression of myopia.

The rebound results also need to be evaluated with caution: clinicians do not prescribe atropine 1% for 2 years and then stop treatment. Patients are treated with atropine for years without interruptions. Studies in which 1% atropine was prescribed for many years found that atropine did not become less effective over time. The subjects who had a reduced response to atropine treatment had the following characteristics: (1) 2 myopic parents, (2) developed myopia earlier, and (3) progressed more than the average of 0.66 D/y.

Recently, low-concentration atropine eye drops (0.05%, 0.025%, and 0.01%) were compared with placebo for 1 year in 438 children aged 4 to 12 years with myopia [214]. After 1 year, the mean refractive change and axial length change was −0.27 D or 0.20 mm for 0.05%, −0.46 D or 0.29 mm for 0.025%, −0.5 D or 0.36 mm for 0.01%, and −0.81 D or 0.41 mm for the placebo groups. The Low-Concentration Atropine for Myopia Progression (LAMP) study concluded that the reduced progression was directly related to concentration, with no real difference between atropine 0.01% and placebo. (Because of this study, and our own observations, the authors begin treatment with atropine 0.02%for a minimum of 5 years before tapering higher dosages, and, if progression recurs, treatment with 0.02% atropine can be resumed. If higher concentrations of atropine are required then atropine 0.05% may be used [208].)

Time spent outdoors

Several recent studies suggest that time spent outdoors slows both onset and progression of myopia in children [215–224]. The effect of outdoor activities on myopia is not necessarily related to physical activity and that the shear exposure to outdoor environment has the therapeutic effect [217]. Several studies suggested that exposure to brighter light, increased levels of vitamin D, increased levels of dopamine, or UV light by itself are responsible for the effect of the outdoors on myopia onset and progression [225–234]. Other studies have ruled out the role of vitamin D and UV light in the inhibition of myopia development by exposure to the outdoors [235,236].

Recently Torii and colleagues [234] showed that violet light (VL) (wavelength 360–400 nm) suppresses myopia progression in chicks and humans. They retrospectively measured the axial length elongation among myopic children, who wore either VL-blocked eyeglasses or 1 of 2 types of contact lenses (partially VL blocking and VL transmitting). They reported that VL-transmitting contact lenses suppressed myopia progression more than VL-blocking lenses. They suggested that because VL exposure is limited by UV protection from being indoors and UV being filtered out by panel window glass, UV-filtering glasses, some contact lenses, and sunglasses, increased VL exposure may be a preventive strategy against myopia progression.

There is also evidence that increasing the illumination in classrooms decreases the incidence of myopia [237]. Bright light has been shown to inhibit form-deprivation myopia and reduce lens-induced (defocus-induced) myopia in animal studies [227–231]. However, there is no information about whether bright light might have caused animals to close their eyes because of photophobia, nor was the use of sunglasses in bright light taken into account, which might account for substantial differences in the visual environment between indoors and outdoors [238]. Indoor activities create far more peripheral hyperopic defocus (causing myopia) than any outdoors activities. Outdoor activities decrease any peripheral defocus and that serves as a stop signal for eye growth (thus inhibiting development of myopia). Brighter light intensity leads to pupil constriction and increased depth of focus, which reduces optical blur and increases contrast. Change in contrast, in turn, affects the function of amacrine cells, which might explain the role of dopamine in myopia development in animal models. Although the exact mechanism responsible for the effect of outdoor activities on myopia is unknown, spending more time outdoors clearly has a therapeutic effect on myopia onset and is associated with an 11% to 33% reduction in myopic progression. Thus, children, especially those who have 2 myopic parents and/or show signs of myopia development or progression, should spend more time outdoors to help prevent myopia from developing.

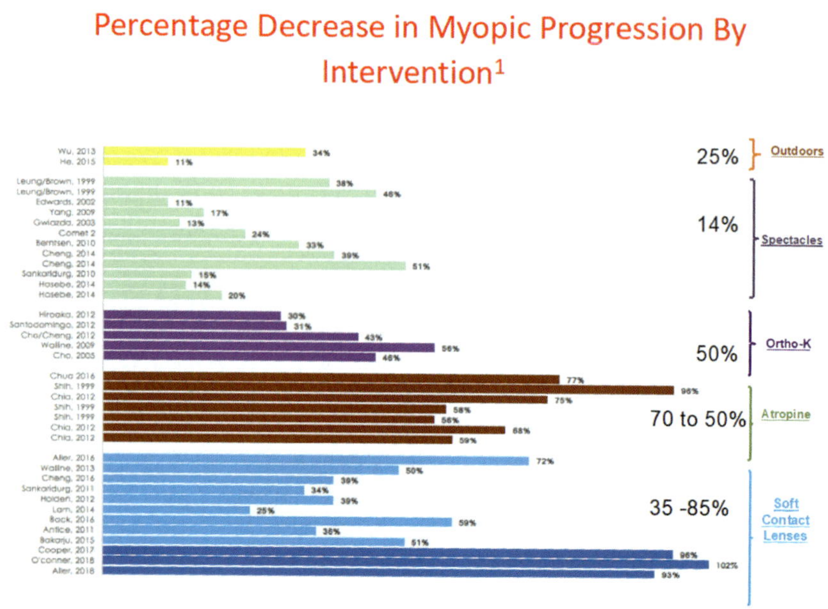

Fig. 4. Studies in yellow, concerning the influence of outdoors exposure in slowing the progression of myopia, have a mean effect of approximately 25%. Spectacle studies, depicted in green by meta-analysis, slow the progression by approximately 14%. A greater effect is found in higher myopes who are of Asian origin. Ortho-k, depicted in violet, reduces the progression of myopia by 50%. Atropine, depicted in brown, must be broken down into high concentrations (>0.5%) and low concentrations. The ability of atropine to slow myopia seems to be concentration related. Atropine 1% slows the progression by almost 70%, whereas low concentrations, such as atropine 0.01%, only slow the progression by 50%. There are also the multiple soft, multifocal lenses, which have various designs and are depicted in blue. The multiple designs are probably the cause of the high variance in multifocal soft lenses slowing the progression of myopia. The more plus there is in the peripheral, which covers a larger area, seems to be related to how effective soft multifocal lenses are in slowing the progression of myopia. As an average amount, soft multifocal contact lenses slow the progression by 40%. The darker blue bars at the bottom are from studies using NaturalVue by VTI, which has the most plus in the midperiphery and seems to be the most effective in slowing the progression of myopia. (*Data from* Sankaridurg P. Contact lenses to slow progression of myopia. Clin Exp Optom 2017; and Cooper J, Tkatchenko AV. A review of current concepts of the etiology and treatment of myopia. Eye Contact Lens 2018;44(4):231–247.)

SUMMARY

There is strong evidence that myopia is a result of an interaction between genes and environment and can be slowed by a variety of treatments. Parents should be aware of what is and is not effective, including the risks and benefits associated with each treatment option (Fig. 4). Despite none of these interventions having US Food and Drug Administration approval/clearance at this time to treat myopia progression, the authors believe that, with informed consent, an appropriate treatment plan should be discussed with risks and benefits described. Treatment preferences now seem to vary by country and profession. More eye care professionals in China advocate the use of ortho-k; in Taiwan and Singapore, more advocate atropine; and in the United States some eye care professionals prescribe soft multifocal contact lenses, and/or advocate ortho-k, and some ophthalmologists advocate atropine. In Taiwan, more than 60% of the children with myopia are on atropine [239]. There are data supporting the additive effects of optically correcting myopic children with ortho-k and low dosages of atropine; after a year in the study, ortho-k–only patients increased axial length by 0.19 mm, whereas ortho-k and atropine increased axial length by 0.09 mm [240]. Because they use different stop mechanisms, it is not surprising that their effects are additive. There is a need for more studies into the mechanisms of myopia and refractive eye development, but the future is encouraging.

Ongoing research has already provided some insights into molecular pathways underlying the development of myopia and might produce new treatment regiments to slow the progression of myopia. In the meantime, children who are at high risk for very progressive myopia (myopia first noted around 4 or 5 years of age, progressing more than 1 D/y, and parental myopia) should probably be started with 1% atropine. Clinicians might consider the prophylactic use of atropine 0.01% in children with a strong risk of development of myopia (ie, 2 parents being myopic and decreasing hyperopia of 0.5 D/y). In contrast, children who become myopic after the age of 8 years can be treated with 0.02% atropine, soft multifocal contact lenses, or ortho-k. In addition, patients with more than 6 D of myopia can wear soft multifocal contact lenses or a combination of ortho-k contact lenses and glasses to obtain an effective treatment result [241]. Because soft multifocal contact lenses, ortho-k, and low dosage of atropine seem to be equally effective [242], patient concerns and compliance may help guide treatment selection.

Some children prefer their glasses and thus require atropine. Children who are more athletic usually prefer ortho-k or soft multifocal contact lenses. Parents who are fearful of overnight contact lens wear often choose low concentrations of atropine or soft multifocal contact lenses, whereas parents/patients concerned about the long-term effects of atropine usually choose ortho-k. Some patients are concerned with the risks of ortho-k associated with sleeping in lenses, whereas others are concerned about the long-term effects of atropine even at low dosages. In addition, distance center soft contact lenses may have a better indication in myopes with less than −2.00 D because effectiveness is related to the initial refractive error. The authors often prescribe distance center soft multifocal contact lenses that have the largest peripheral plus, even though the published clinical evidence only includes case series analysis, because the perceived risk of treatment with this modality is low [179]. In addition, children should be encouraged to spend more time outside and the public and policymakers should be informed of the potential benefits of outdoor activities so that schools might schedule more time for outdoor activities during school hours and after school.

Our office uses an extend-and-treat approach, in which we prescribe a primary treatment, either atropine or lenses, and have the patient return in 3 months. At that examination, we measure axial length 20 times using an IOL Master [243]. If progression is greater than normal growth amounts, we either increase the concentration of atropine (ie, 0.01% to 0.02% to 0.05% to 0.1% to 1%) or add atropine to optical treatments and see the patient again in 3 months. If at the follow-up examination progression occurs, the dosage is increased and the patient is seen again in 3 months. Patients who do not progress are seen in 4 months; if at that visit no progression occurs, then the next visit is at 6 months. Patients are maintained on the regimen for 5 years or until their early 20s, at which time treatment is evaluated for discontinuation by tapering down the atropine. As a final note, every clinician can institute simple and effective treatment by using either low-dosage atropine or multifocal soft contact lenses with a distance center.

References

[1] Flitcroft DI. The complex interactions of retinal, optical and environmental factors in myopia aetiology. Prog Retin Eye Res 2012;31(6):622–60.

[2] Holden BA. The Charles F. Prentice award lecture 2014: a 50-year research journey: giants and great collaborators. Optom Vis Sci 2015;92(7):741–9.

[3] Tkatchenko AV, Tkatchenko TV, Guggenheim JA, et al. APLP2 regulates refractive error and myopia development in mice and humans. PLoS Genet 2015;11(8):e1005432.

[4] Cooper J, Schulman E, Jamal N. Current status on the development and treatment of myopia. Optometry 2012;83(5):179–99.

[5] Cooper J, Weibel K, Borukhov G. Use of atropine to slow the progression of myopia: a literature review and guidelines for clinical use. Vision Development & Rehabilitation 2018;4(1):12–28.

[6] Cooper J, Tkatchenko AV. A review of current concepts of the etiology and treatment of myopia. Eye Contact Lens 2018;44(4):231–47.

[7] Pararajasegaram R. VISION 2020-the right to sight: from strategies to action. Am J Ophthalmol 1999;128(3):359–60.

[8] Kempen JH, Mitchell P, Lee KE, et al. The prevalence of refractive errors among adults in the United States, Western Europe, and Australia. Arch Ophthalmol 2004;122(4):495–505.

[9] Javitt JC, Chiang YP. The socioeconomic aspects of laser refractive surgery. Arch Ophthalmol 1994;112(12):1526–30.

[10] Vitale S, Sperduto RD, Ferris FL 3rd. Increased prevalence of myopia in the United States between 1971-1972 and 1999-2004. Arch Ophthalmol 2009;127(12):1632–9.

[11] Lin LL, Shih YF, Hsiao CK, et al. Prevalence of myopia in Taiwanese schoolchildren: 1983 to 2000. Ann Acad Med Singapore 2004;33(1):27–33.

[12] Lam CS, Goldschmidt E, Edwards MH. Prevalence of myopia in local and international schools in Hong Kong. Optom Vis Sci 2004;81(5):317–22.

[13] Niroula DR, Saha CG. Study on the refractive errors of school going children of Pokhara city in Nepal. Kathmandu Univ Med J (KUMJ) 2009;7(25):67–72.

[14] Saw SM, Gazzard G, Shih-Yen EC, et al. Myopia and associated pathological complications. Ophthalmic Physiol Opt 2005;25(5):381–91.

[15] Pesudovs K, Garamendi E, Elliott DB. A quality of life comparison of people wearing spectacles or contact lenses or having undergone refractive surgery. J Refract Surg 2006;22(1): 19–27.

[16] Rose K, Harper R, Tromans C, et al. Quality of life in myopia. Br J Ophthalmol 2000;84(9): 1031–4.

[17] Takashima T, Yokoyama T, Futagami S, et al. The quality of life in patients with pathologic myopia. Jpn J Ophthalmol 2001;45(1):84–92.
[18] Holden B, Sankaridurg P, Smith E, et al. Myopia, an underrated global challenge to vision: where the current data takes us on myopia control. Eye (Lond) 2014;28(2):142–6.
[19] Arevalo JF, Ramirez E, Suarez E, et al. Rhegmatogenous retinal detachment after laser-assisted in situ keratomileusis (LASIK) for the correction of myopia. Retina 2000;20(4):338–41.
[20] Arevalo JF, Azar-Arevalo O. Retinal detachment in myopic eyes after laser in situ keratomileusis. Am J Ophthalmol 2000;129(6):825–6.
[21] Steidl SM, Pruett RC. Macular complications associated with posterior staphyloma. Am J Ophthalmol 1997;123(2):181–7.
[22] Holden BA, Fricke TR, Wilson DA, et al. Global Prevalence of Myopia and High Myopia and Temporal Trends from 2000 through 2050. Ophthalmology 2016;123(5):1036–42.
[23] Wu PC, Tsai CL, Gordon GM, et al. Chondrogenesis in scleral stem/progenitor cells and its association with form-deprived myopia in mice. Mol Vis 2015;21:138–47.
[24] Morgan IG. The biological basis of myopic refractive error. Clin Exp Optom 2003;86(5):276–88.
[25] Young TL. Molecular genetics of human myopia: an update. Optom Vis Sci 2009;86(1):E8–22.
[26] Baird PN, Schache M, Dirani M. The GEnes in Myopia (GEM) study in understanding the aetiology of refractive errors. Prog Retin Eye Res 2010;29(6):520–42.
[27] Wojciechowski R. Nature and nurture: the complex genetics of myopia and refractive error. Clin Genet 2011;79(4):301–20.
[28] Parssinen O, Lyyra AL. Myopia and myopic progression among schoolchildren: a three-year follow-up study. Invest Ophthalmol Vis Sci 1993;34(9):2794–802.
[29] Goss DA. Nearwork and myopia. Lancet 2000;356(9240):1456–7.
[30] Hepsen IF, Evereklioglu C, Bayramlar H. The effect of reading and near-work on the development of myopia in emmetropic boys: a prospective, controlled, three-year follow-up study. Vision Res 2001;41(19):2511–20.
[31] Saw SM, Chua WH, Hong CY, et al. Nearwork in early-onset myopia. Invest Ophthalmol Vis Sci 2002;43(2):332–9.
[32] Wong L, Coggon D, Cruddas M, et al. Education, reading, and familial tendency as risk factors for myopia in Hong Kong fishermen. J Epidemiol Community Health 1993;47(1):50–3.
[33] Saw SM, Wu HM, Seet B, et al. Academic achievement, close up work parameters, and myopia in Singapore military conscripts. Br J Ophthalmol 2001;85(7):855–60.
[34] Li SM, Li SY, Kang MT, et al. Near work related parameters and myopia in Chinese children: the Anyang Childhood Eye Study. PLoS One 2015;10(8):e0134514.
[35] Mutti DO, Zadnik K. Has near work's star fallen? Optom Vis Sci 2009;86(2):76–8.
[36] Zylbermann R, Landau D, Berson D. The influence of study habits on myopia in Jewish teenagers. J Pediatr Ophthalmol Strabismus 1993;30(5):319–22.
[37] Saw SM, Tan SB, Fung D, et al. IQ and the association with myopia in children. Invest Ophthalmol Vis Sci 2004;45(9):2943–8.
[38] Williams C, Miller LL, Gazzard G, et al. A comparison of measures of reading and intelligence as risk factors for the development of myopia in a UK cohort of children. Br J Ophthalmol 2008;92(8):1117–21.
[39] Czepita D, Lodygowska E, Czepita M. Are children with myopia more intelligent? A literature review. Ann Acad Med Stetin 2008;54(1):13–6 [discussion: 16].
[40] Pan CW, Ramamurthy D, Saw SM. Worldwide prevalence and risk factors for myopia. Ophthalmic Physiol Opt 2012;32(1):3–16.
[41] Lee YY, Lo CT, Sheu SJ, et al. What factors are associated with myopia in young adults? A survey study in Taiwan military conscripts. Invest Ophthalmol Vis Sci 2013;54(2):1026–33.

[42] Saw SM, Cheng A, Fong A, et al. School grades and myopia. Ophthalmic Physiol Opt 2007;27(2):126–9.
[43] Zadnik K, Mutti DO. Refractive error changes in law students. Am J Optom Physiol Opt 1987;64(7):558–61.
[44] Ip JM, Rose KA, Morgan IG, et al. Myopia and the urban environment: findings in a sample of 12-year-old Australian school children. Invest Ophthalmol Vis Sci 2008;49(9): 3858–63.
[45] Cortinez MF, Chiappe JP, Iribarren R. Prevalence of refractive errors in a population of office-workers in Buenos Aires, Argentina. Ophthalmic Epidemiol 2008;15(1):10–6.
[46] Ip JM, Saw SM, Rose KA, et al. Role of near work in myopia: findings in a sample of Australian school children. Invest Ophthalmol Vis Sci 2008;49(7):2903–10.
[47] Ting PW, Lam CS, Edwards MH, et al. Prevalence of myopia in a group of Hong Kong microscopists. Optom Vis Sci 2004;81(2):88–93.
[48] Gwiazda J, Thorn F, Bauer J, et al. Myopic children show insufficient accommodative response to blur. Invest Ophthalmol Vis Sci 1993;34(3):690–4.
[49] Seidemann A, Schaeffel F. An evaluation of the lag of accommodation using photorefraction. Vision Res 2003;43(4):419–30.
[50] Gwiazda J, Bauer J, Thorn F, et al. A dynamic relationship between myopia and blur-driven accommodation in school-aged children. Vision Res 1995;35(9):1299–304.
[51] Abbott ML, Schmid KL, Strang NC. Differences in the accommodation stimulus response curves of adult myopes and emmetropes. Ophthalmic Physiol Opt 1998;18(1):13–20.
[52] Charman WN. Near vision, lags of accommodation and myopia. Ophthalmic Physiol Opt 1999;19(2):126–33.
[53] Gwiazda JE, Hyman L, Norton TT, et al. Accommodation and related risk factors associated with myopia progression and their interaction with treatment in COMET children. Invest Ophthalmol Vis Sci 2004;45(7):2143–51.
[54] Shen W, Sivak JG. Eyes of a lower vertebrate are susceptible to the visual environment. Invest Ophthalmol Vis Sci 2007;48(10):4829–37.
[55] Shen W, Vijayan M, Sivak JG. Inducing form-deprivation myopia in fish. Invest Ophthalmol Vis Sci 2005;46(5):1797–803.
[56] Kroger RH, Wagner HJ. The eye of the blue acara (*Aequidens pulcher*, Cichlidae) grows to compensate for defocus due to chromatic aberration. J Comp Physiol A 1996;179(6): 837–42.
[57] Wallman J, Turkel J, Trachtman J. Extreme myopia produced by modest change in early visual experience. Science 1978;201(4362):1249–51.
[58] Irving EL, Sivak JG, Callender MG. Refractive plasticity of the developing chick eye. Ophthalmic Physiol Opt 1992;12(4):448–56.
[59] Irving EL, Callender MG, Sivak JG. Inducing myopia, hyperopia, and astigmatism in chicks. Optom Vis Sci 1991;68(5):364–8.
[60] Sherman SM, Norton TT, Casagrande VA. Myopia in the lid-sutured tree shrew (*Tupaia glis*). Brain Res 1977;124(1):154–7.
[61] Cottriall CL, McBrien NA. The M1 muscarinic antagonist pirenzepine reduces myopia and eye enlargement in the tree shrew. Invest Ophthalmol Vis Sci 1996;37(7):1368–79.
[62] Raviola E, Wiesel TN. An animal model of myopia. N Engl J Med 1985;312(25): 1609–15.
[63] Wiesel TN, Raviola E. Myopia and eye enlargement after neonatal lid fusion in monkeys. Nature 1977;266(5597):66–8.
[64] Whatham AR, Judge SJ. Compensatory changes in eye growth and refraction induced by daily wear of soft contact lenses in young marmosets. Vision Res 2001;41(3):267–73.
[65] Smith EL 3rd, Bradley DV, Fernandes A, et al. Form deprivation myopia in adolescent monkeys. Optom Vis Sci 1999;76(6):428–32.
[66] Smith EL 3rd, Hung LF. The role of optical defocus in regulating refractive development in infant monkeys. Vision Res 1999;39(8):1415–35.

[67] Howlett MH, McFadden SA. Spectacle lens compensation in the pigmented guinea pig. Vision Res 2009;49(2):219–27.
[68] Howlett MH, McFadden SA. Form-deprivation myopia in the guinea pig (*Cavia porcellus*). Vision Res 2006;46(1–2):267–83.
[69] Tkatchenko TV, Shen Y, Tkatchenko AV. Mouse experimental myopia has features of primate myopia. Invest Ophthalmol Vis Sci 2010;51(3):1297–303.
[70] Raviola E, Wiesel TN. Effect of dark-rearing on experimental myopia in monkeys. Invest Ophthalmol Vis Sci 1978;17(6):485–8.
[71] Wallman J, Gottlieb MD, Rajaram V, et al. Local retinal regions control local eye growth and myopia. Science 1987;237(4810):73–7.
[72] Smith EL, Hung LF, Huang J, et al. Effects of optical defocus on refractive development in monkeys: evidence for local, regionally selective mechanisms. Invest Ophthalmol Vis Sci 2010;51(8):3864–73.
[73] Smith EL 3rd, Hung LF, Huang J, et al. Effects of optical defocus on refractive development in monkeys: evidence for local, regionally selective mechanisms. Invest Ophthalmol Vis Sci 2010;51(8):3864–73.
[74] Troilo D, Wallman J. The regulation of eye growth and refractive state: an experimental study of emmetropization. Vision Res 1991;31(7–8):1237–50.
[75] Zhou X, Lu F, Xie R, et al. Recovery from axial myopia induced by a monocularly deprived facemask in adolescent (7-week-old) guinea pigs. Vision Res 2007;47(8):1103–11.
[76] Troilo D, Gottlieb MD, Wallman J. Visual deprivation causes myopia in chicks with optic nerve section. Curr Eye Res 1987;6(8):993–9.
[77] Smith EL 3rd, Huang J, Hung LF, et al. Hemiretinal form deprivation: evidence for local control of eye growth and refractive development in infant monkeys. Invest Ophthalmol Vis Sci 2009;50(11):5057–69.
[78] Rada JA, Shelton S, Norton TT. The sclera and myopia. Exp Eye Res 2006;82(2): 185–200.
[79] Smith EL 3rd, Hung LF, Huang J. Relative peripheral hyperopic defocus alters central refractive development in infant monkeys. Vision Res 2009;49(19):2386–92.
[80] Smith EL 3rd. Prentice award lecture 2010: a case for peripheral optical treatment strategies for myopia. Optom Vis Sci 2011;88(9):1029–44.
[81] Smith EL 3rd, Ramamirtham R, Qiao-Grider Y, et al. Effects of foveal ablation on emmetropization and form-deprivation myopia. Invest Ophthalmol Vis Sci 2007;48(9):3914–22.
[82] Wildsoet C, Pettigrew J. Experimental myopia and anomalous eye growth patterns unaffected by optic nerve section in chickens: evidence for local control of eye growth. Clinical Vision Science 1988;3:99–107.
[83] Tan NW, Saw SM, Lam DS, et al. Temporal variations in myopia progression in Singaporean children within an academic year. Optom Vis Sci 2000;77(9):465–72.
[84] Fan DS, Lam DS, Lam RF, et al. Prevalence, incidence, and progression of myopia of school children in Hong Kong. Invest Ophthalmol Vis Sci 2004;45(4):1071–5.
[85] Donovan L, Sankaridurg P, Ho A, et al. Myopia progression rates in urban children wearing single-vision spectacles. Optom Vis Sci 2012;89(1):27–32.
[86] Mutti DO, Hayes JR, Mitchell GL, et al. Refractive error, axial length, and relative peripheral refractive error before and after the onset of myopia. Invest Ophthalmol Vis Sci 2007;48(6):2510–9.
[87] Donovan L, Sankaridurg P, Ho A, et al. Myopia progression in Chinese children is slower in summer than in winter. Optom Vis Sci 2012;89(8):1196–202.
[88] Fulk GW, Cyert LA, Parker DA. Seasonal variation in myopia progression and ocular elongation. Optom Vis Sci 2002;79(1):46–51.
[89] Group C. Myopia stabilization and associated factors among participants in the Correction of Myopia Evaluation Trial (COMET). Invest Ophthalmol Vis Sci 2013;54(13): 7871–84.

[90] Fernandez-Montero A, Olmo-Jimenez JM, Olmo N, et al. The impact of computer use in myopia progression: a cohort study in Spain. Prev Med 2015;71:67–71.
[91] Bullimore MA, Jones LA, Moeschberger ML, et al. A retrospective study of myopia progression in adult contact lens wearers. Invest Ophthalmol Vis Sci 2002;43(7):2110–3.
[92] Lyhne N, Sjolie AK, Kyvik KO, et al. The importance of genes and environment for ocular refraction and its determiners: a population based study among 20-45 year old twins. Br J Ophthalmol 2001;85(12):1470–6.
[93] Hammond CJ, Snieder H, Gilbert CE, et al. Genes and environment in refractive error: the twin eye study. Invest Ophthalmol Vis Sci 2001;42(6):1232–6.
[94] Dirani M, Chamberlain M, Shekar SN, et al. Heritability of refractive error and ocular biometrics: the Genes in Myopia (GEM) twin study. Invest Ophthalmol Vis Sci 2006;47(11): 4756–61.
[95] Teikari JM, Kaprio J, Koskenvuo MK, et al. Heritability estimate for refractive errors–a population-based sample of adult twins. Genet Epidemiol 1988;5(3):171–81.
[96] Lopes MC, Andrew T, Carbonaro F, et al. Estimating heritability and shared environmental effects for refractive error in twin and family studies. Invest Ophthalmol Vis Sci 2009;50(1): 126–31.
[97] Pacella R, McLellan J, Grice K, et al. Role of genetic factors in the etiology of juvenile-onset myopia based on a longitudinal study of refractive error. Optom Vis Sci 1999;76(6): 381–6.
[98] Dirani M, Shekar SN, Baird PN. Evidence of shared genes in refraction and axial length: the Genes in Myopia (GEM) twin study. Invest Ophthalmol Vis Sci 2008;49(10):4336–9.
[99] Jones-Jordan LA, Sinnott LT, Manny RE, et al. Early childhood refractive error and parental history of myopia as predictors of myopia. Invest Ophthalmol Vis Sci 2010;51(1): 115–21.
[100] Dirani M, Shekar SN, Baird PN. Adult-onset myopia: the Genes in Myopia (GEM) twin study. Invest Ophthalmol Vis Sci 2008;49(8):3324–7.
[101] Teikari J, Koskenvuo M, Kaprio J, et al. Study of gene-environment effects on development of hyperopia: a study of 191 adult twin pairs from the Finnish Twin Cohort Study. Acta Genet Med Gemellol (Roma) 1990;39(1):133–6.
[102] Tsai MY, Lin LL, Lee V, et al. Estimation of heritability in myopic twin studies. Jpn J Ophthalmol 2009;53(6):615–22.
[103] Young TL, Ronan SM, Drahozal LA, et al. Evidence that a locus for familial high myopia maps to chromosome 18p. Am J Hum Genet 1998;63(1):109–19.
[104] Young TL, Ronan SM, Alvear AB, et al. A second locus for familial high myopia maps to chromosome 12q. Am J Hum Genet 1998;63(5):1419–24.
[105] Naiglin L, Gazagne C, Dallongeville F, et al. A genome wide scan for familial high myopia suggests a novel locus on chromosome 7q36. J Med Genet 2002;39(2):118–24.
[106] Lam DS, Tam PO, Fan DS, et al. Familial high myopia linkage to chromosome 18p. Ophthalmologica 2003;217(2):115–8.
[107] Paluru P, Ronan SM, Heon E, et al. New locus for autosomal dominant high myopia maps to the long arm of chromosome 17. Invest Ophthalmol Vis Sci 2003;44(5):1830–6.
[108] Farbrother JE, Kirov G, Owen MJ, et al. Linkage analysis of the genetic loci for high myopia on 18p, 12q, and 17q in 51 U.K. families. Invest Ophthalmol Vis Sci 2004;45(9): 2879–85.
[109] Stambolian D, Ibay G, Reider L, et al. Genomewide linkage scan for myopia susceptibility loci among Ashkenazi Jewish families shows evidence of linkage on chromosome 22q12. Am J Hum Genet 2004;75(3):448–59.
[110] Zhang Q, Guo X, Xiao X, et al. A new locus for autosomal dominant high myopia maps to 4q22-q27 between D4S1578 and D4S1612. Mol Vis 2005;11:554–60.
[111] Paluru PC, Nallasamy S, Devoto M, et al. Identification of a novel locus on 2q for autosomal dominant high-grade myopia. Invest Ophthalmol Vis Sci 2005;46(7):2300–7.

[112] Stambolian D, Ciner EB, Reider LC, et al. Genome-wide scan for myopia in the Old Order Amish. Am J Ophthalmol 2005;140(3):469–76.
[113] Zhang Q, Guo X, Xiao X, et al. Novel locus for X linked recessive high myopia maps to Xq23-q25 but outside MYP1. J Med Genet 2006;43(5):e20.
[114] Nallasamy S, Paluru PC, Devoto M, et al. Genetic linkage study of high-grade myopia in a Hutterite population from South Dakota. Mol Vis 2007;13:229–36.
[115] Yu ZQ, Li YB, Huang CX, et al. A genome-wide screening for pathological myopia suggests a novel locus on chromosome 15q12 - 13. Zhonghua Yan Ke Za Zhi 2007;43(3):233–8 [in Chinese].
[116] Paget S, Julia S, Vitezica ZG, et al. Linkage analysis of high myopia susceptibility locus in 26 families. Mol Vis 2008;14:2566–74.
[117] Ciner E, Wojciechowski R, Ibay G, et al. Genomewide scan of ocular refraction in African-American families shows significant linkage to chromosome 7p15. Genet Epidemiol 2008;32(5):454–63.
[118] Lam CY, Tam PO, Fan DS, et al. A genome-wide scan maps a novel high myopia locus to 5p15. Invest Ophthalmol Vis Sci 2008;49(9):3768–78.
[119] Schache M, Chen CY, Pertile KK, et al. Fine mapping linkage analysis identifies a novel susceptibility locus for myopia on chromosome 2q37 adjacent to but not overlapping MYP12. Mol Vis 2009;15:722–30.
[120] Yang Z, Xiao X, Li S, et al. Clinical and linkage study on a consanguineous Chinese family with autosomal recessive high myopia. Mol Vis 2009;15:312–8.
[121] Nishizaki R, Ota M, Inoko H, et al. New susceptibility locus for high myopia is linked to the uromodulin-like 1 (UMODL1) gene region on chromosome 21q22.3. Eye (Lond) 2009;23(1):222–9.
[122] Ciner E, Ibay G, Wojciechowski R, et al. Genome-wide scan of African-American and white families for linkage to myopia. Am J Ophthalmol 2009;147(3):512–7.e512.
[123] Li YJ, Guggenheim JA, Bulusu A, et al. An international collaborative family-based whole-genome linkage scan for high-grade myopia. Invest Ophthalmol Vis Sci 2009;50(7):3116–27.
[124] Nakanishi H, Yamada R, Gotoh N, et al. A genome-wide association analysis identified a novel susceptible locus for pathological myopia at 11q24.1. PLoS Genet 2009;5(9):e1000660.
[125] Ma JH, Shen SH, Zhang GW, et al. Identification of a locus for autosomal dominant high myopia on chromosome 5p13.3-p15.1 in a Chinese family. Mol Vis 2010;16:2043–54.
[126] Li YJ, Goh L, Khor CC, et al. Genome-wide association studies reveal genetic variants in CTNND2 for high myopia in Singapore Chinese. Ophthalmology 2011;118(2):368–75.
[127] Solouki AM, Verhoeven VJ, van Duijn CM, et al. A genome-wide association study identifies a susceptibility locus for refractive errors and myopia at 15q14. Nat Genet 2010;42(10):897–901.
[128] Hysi PG, Young TL, Mackey DA, et al. A genome-wide association study for myopia and refractive error identifies a susceptibility locus at 15q25. Nat Genet 2010;42(10):902–5.
[129] Verhoeven VJ, Hysi PG, Wojciechowski R, et al. Genome-wide meta-analyses of multiancestry cohorts identify multiple new susceptibility loci for refractive error and myopia. Nat Genet 2013;45(3):314–8.
[130] Lango Allen H, Estrada K, Lettre G, et al. Hundreds of variants clustered in genomic loci and biological pathways affect human height. Nature 2010;467(7317):832–8.
[131] Tkatchenko TV, Troilo D, Benavente-Perez A, et al. Gene expression in response to optical defocus of opposite signs reveals bidirectional mechanism of visually guided eye growth. PLoS Biol 2018;16(10):e2006021.
[132] Brennan NA. Predicted reduction in high myopia for various degrees of myopia control. Cont Lens Anterior Eye 2012;35(Suppl):14–5.
[133] Rosenfield M, Gilmartin B. Accommodative error, adaptation and myopia. Ophthalmic Physiol Opt 1999;19(2):159–64.

[134] Gwiazda J, Thorn F, Held R. Accommodation, accommodative convergence, and response AC/A ratios before and at the onset of myopia in children. Optom Vis Sci 2005;82(4):273–8.

[135] Goss DA. Variables related to the rate of childhood myopia progression. Optom Vis Sci 1990;67(8):631–6.

[136] Parssinen O, Hemminki E. Spectacle-use, bifocals and prevention of myopic progression. The two-years results of a randomized trial among schoolchildren. Acta Ophthalmol Suppl 1988;185:156–61.

[137] Goss DA, Grosvenor T. Rates of childhood myopia progression with bifocals as a function of nearpoint phoria: consistency of three studies. Optom Vis Sci 1990;67(8):637–40.

[138] Gwiazda JE, Hyman L, Everett D, et al. Five-year results from the correction of myopia evaluation trial (COMET). Invest Ophthalmol Vis Sci 2006;47 [E–abstract: 1166].

[139] Kurtz D, Hyman L, Gwiazda JE, et al. Role of parental myopia in the progression of myopia and its interaction with treatment in COMET children. Invest Ophthalmol Vis Sci 2007;48(2):562–70.

[140] Cheng D, Schmid KL, Woo GC, et al. Randomized trial of effect of bifocal and prismatic bifocal spectacles on myopic progression: two-year results. Arch Ophthalmol 2010;128(1):12–9.

[141] Li SM, Ji YZ, Wu SS, et al. Multifocal versus single vision lenses intervention to slow progression of myopia in school-age children: a meta-analysis. Surv Ophthalmol 2011;56(5):451–60.

[142] Sankaridurg P, Donovan L, Varnas S, et al. Spectacle lenses designed to reduce progression of myopia: 12-month results. Optom Vis Sci 2010;87(9):631–41.

[143] Chung K, Mohidin N, O'Leary DJ. Undercorrection of myopia enhances rather than inhibits myopia progression. Vision Res 2002;42(22):2555–9.

[144] Adler D, Millodot M. The possible effect of undercorrection on myopic progression in children. Clin Exp Optom 2006;89(5):315–21.

[145] Walline JJ, Jones LA, Mutti DO, et al. A randomized trial of the effects of rigid contact lenses on myopia progression. Arch Ophthalmol 2004;122(12):1760–6.

[146] Walline JJ, Jones LA, Sinnott L, et al. A randomized trial of the effect of soft contact lenses on myopia progression in children. Invest Ophthalmol Vis Sci 2008;49(11):4702–6.

[147] Reim T, Lund M, Wu R. Orthokeratology and adolescent myopia control. Contact Lens Spectrum 2003;18:40–2.

[148] Lui WO, Edwards MH. Orthokeratology in low myopia. Part 1: efficacy and predictability. Cont Lens Anterior Eye 2000;23(3):77–89.

[149] Walline JJ, Rah MJ, Jones LA. The Children's Overnight Orthokeratology Investigation (COOKI) pilot study. Optom Vis Sci 2004;81(6):407–13.

[150] Cho P, Cheung SW, Edwards M. The longitudinal orthokeratology research in children (LORIC) in Hong Kong: a pilot study on refractive changes and myopic control. Curr Eye Res 2005;30(1):71–80.

[151] Walline JJ, Jones LA, Sinnott LT. Corneal reshaping and myopia progression. Br J Ophthalmol 2009;93(9):1181–5.

[152] Kakita T, Hiraoka T, Oshika T. Influence of overnight orthokeratology on axial elongation in childhood myopia. Invest Ophthalmol Vis Sci 2011;52(5):2170–4.

[153] Santodomingo-Rubido J, Villa-Collar C, Gilmartin B, et al. Myopia control with orthokeratology contact lenses in Spain (MCOS): refractive and biometric changes. Invest Ophthalmol Vis Sci 2012;53(8):5060–5.

[154] Swarbrick HA, Alharbi A, Watt K, et al. Myopia control during orthokeratology lens wear in children using a novel study design. Ophthalmology 2015;122(3):620–30.

[155] Mok A, Chung CS. Seven-year retrospective analysis of the myopic control effect of orthokeratology in children: a pilot study. Clin Optom 2011;3:1–4.

[156] Hiraoka T, Kakita T, Okamoto F, et al. Long-term effect of overnight orthokeratology on axial length elongation in childhood myopia: a 5-year follow-up study. Invest Ophthalmol Vis Sci 2012;53(7):3913–9.
[157] Sun Y, Xu F, Zhang T, et al. Orthokeratology to control myopia progression: a meta-analysis. PLoS One 2015;10(4):e0124535.
[158] Si JK, Tang K, Bi HS, et al. Orthokeratology for myopia control: a meta-analysis. Optom Vis Sci 2015;92(3):252–7.
[159] Rah MJ, Jackson JM, Jones LA, et al. Overnight orthokeratology: preliminary results of the Lenses and Overnight Orthokeratology (LOOK) study. Optom Vis Sci 2002;79(9): 598–605.
[160] Van Meter WS, Musch DC, Jacobs DS, et al. Safety of overnight orthokeratology for myopia: a report by the American Academy of Ophthalmology. Ophthalmology 2008;115(12):2301–13.e1.
[161] Bullimore MA. What can be done for my child? Optom Vis Sci 2000;77(8):381.
[162] Stapleton F, Keay L, Edwards K, et al. The incidence of contact lens-related microbial keratitis in Australia. Ophthalmology 2008;115(10):1655–62.
[163] Bullimore MA, Sinnott LT, Jones-Jordan LA. The risk of microbial keratitis with overnight corneal reshaping lenses. Optom Vis Sci 2013;90(9):937–44.
[164] Liu YM, Xie P. The safety of orthokeratology–a systematic review. Eye Contact Lens 2016;42(1):35–42.
[165] Li SM, Kang MT, Wu SS, et al. Efficacy, safety and acceptability of orthokeratology on slowing axial elongation in myopic children by meta-analysis. Curr Eye Res 2016;41(5):600–8.
[166] Fu AC, Chen XL, Lv Y, et al. Higher spherical equivalent refractive errors is associated with slower axial elongation wearing orthokeratology. Cont Lens Anterior Eye 2016;39(1): 62–6.
[167] Wang B, Naidu RK, Qu X. Factors related to axial length elongation and myopia progression in orthokeratology practice. PLoS One 2017;12(4):e0175913.
[168] Cho P, Cheung SW. Discontinuation of orthokeratology on eyeball elongation (DOEE). Cont Lens Anterior Eye 2017;40(2):82–7.
[169] Anstice NS, Phillips JR. Effect of dual-focus soft contact lens wear on axial myopia progression in children. Ophthalmology 2011;118(6):1152–61.
[170] Sankaridurg P, Holden B, Smith E 3rd, et al. Decrease in rate of myopia progression with a contact lens designed to reduce relative peripheral hyperopia: one-year results. Invest Ophthalmol Vis Sci 2011;52(13):9362–7.
[171] Holden B, Sankaridurg P, Lazon P, et al. Central and peripheral visual performance of a novel contact lens designed to control progression of myopia. Invest Ophthalmol Vis Sci 2011;52 [E-abstract: 6518].
[172] Woods J, Guthrie SE, Keir N, et al. Inhibition of defocus-induced myopia in chickens. Invest Ophthalmol Vis Sci 2013;54(4):2662–8.
[173] Woods J, Guthrie S, Keir N, et al. The effect of a unique lens designed for myopia progression control (MPC) on the level of induced myopia in chicks. Invest Ophthalmol Vis Sci 2011;52 [E-abstract: 6651].
[174] Walline JJ, Greiner KL, McVey ME, et al. Multifocal contact lens myopia control. Optom Vis Sci 2013;90(11):1207–14.
[175] Paune J, Morales H, Armengol J, et al. Myopia control with a novel peripheral gradient soft lens and orthokeratology: a 2-year clinical trial. Biomed Res Int 2015;2015:507572.
[176] Aller TA, Liu M, Wildsoet CF. Myopia control with bifocal contact lenses: a randomized clinical trial. Optom Vis Sci 2016;93(4):344–52.
[177] Li SM, Kang MT, Wu SS, et al. Studies using concentric ring bifocal and peripheral add multifocal contact lenses to slow myopia progression in school-aged children: a meta-analysis. Ophthalmic Physiol Opt 2017;37(1):51–9.

[178] Turnbull PR, Munro OJ, Phillips JR. Contact lens methods for clinical myopia control. Optom Vis Sci 2016;93(9):1120–6.
[179] Cooper J, O'Connor B, Watanabe R, et al. Case series analysis of myopic progression control with a unique extended depth of focus multifocal contact lens. Eye Contact Lens 2018;44(5):e16–24.
[180] Gimbel HV. The control of myopia with atropine. Can J Ophthalmol 1973;8(4):527–32.
[181] Kelly TS, Chatfield C, Tustin G. Clinical assessment of the arrest of myopia. Br J Ophthalmol 1975;59(10):529–38.
[182] Dyer JA. Role of cyclopegics in progressive myopia. Ophthalmology 1979;86(5):692–4.
[183] Sampson WG. Role of cycloplegia in the management of functional myopia. Ophthalmology 1979;86(5):695–7.
[184] Bedrossian RH. The treatment of myopia with atropine and bifocals: a long-term prospective study. Ophthalmology 1985;92(5):716.
[185] Bedrossian RH. The effect of atropine on myopia. Ophthalmology 1979;86(5):713–9.
[186] Bedrossian RH. The effect of atropine on myopia. Ann Ophthalmol 1971;3(8):891–7.
[187] Gruber E. Treatment of myopia with atropine and bifocals. Ophthalmology 1985;92(7):985.
[188] Brodstein RS, Brodstein DE, Olson RJ, et al. The treatment of myopia with atropine and bifocals. A long-term prospective study. Ophthalmology 1984;91(11):1373–9.
[189] Brenner RL. Further observations on use of atropine in the treatment of myopia. Ann Ophthalmol 1985;17(2):137–40.
[190] Yen MY, Liu JH, Kao SC, et al. Comparison of the effect of atropine and cyclopentolate on myopia. Ann Ophthalmol 1989;21(5):180–2, 187.
[191] Kennedy RH, Dyer JA, Kennedy MA, et al. Reducing the progression of myopia with atropine: a long term cohort study of Olmsted County students. Binocul Vis Strabismus Q 2000;15(3 Suppl):281–304.
[192] Kennedy RH. Progression of myopia. Trans Am Ophthalmol Soc 1995;93:755–800.
[193] McBrien NA, Moghaddam HO, Reeder AP. Atropine reduces experimental myopia and eye enlargement via a nonaccommodative mechanism. Invest Ophthalmol Vis Sci 1993;34(1):205–15.
[194] Schaeffel F, Troilo D, Wallman J, et al. Developing eyes that lack accommodation grow to compensate for imposed defocus. Vis Neurosci 1990;4(2):177–83.
[195] Zou L, Liu R, Zhang X, et al. Upregulation of regulator of G-protein signaling 2 in the sclera of a form deprivation myopic animal model. Mol Vis 2014;20:977–87.
[196] Gallego P, Martinez-Garcia C, Perez-Merino P, et al. Scleral changes induced by atropine in chicks as an experimental model of myopia. Ophthalmic Physiol Opt 2012;32(6):478–84.
[197] Barathi VA, Beuerman RW. Molecular mechanisms of muscarinic receptors in mouse scleral fibroblasts: Prior to and after induction of experimental myopia with atropine treatment. Mol Vis 2011;17:680–92.
[198] Prepas SB. Light, literacy and the absence of ultraviolet radiation in the development of myopia. Med Hypotheses 2008;70(3):635–7.
[199] Chia A, Chua WH, Cheung YB, et al. Atropine for the treatment of childhood myopia: safety and efficacy of 0.5%, 0.1%, and 0.01% doses (Atropine for the Treatment of Myopia 2). Ophthalmology 2012;119(2):347–54.
[200] North RV, Kelly ME. A review of the uses and adverse effects of topical administration of atropine. Ophthalmic Physiol Opt 1987;7(2):109–14.
[201] Luu CD, Lau AM, Koh AH, et al. Multifocal electroretinogram in children on atropine treatment for myopia. Br J Ophthalmol 2005;89(2):151–3.
[202] Chia A, Li W, Tan D, et al. Full-field electroretinogram findings in children in the atropine treatment for myopia (ATOM2) study. Doc Ophthalmol 2013;126(3):177–86.
[203] Chiang MF, Kouzis A, Pointer RW, et al. Treatment of childhood myopia with atropine eyedrops and bifocal spectacles. Binocul Vis Strabismus Q 2001;16(3):209–15.

[204] Chua WH, Balakrishnan V, Chan YH, et al. Atropine for the treatment of childhood myopia. Ophthalmology 2006;113(12):2285–91.
[205] Shih YF, Chen CH, Chou AC, et al. Effects of different concentrations of atropine on controlling myopia in myopic children. J Ocul Pharmacol Ther 1999;15(1):85–90.
[206] Lu P, Chen J. Retarding progression of myopia with seasonal modification of topical atropine. J Ophthalmic Vis Res 2010;5:75–81.
[207] Fang PC, Chung MY, Yu HJ, et al. Prevention of myopia onset with 0.025% atropine in premyopic children. J Ocul Pharmacol Ther 2010;26(4):341–5.
[208] Cooper J, Eisenberg N, Schulman E, et al. Maximum atropine dose without clinical signs or symptoms. Optom Vis Sci 2013;90(12):1467–72.
[209] Chia A, Chua WH, Wen L, et al. Atropine for the treatment of childhood myopia: changes after stopping atropine 0.01%, 0.1% and 0.5%. Am J Ophthalmol 2014;157(2):451–7.e1.
[210] Lee CY, Sun CC, Lin YF, et al. Effects of topical atropine on intraocular pressure and myopia progression: a prospective comparative study. BMC Ophthalmol 2016;16:114.
[211] Chia A, Lu QS, Tan D. Five-year clinical trial on atropine for the treatment of myopia 2: myopia control with atropine 0.01% eyedrops. Ophthalmology 2016;123(2):391–9.
[212] Saw SM, Chua WH, Wu HM, et al. Myopia: gene-environment interaction. Ann Acad Med Singapore 2000;29(3):290–7.
[213] Gong Q, Janowski M, Luo M, et al. Efficacy and adverse effects of atropine in childhood myopia: a meta-analysis. JAMA Ophthalmol 2017;135(6):624–30.
[214] Yam JC, Jiang Y, Tang SM, et al. Low-concentration atropine for myopia progression (LAMP) study: a randomized, double-blinded, placebo-controlled trial of 0.05%, 0.025%, and 0.01% atropine eye drops in myopia control. Ophthalmology 2019;126(1):113–24.
[215] Rose KA, Morgan IG, Ip J, et al. Outdoor activity reduces the prevalence of myopia in children. Ophthalmology 2008;115(8):1279–85.
[216] Dirani M, Tong L, Gazzard G, et al. Outdoor activity and myopia in Singapore teenage children. Br J Ophthalmol 2009;93(8):997–1000.
[217] Guggenheim JA, Northstone K, McMahon G, et al. Time outdoors and physical activity as predictors of incident myopia in childhood: a prospective cohort study. Invest Ophthalmol Vis Sci 2012;53(6):2856–65.
[218] He M, Xiang F, Zeng Y, et al. Effect of time spent outdoors at school on the development of myopia among children in china: a randomized clinical trial. JAMA 2015;314(11):1142–8.
[219] Jones LA, Sinnott LT, Mutti DO, et al. Parental history of myopia, sports and outdoor activities, and future myopia. Invest Ophthalmol Vis Sci 2007;48(8):3524–32.
[220] Deng L, Gwiazda J, Thorn F. Children's refractions and visual activities in the school year and summer. Optom Vis Sci 2010;87(6):406–13.
[221] Guo Y, Liu LJ, Xu L, et al. Myopic shift and outdoor activity among primary school children: one-year follow-up study in Beijing. PLoS One 2013;8(9):e75260.
[222] Guo Y, Liu LJ, Xu L, et al. Outdoor activity and myopia among primary students in rural and urban regions of Beijing. Ophthalmology 2013;120(2):277–83.
[223] Wu PC, Tsai CL, Wu HL, et al. Outdoor activity during class recess reduces myopia onset and progression in school children. Ophthalmology 2013;120(5):1080–5.
[224] Jin JX, Hua WJ, Jiang X, et al. Effect of outdoor activity on myopia onset and progression in school-aged children in northeast China: the Sujiatun Eye Care Study. BMC Ophthalmol 2015;15:73.
[225] Mutti DO. Vitamin D may reduce the prevalence of myopia in Korean adolescents. Invest Ophthalmol Vis Sci 2014;55(4):2048.
[226] Mutti DO, Marks AR. Blood levels of vitamin D in teens and young adults with myopia. Optom Vis Sci 2011;88(3):377–82.

[227] Ashby R, Ohlendorf A, Schaeffel F. The effect of ambient illuminance on the development of deprivation myopia in chicks. Invest Ophthalmol Vis Sci 2009;50(11):5348–54.
[228] Karouta C, Ashby RS. Correlation between light levels and the development of deprivation myopia. Invest Ophthalmol Vis Sci 2014;56(1):299–309.
[229] Smith EL 3rd, Hung LF, Huang J. Protective effects of high ambient lighting on the development of form-deprivation myopia in rhesus monkeys. Invest Ophthalmol Vis Sci 2012;53(1):421–8.
[230] Ashby RS, Schaeffel F. The effect of bright light on lens compensation in chicks. Invest Ophthalmol Vis Sci 2010;51(10):5247–53.
[231] Smith EL 3rd, Hung LF, Arumugam B, et al. Negative lens-induced myopia in infant monkeys: effects of high ambient lighting. Invest Ophthalmol Vis Sci 2013;54(4):2959–69.
[232] Feldkaemper M, Schaeffel F. An updated view on the role of dopamine in myopia. Exp Eye Res 2013;114:106–19.
[233] Zhou X, Pardue MT, Iuvone PM, et al. Dopamine signaling and myopia development: what are the key challenges. Prog Retin Eye Res 2017;61:60–71.
[234] Torii H, Kurihara T, Seko Y, et al. Violet light exposure can be a preventive strategy against myopia progression. EBioMedicine 2017;15:210–9.
[235] Rose KA, French AN, Morgan IG. Environmental factors and myopia: paradoxes and prospects for prevention. Asia Pac J Ophthalmol (Phila) 2016;5(6):403–10.
[236] Schaeffel F, Smith EL 3rd. Inhibiting myopia by (nearly) invisible light? EBioMedicine 2017;16:27–8.
[237] Hua WJ, Jin JX, Wu XY, et al. Elevated light levels in schools have a protective effect on myopia. Ophthalmic Physiol Opt 2015;35(3):252–62.
[238] Ngo C, Saw SM, Dharani R, et al. Does sunlight (bright lights) explain the protective effects of outdoor activity against myopia? Ophthalmic Physiol Opt 2013;33(3):368–72.
[239] Fang YT, Chou YJ, Pu C, et al. Prescription of atropine eye drops among children diagnosed with myopia in Taiwan from 2000 to 2007: a nationwide study. Eye (Lond) 2013;27(3):418–24.
[240] Kakehashi NKYKNHA. Suppressive effect of combined treatment of orthokeratology and 0.01% atropine instillation on axial length elongation in childhood myopia. Invest Ophthalmol Vis Sci 2017;58:2386.
[241] Charm J, Cho P. High myopia-partial reduction ortho-k: a 2-year randomized study. Optom Vis Sci 2013;90(6):530–9.
[242] Lin HJ, Wan L, Tsai FJ, et al. Overnight orthokeratology is comparable with atropine in controlling myopia. BMC Ophthalmol 2014;14:40.
[243] Dillehay S, Cooper J, Eiden S, et al. Determination of IOLMaster number of measurements for tracking axial length changes in myopia. Invest Ophthalmol Vis Sci 2018;59(9):2133.

Section II: Pediatric

Advances in Ophthalmology and Optometry 4 (2019) 65–73

ADVANCES IN OPHTHALMOLOGY AND OPTOMETRY

Binocular Treatment for Amblyopia

Osama Mufti, MD, Aparna Ramasubramanian, MD*

Kentucky Lions Eye Center, University of Louisville, Louisville, KY, USA

Keywords

• Binocular treatment • Amblyopia • Lazy eye

Key points

- Amblyopia affects 1-4% of pediatric population and the traditional treatments have focused on monocular treatments like patching and atropine.
- The newer approach to treatment involves binocular treatment where the focus is on restoring binocular vision and stereoacuity.
- Binocular treatment can also be utilized in adults with amblyopia with some benefit.
- The technologies involving binocular treatment still need to be modified to impart sustained and consistent visual outcome.

INTRODUCTION

Amblyopia is a functional reduction in visual acuity caused by abnormal visual development early in life. Clinically, amblyopia can be considered when the best-corrected visual acuity of 1 eye is 2 lines or worse in the absence of known or obvious pathologic condition. It is an exceedingly common cause of visual impairment in children, estimated at 1% to 4% of the pediatric population [1,2]. Estimations for the cost of burden of general visual loss have been assessed at more than $27 billion, with amblyopia a major percentage [2]. Amblyopia can be subclassified based on the cause of the disturbance, including strabismic, deprivational, and refractive amblyopic subtypes [3]. Treatment

The authors have nothing to disclose.

This work was supported in part by an unrestricted institutional grant from Research to Prevent Blindness, New York, NY.

*Corresponding author. 301 East Muhammad Ali Blvd, Louisville, KY, 40202. *E-mail address:* aparna.ramasubramanian@louisville.edu

https://doi.org/10.1016/j.yaoo.2019.04.003

2452-1760/19/

generally is recommended before the age of 7 years. Common thought has been that correcting amblyopia before the brain and visual pathways have fully matured will lead to optimal results. In older children and adolescents, however, treatment was generally not recommended because the "lazy eye" had already fixated. Historically, treatment options have been cycloplegic blurring typically via atropine eye drops versus patching therapy. The idea behind this is that by limiting visual exposure in the dominant eye, the amblyopic eye is forced to do the heavy burden of the seeing, thus helping reinforce the visual pathways of the amblyopic eye. Although traditionally a monocular approach where negative reinforcement of the sound eye was done (ie, removing visual stimulation such as with blurring or patching), a novel approach was started in 1978, whereby binocular therapy was considered using electronic devices. This first attempt to provide the combination of short-term occlusion (20 minutes), controlled visual stimulation, and attentive game play was the e CAM visual stimulator (Clemente Clarke International, Harlow, England) treatment [4,5].

BURDEN OF THE PROBLEM

Amblyopia, or as it is more commonly referred to as "lazy eye," is decreased vision in 1 or both eyes due to any number of abnormal development of the visual pathways in conjunction with the brain. Because the nerves in the pathways are not properly stimulating the brain, and the brain sees these blurry images during major developmental years, the vision in the eye becomes compromised [2]. A critical period of growth occurs within the first few years of life. If the infant is unable to properly see during this time, the pathways become underdeveloped and lead to poor visual potential usually despite the relatively normal appearance of the eye. Dissimilar refractive error called refractive amblyopia is the most common cause [6].

Because epidemiologic studies have estimated that 1% to 4% of the pediatric population suffer from amblyopia, this condition has major economic impacts. A 2012 study estimated that the economic burden of vision loss and eye disorders among the United States population younger than 40 years was $27.5 billion (95% confidence interval, $21.5–$37.2 billion), including $5.9 billion for children and $21.6 billion for adults (defined as 18–39 years of age). Direct costs were calculated at $14.5 billion and indirect costs were $13 billion, of which $12.2 billion was a loss of productivity [7,8].

PHYSIOLOGY OF AMBLYOPIA

Amblyopia is the most common cause of visual impairment in childhood and can occur whenever there is a misalignment between what the 2 eyes see, for example, if 1 eye is clouded by a cataract, if there is refractive error, or if the eyes are positioned at different angles. When the eyes have exact balance, they are said to be orthophoric. The brain at first has a slight preference for the more functional eye, and over time as that eye continues to send the brain useful information, the brain's preference for that eye gets stronger at the expense of the other eye. Although the concept of 1 eye facing a restrictive visual field leading to impaired visual pathways is simple, the mechanisms underlying this process are not clearly understood. Recent research aimed at identifying the mechanisms have proposed that within the brain, in a limited region called the binocular zone, cells can receive input from both eyes. During brain development, the eyes compete to connect within this zone, and sometimes 1 eye prevails, a process known as ocular dominance. Ocular dominance is a normal process and is an example of the brain's ability to adapt based on experience-termed plasticity, but it also can set the stage for amblyopia. If 1 eye is impaired and cannot effectively compete, it will lose space in the binocular zone to the other eye [9].

This competition takes place during a limited time called the critical period. The critical period is seen as the period of time during which abnormal visual inputs can result in amblyopia, but it is also the time during which amblyopia can be reversed by eliminating the abnormal visual inputs and, usually, occluding the normal eye for some periods of time [10]. Once the critical period closes, which current literature suggests is around 7 years of age, connections are difficult to change. Some studies have shown, however, that it is possible to partially correct amblyopia in the teenage years [11]. Specifically, a nationwide trial showed that 53% of children aged 7 to 12 and 47% of children aged 13 to 17 showed improvement in glasses fitted with daily patching versus glasses alone, challenging the previously held notion of treatment futility after the critical period closes [12].

TRADITIONAL APPROACHES TO TREATMENT

For hundreds of years, the mainstays of amblyopic treatments have consisted of patching versus cycloplegics. Patching therapy typically is the first-line procedure, because a patch is easy to implement and a cost-effective solution. However, the shortcomings are abundant because problems with compliance can arise due to the psychological and social implications of wearing a patch. The shortcomings in conjunction with the discomfort of decreasing a child's visual field via the patch has made patching therapy difficult to adhere to for parents [12,13]. A 2003 study by Repka and colleagues [14] found that 79% of children after 4 months with 2 hours of patching showed improved visual acuity by at least 2 lines. A follow-up study in 2004, however, showed up to 25% regression of those children. Further studies have shown that even when visual acuity increases in the amblyopic eye, the binocular vision remains underutilized. Binocular vision is the overlapping of visual fields between the 2 eyes, permitting enhanced depth perception. The idea of binocular vision in amblyopia is important to recognize because the amblyopic eye usage is forced with a patch, thus increasing its visual potential; however, because the opposing eye is patched, the 2 eyes do not develop in synchrony. Ultimately, although patching therapy has had some success, an apparent need exists for more successful alternatives.

Multiple studies aimed at improving the patching model to make it more convenient have been attempted. Before the prospective trials by the Pediatric

Eye Disease Investigator Group (PEDIG), patching therapy was recommended full time. The social stigma of a patch in addition to the discomfort of wearing a full-time patch led to frustration and poor compliance among families for whom patching therapy was recommended. Also, a risk of reverse amblyopia in the better-seeing eye occurred. The PEDIG studies supported a change in this practice, suggesting that mild to moderate amblyopia (defined as best-corrected visual acuity of 20/40 to 20/100) had an equivocal response to patching for 2 hours every day compared with full-time patching, which was previously the standard.

The alternative approach to patching has been atropine eye drops. Atropine blocks muscarinic receptors in the eye, which control the size and shape of the pupil and lens. Atropine causes a mydriatic (increased size of the pupil) and cycloplegic effect (paralysis of the fibers controlling accommodation of the lens), which serves as a penalization therapy blurring the well-seeing eye. The PEDIG trials showed that atropine eye drops were equally effective as patching for moderate amblyopia; however, when taking into consideration the ease of applying an eye patch compared with the inconvenience of putting in drops that cause a strange blurring sensation, it is no wonder that patching therapy is preferred for both parents and practitioners [7,13,14].

A NOVEL APPROACH TO TREATMENT: BINOCULAR TREATMENT

Although it has been accepted for many years that amblyopia is a binocular problem, the traditional approach has always targeted monocular vision. The potential for binocular approaches to amblyopic vision is a more recent endeavor. Suggestions for novel therapeutic approaches recently have been making strides in amblyopic literature. The approaches discussed range from pure monocular therapy, pure binocular therapy, and a combination therapy consisting of both. While the monocular approaches have already been discussed, we will now shift our focus to the binocular approach.

A new treatment regimen, using dichoptic glasses while playing electronic games, incorporates a binocular stimulation that was previously missing in amblyopic treatment methodologies [7,15]. This dichoptic manipulation of different contrasts enables the stimulation for both eyes. The approach trains the eyes by presenting a high-contrast image to the amblyopic eye. A key distinguishing feature of this approach is that it is not designed to cause suppression of the fixing eye, but rather causes strengthening of neural connections in the amblyopic eye, thereby promoting binocular vision.

The primary aim of this approach is not the improvement of visual acuity in the amblyopic eye (however, that is a preferred secondary outcome), but rather to restore binocular fusion and stereopsis. To achieve this, complementary dichoptic stimuli are used such that the visual task only can be solved if both left and right information eye is combined (the binocular criterion). To achieve this, the contrast of the signal seen by the fixing eye is reduced (to negate suppression) to a point where binocular combination is achievable. This "balance point" is determined individually for each patient. With time, the treatment strengthens and extends the contrast range over which binocular fusion can occur until it includes images of the same contrast in each eye (comparable to natural viewing). Numerous clinical trials have demonstrated the efficacy of binocular game treatment over patching, as a treatment for amblyopia. The game therapy requires less time commitment and achieves a better best corrected visual acuity than patching.

When discussing binocular treatment, clinical suppression must be assessed. Clinical suppression refers to the lack of contribution of an amblyopic and/or strabismic eye under binocular viewing conditions. The most common tool for assessing this clinically is the Worth 4-dot test in which stimuli of different colors are presented anaglyphically, and the degree to which each eye contributes to perception is assessed subjectively. Until recently, no gold standard has been adopted to quantify the degree of clinical suppression. Recent studies have suggested that there is a direct relationship between the strength of suppression and the depth of amblyopia present [7,15–17].

UNDERSTANDING THE THEORY OF THE BINOCULAR TREATMENT MODEL

Current evidence suggests that binocular rebalancing works; however, much debate exists on the neural mechanisms at work. In cats, research has shown that the suppression in the amblyopic eye is mediated by inhibitory GABAergic inputs. Several studies of suppression have supported the theory for a passive attenuation, rather than for an active inhibition in the amblyopic eye [18]. These results argue that although the dichoptic interactions themselves are normal in amblyopes (ie, each eye can appreciate an image in isolation), the fact that the amblyopic eye needs more contrast to detect stimuli means that stimuli of a fixed suprathreshold contrast will produce less masking from the amblyopic to the fellow fixing eye. The resultant interocular imbalance in dichoptic masking will allow the fellow fixing eye to always dominate in binocular viewing [7]. Although binocular interaction does not normally occur in amblyopia, it can occur when fellow-eye contrast is reduced. Recent physiologic evidence also suggests that weak, noisy signals from the amblyopic eye can contribute to binocular vision if suppression by the fellow eye is reduced by signal attenuation.

The neural connections underlying amblyopia may be able to undergo synaptic plasticity. Under typical conditions, the fixing eye has a lower threshold for activation and typically will govern the inputs received, meaning that even under strong stimulation, the amblyopic eye will be unable to take advantage of the neural activity. However, with dichoptic therapy, when the fixing eye activation is driven down (via manipulation of contrasts), the modification thresholds may shift in favor of long-term potentiation and the weak inputs from the amblyopic eye. These inputs may be able to initiate potentiation via synaptic metaplasticity [7,11,15–18].

As binocular therapy is further studied, answers to the specific pathophysiologic mechanisms that govern the development of amblyopia will be unearthed.

Table 1
Summary of current literature involving a binocular approach to amblyopic therapy

	Study, year of study	Participants	Treatment hours	Intervention type	Improvement (LogMAR)	Stereopsis improvement
Adults	Hess et al [16], 2010	9	5–52	Dichoptic global motion	0.26	8/9 improved
	To et al [36], 2011	9	6–35	Falling blocks	0.19	5/9 improved
	Li et al [35], 2013	18	10	Falling blocks	0.18	15/18 improved
	Spiegel et al [29], 2013	16	11	Falling blocks	0.34	14/16 improved
	Vedamurthy et al [19], 2015	23	40	Action video game	0.14	9/23 improved
	Žiak et al [20], 2017	17	5–6	Virtual reality	0.43 ± 0.38	13/17 improved
Mixed	Hess et al [30], 2014	14	22–108	Falling blocks	0.11	11/14 improved
	Mansouri et al [31], 2014	22	10–64	Dichoptic global motion	0.34	N/A
	Gao et al [21], 2018	56	42	Falling blocks	0.06	No difference between binocular and monocular approach
Children	Knox et al [33], 2012	14	5	Falling blocks	0.09	7/14
	Li et al [32], 2014	45	16–32	4 dichoptic games	0.08	5/45 improved
	Birch et al [34], 2014	45	16–32	4 dichoptic games	0.09	3/45 improved
	Li et al [22], 2015	8	8–10	Movie watching	0.20	No significant improvement
	Herbison et al [23], 2016	75	3	DVD and modified shooting game	0.07	No significant improvement
	Webber et al [24], 2016	18	25	Dichoptic iPod game play	0.09	9/18 improved
	Bossi et al [25], 2017	22	56–196	Dichoptic movies and game play	0.27	N/A
	Mezad-Koursh et al [26], 2018	19	48–72	animated shows using BinoVision device	0.26	N/A
	Gambacorta et al [27], 2018	21	20	Custom-made action video game	0.14	8/21 improved
	Holmes et al [28], 2018	138	40	Dichoptic binocular Dig Rush iPad game	0.026	N/A

Abbreviation: N/A, not applicable.

Clinical trials have proven the effectiveness of using binocular therapy over the traditional approaches, such as patching and cycloplegics. Perhaps a combination of the 2 methods will be the mainstay of treatment in the coming years. Binocular treatment of amblyopia is novel, and many questions remain. It needs to be determined how to convert binocular games to longer-term amblyopia treatment (eg, development of a variety of engaging games, adjustment of contrast levels, and maintenance treatment). A crossover between patching and game-phase therapy proved to be the most significantly improved group in 1 study, suggesting that investigation of a combination treatment would be worthwhile.

REVIEW OF CURRENT LITERATURE

The review of current literature published on binocular treatment is presented in Table 1.

SUMMARY

In the past few years, there has been an apparent shift in amblyopic literature, going away from the previous trend of monocular suppression therapy. In addition to enhancing visual acuity, binocular therapy has an additional component of heightened stereopsis. Although previously it had been thought that adults with amblyopia should not be treated, recent literature has challenged that notion, suggesting evidence that there may be some benefit to treating amblyopic adults. Many of the previously held ideas relating to amblyopia are being reexamined, and as research trials continue to showcase the potential of dichoptic therapy, it may soon become the standard of care.

References

[1] Prevalence and impact of vision disorders in U.S. children | The National Center for Children's Vision Health. Available at: https://nationalcenter.preventblindness.org/content/prevalence-and-impact-vision-disorders-us-children. Accessed November 30, 2018.

[2] Wittenborn JS, Zhang X, Feagan CW, et al. The economic burden of vision loss and eye disorders among the United States population younger than 40 years. Ophthalmology 2013;120(9):1728–35.

[3] "Types of Amblyopia." American Academy of Ophthalmology. 2015. Available at: https://www.aao.org/disease-review/types-of-amblyopia. Accessed November 30, 2018.

[4] Nyman KG, Singh G, Rydberg A, et al. Controlled study comparing CAM treatment with occlusion therapy. Br J Ophthalmol 1983;67(3):178–80.

[5] Evaluation of the CAM Treatment for Amblyopia: A Controlled Study. | IOVS | ARVO Journals. Available at: https://iovs.arvojournals.org/article.aspx?articleid=2159274. Accessed October 7, 2018.

[6] Amblyopia — AAPOS. Available at: https://www.aapos.org/terms/conditions/21. Accessed November 30, 2018.

[7] Hess RF, Thompson B. Amblyopia and the binocular approach to its therapy. Vision Res 2015;114:4–16, ScienceDirect.

[8] Levin AV, Wilson TW, Kraft SP, et al. Strabismus. In: Wilson TW, editor. The hospital for sick children's atlas of pediatric ophthalmology and strabismus. Philadelphia: Lippincott Williams & Wilkins; 2005. p. 3–31.

[9] Kuhlman SJ, Olivas ND, Tring E, et al. A disinhibitory microcircuit initiates critical-period plasticity in the visual cortex. Nature 2013;501(7468):543–6.

[10] Hoyt C. Amblyopia. Br J Ophthalmol 2000;84(9):944–5. Available at: bjo.bmj.com.
[11] Birch EE, Li SL, Jost RM, et al. Binocular iPad treatment for amblyopia in preschool children. J AAPOS 2015;19(1):6–11.
[12] Older children can benefit from treatment for childhood's most common eye disorder National Eye Institute. Available at: https://nei.nih.gov/news/pressreleases/041105. Accessed September 11, 2018.
[13] Chen AM, Cotter SA. The amblyopia treatment studies: implications for clinical practice. Adv Ophthalmol Optom 2016;1(1):287–305.
[14] Repka MX, Beck RW, Holmes JM, et al. Pediatric Eye Disease Investigator Group. A randomized trial of patching regimens for treatment of moderate amblyopia in children. Arch Ophthalmol 2003;121(5):603–11.
[15] Atropine vs Patching for Treatment of Moderate Amblyopia: Follow-up at 15 Years of Age of a Randomized Clinical Trial | Neuro-Ophthalmology | JAMA Ophthalmology | JAMA Network. Available at: https://jamanetwork.com/journals/jamaophthalmology/fullarticle/1865505. Accessed September 11, 2018.
[16] Hess RF, Mansouri B, Thompson B. A new binocular approach to the treatment of amblyopia in adults well beyond the critical period of visual development. Restor Neurol Neurosci 2010;28:793–802.
[17] Kelly KR, Jost RM, Dao L, et al. Binocular iPad game vs patching for treatment of amblyopia in children: a randomized clinical trial. JAMA Ophthalmol 2016;134(12):1402–8. jamanetwork.com.
[18] Heimel JA, van Versendaal D, Levelt CN, et al. The role of GABAergic inhibition in ocular dominance plasticity. Neural Plast 2011;2011; https://doi.org/10.1155/2011/391763.
[19] Vedamurthy I, Nahum M, Huang SJ, et al. A dichoptic custom-made action video game as a treatment for adult amblyopia. Vision Res 2015;114:173–87.
[20] Žiak P, Holm A, Halička J, et al. Amblyopia treatment of adults with dichoptic training using the virtual reality oculus rift head mounted display: preliminary results. BMC Ophthalmol 2017;17; https://doi.org/10.1186/s12886-017-0501-8.
[21] Gao TY, Guo CX, Babu RJ, et al. Effectiveness of a binocular video game vs placebo video game for improving visual functions in older children, teenagers, and adults with amblyopia: a randomized clinical trial. JAMA Ophthalmol 2018;136(2):172–81.
[22] Li SL, Reynaud A, Hess RF, et al. Dichoptic movie viewing treats childhood amblyopia. J AAPOS 2015;19(5):401–5.
[23] Herbison N, MacKeith D, Vivian A, et al. Randomised controlled trial of video clips and interactive games to improve vision in children with amblyopia using the I-BiT system. Br J Ophthalmol 2016;100(11):1511–6.
[24] Webber AL, Wood JM, Thompson B. Fine motor skills of children with amblyopia improve following binocular treatment. Invest Ophthalmol Vis Sci 2016;57(11):4713–20. Available at: iovs.arvojournals.org.
[25] Bossi M, Tailor VK, Anderson EJ, et al. Binocular therapy for childhood amblyopia improves vision without breaking interocular suppression. Invest Ophthalmol Vis Sci 2017;58(7):3031–43. Available at: iovs.arvojournals.org.
[26] Mezad-Koursh D, Rosenblatt A, Newman H, et al. Home use of binocular dichoptic video content device for treatment of amblyopia: a pilot study. J AAPOS 2018;22(2):134–8.e4.
[27] Gambacorta C, Nahum M, Vedamurthy I, et al. An action video game for the treatment of amblyopia in children: a feasibility study. Vision Res 2018;148:1–14.
[28] Holmes JM, Manny RE, Lazar EL, et al. A randomized trial of binocular dig rush game treatment for amblyopia in children aged 7 to 12 years of age. Ophthalmology 2018; https://doi.org/10.1016/j.ophtha.2018.10.032.
[29] Spiegel DP, Li J, Hess RF, et al. Transcranial direct current stimulation enhances recovery of stereopsis in adults with amblyopia. Neurotherapeutics 2013;10(4):831–9.

[30] Hess RF, Babu RJ, Clavagnier S, et al. The iPod binocular home-based treatment for amblyopia in adults: efficacy and compliance. Clin Exp Optom 2014;97(5):389–98.
[31] Mansouri B, Singh P, Globa A, et al. Binocular training reduces amblyopic visual acuity impairment. Strabismus 2014;22(1):1–6.
[32] Li SL, Jost RM, Morale SE, et al. A binocular iPad treatment for amblyopic children. Eye (Lond) 2014;28(10):1246–53.
[33] Knox PJ, Simmers AJ, Gray LS, et al. An exploratory study: prolonged periods of binocular stimulation can provide an effective treatment for childhood amblyopia. Invest Ophthalmol Vis Sci 2012;53(2):817–24.
[34] Birch EE, Li SL, Jost RM, et al. Binocular iPad treatment for amblyopia in preschool children. J AAPOS 2015;19(1):6–11.
[35] Li J, Thompson B, Deng D, et al. Dichoptic training enables the adult amblyopic brain to learn. Curr Biol 2013;23(8):R308–9.
[36] To L, Thompson B, Blum JR, et al. A game platform for treatment of amblyopia. IEEE Trans Neural Syst Rehabil Eng 2011;19(3):280–9.

Advances in Ophthalmology and Optometry 4 (2019) 75–87

ADVANCES IN OPHTHALMOLOGY AND OPTOMETRY

Orthokeratology for Managing Myopia Progression in Children

Michael J. Lipson, OD, FAOO, FSLS[a], Bruce H. Koffler, MD[b,*]

[a]Department of Ophthalmology and Visual Science, University of Michigan, Northville Health Center, 39901 Traditions Dr. #230, Northville, MI 48168, USA; [b]Department of Ophthalmology, University of Kentucky, Lexington, KY, USA

Keywords

• Myopia • Orthokeratology • Myopia progression • Myopia management • Myopia control • Axial length • Peripheral refraction • Hyperopic defocus

Key points

- Orthokeratology (OrthoK) consists of fitting specially designed gas-permeable contact lenses that are worn overnight.
- Children using OrthoK show a slower rate of myopia progression than those wearing spectacles or soft contact lenses.
- Incidence, prevalence, and degree of myopia are increasing in the United States and worldwide.
- Myopia is a disease process characterized by increasing axial length that creates higher risk of glaucoma, cataract, retinal detachment, and myopic macular degeneration.
- OrthoK is safe and efficacious in correcting myopic refractive error and in slowing myopic progression.

INTRODUCTION

Myopia is the most common eye condition in the world [1]. In 2004, the prevalence of myopia in adults in the United States was reported to have grown to 41% from 25% in 1979 [2]. At the current rate, it is estimated that 50% of American adults will be myopic in 2020 [1]. A notable group of world health experts project that with current trends, half of the world population (about 5 billion)

Disclosure: M.J. Lipson is a consultant to Bausch and Lomb's Specialty Vision Products division. B.H. Koffler is on the speakers' bureau for Paragon Vision Sciences and Bausch and Lomb.

*Corresponding author. Koffler Vision Group, 120 N. Eagle Creek Dr. Suite 431, Lexington, Kentucky 40509, USA. *E-mail address:* bkoffler@aol.com

https://doi.org/10.1016/j.yaoo.2019.04.004

will be myopic by 2050 [1]. An alarming 1 billion (20%) of those will be considered "highly myopic" (more than 5.00 diopters [D]) with high associated risk of ocular pathology [3].

Myopia is more than a minor inconvenience requiring vision correction with glasses or contact lenses. It is a disease process creating significant risk of serious vision-threatening eye disease [4]. Although high myopia, associated with longer than average axial length, poses a much higher risk, any amount of myopia increases the risk of developing cataracts, glaucoma, retinal detachment, and myopic macular degeneration [5].

Development of myopia has been described as a complex interaction of genetics, environment, optical, and behavioral influences [5]. Extensive study shows children of myopic parents are at higher risk of becoming myopic [6–8]. A consensus of studies reports that spending more hours outdoors may delay the onset of myopia but may not slow myopic progression once it has been diagnosed [7,9–11]. The effect of extensive near work on myopia is strongly correlated, but causation has not been proved [12]. Also, younger myopic children (7–9 years old) progress in degree of myopia faster than older myopic children (11–15 years old) [13,14]. Historically, eye-care practitioners have prescribed spectacles for myopic children to correct their vision. Numerous studies show that myopic children corrected with spectacles have significant increases in axial length and higher degree of myopia over time [14,15].

Given these serious concerns, intervention by all eye-care practitioners to slow increasing axial length and myopic progression at younger age and at lower levels of myopia may provide significant long-term eye health and vision benefits to these young patients. Various methods of treatment for myopia and myopic progression have been prescribed [16,17]. Recent studies have determined 3 methods to be most effective [16,18]. These include the optical interventions of orthokeratology (OrthoK) and contact lenses of multifocal design and pharmacologic treatment with atropine. Ongoing research and clinical evaluations continue in effort to find the modality, or combination of modalities, that are effective, safe, and that patients will be compliant with. Peer-reviewed studies have shown OrthoK is safe and effective in slowing myopic progression [19,20]. Very recent studies suggest that combining OrthoK with atropine shows greater slowing of myopic progression than either modality alone [21].

OrthoK consists of fitting specially designed gas-permeable contact lenses that are worn overnight. OrthoK creates changes in the corneal topography, characterized by central corneal flattening surrounded by a ring of midperipheral steepening (Fig. 1). A representative photo of an OrthoK lens on the eye is shown in Fig. 2. Detailed optical coherence tomography evaluation of the post-OrthoK cornea reveals slight central epithelial thinning surrounded by a ring of midperipheral epithelial thickening in the areas corresponding to the topographic changes (Fig. 3). At the level of the retina, the induced corneal changes result in reduced myopic refractive error centrally, providing good central visual acuity, combined with relative myopic defocus peripheral to the macular area (Fig. 4) (also, see section on peripheral myopic defocus discussed later).

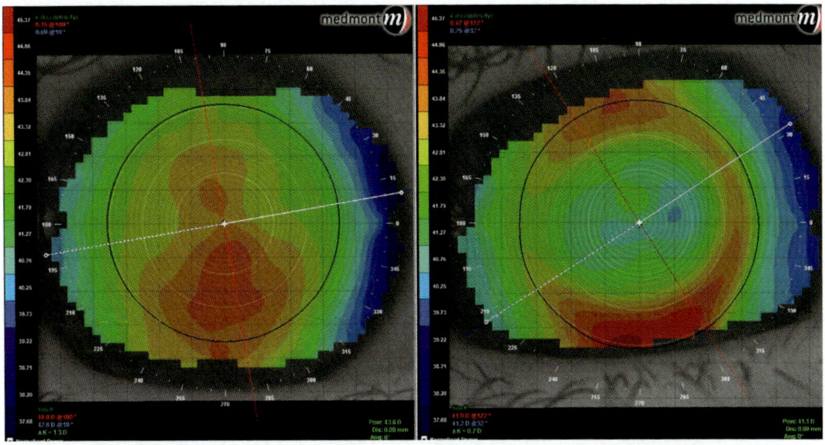

Fig. 1. Pretreatment axial topographic map (*left*). Post-OrthoK axial topographic map (*right*).

SIGNIFICANCE

Who is at risk of becoming myopic?

Significant debate exists about whether development of myopia is genetic or environmental. Both factors have strong scientific support in addition to other factors. Parental history of myopia has long been thought to be a risk factor for the development of myopia [12]. The Orinda Longitudinal Study of Myopia showed an association between parental myopia and a child's refractive error and axial length before the onset of myopia [22,23]. Historically, studies have shown a higher proportion of myopic children among families with 2 myopic parents compared with one and no myopic parent [8]. More recent and more detailed evaluation has shown that a child's risk of future myopia can be predicted in a nonmyopic child using only the single measure of refractive error at a specified age [6]. Currently, we can say that if both parents are

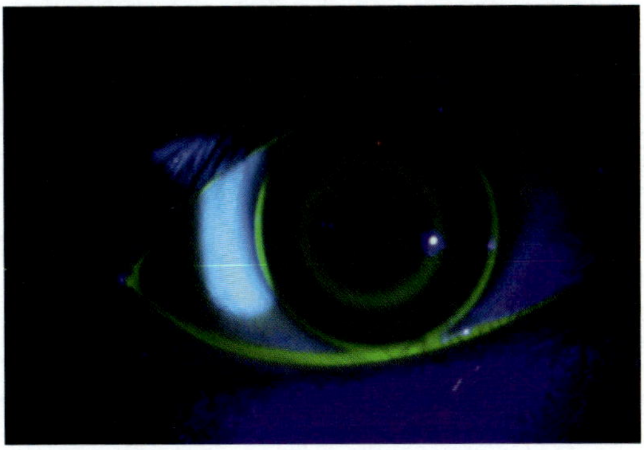

Fig. 2. Typical fluorescein pattern of a well-fit OrthoK lens.

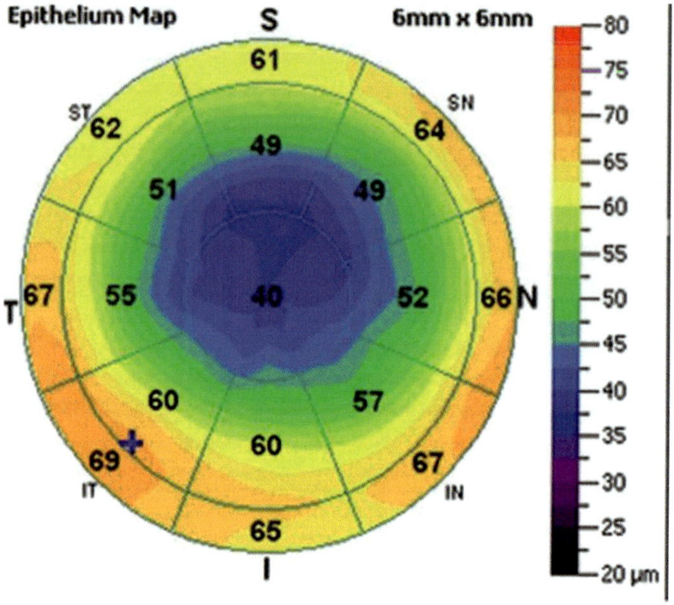

Fig. 3. Optical coherence tomographic mapping of epithelial thickness of post-OrthoK eye. (*From* Yishan Qian, Feng Xue, Jia Huang, Xiaomei Qu, Xingtao Zhou and Devan Van Lanen-Wanek (2014) Pachymetry map of corneal epithelium in children wearing orthokeratology contact lenses. Current Eye Research 39:3:263–70; with permission.)

myopic or if a child is less hyperopic than +0.75D at age 6 years, that child has a high risk of becoming myopic by age 8 years [6].

Although more than 20 chromosomal loci and 100 gene variants have been reported to be associated with myopia, no definite genetic pattern has been

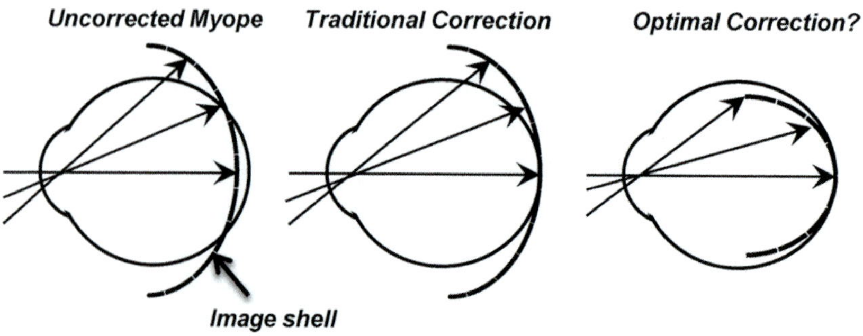

Fig. 4. Peripheral retinal image shell created by uncorrected myopia (*left*), typical spectacle correction (*middle*), and OrthoK (*right*). Note: the labels on the original are uncorrected myope (*left*), traditional correction (*middle*), and optimal correction (*right*). (*From* Smith EL. The Charles F. Prentice Award Lecture 2010: a case for peripheral optical treatment strategies for myopia. Optom Vis Sci 2011;88(9):1029–44, with permission.)

isolated for myopia [24,25]. It is apparent genetic and environmental, and other influences interacting to create the significant increase in myopia prevalence have been seen over the previous 3 to 4 decades [5]. Other influences may include, amount of near work [26], duration of exposure to electronic media (phones, tablets, computer screens, TV, and video games) [27], educational pressures [28], outdoor time [9,11], and sports activities [9,29]. Development of myopia and progression of myopia are complex entities with multifactorial influences. It is prudent to make parents aware of these factors and have their children monitored regularly during this growth/risk period. If progression of myopia is seen, steps to slow that progression should be undertaken.

Safety

Because most OrthoK wearers are children, safety of OrthoK is a prime concern. The authors have a combined 41 years of clinical experience with OrthoK. Neither of them have had a patient with a serious complication (like microbial keratitis [MK]), and no patients have experienced a loss of best-corrected visual acuity. Likewise, an analysis of combined data from 3 ophthalmology offices, including 260 eyes, showed no evidence of documented MK cases [30]. Many years ago, reports of serious complications in OrthoK users occurred in Southeast Asia. Detailed analysis of these case reports showed a lack of compliance with care, limited or no regulation of fitting practices, and inappropriate lens materials or designs used. Recent studies and meta-analyses in the United States and worldwide have shown OrthoK to be safe with very rare reports of complications [19,31,32]. One of the largest of these investigations involved 58 studies in English and 112 in Chinese [32]. This study summarized its findings with the following statement, "There is sufficient evidence to suggest that OrthoK is a safe option for myopia correction and retardation. Long-term success of OrthoK treatment requires a combination of proper lens fitting, rigorous compliance to lens care regimen, good adherence to routine follow-ups, and timely treatment of complications." The authors also reported no long-term effect of OrthoK on corneal endothelium. In a large retrospective study of OrthoK wearers in the United States involving 1316 patients [31], representing about 2600 patient-years of wear, only 2 events of MK occurred; this resulted in an estimated overall incidence of MK with OrthoK of 7.7 per 10,000 years of wear and 13.9 per 10,000 years of wear for children (younger than 18 years). In comparison, the incidence of MK for overnight wear of soft contact lenses was 19.5 per 10,000 wearers for conventional hydrogels and 25.4 per 10,000 wearers for silicone hydrogels. Another retrospective study on OrthoK wearers in the United States involved 296 patients [19], in the practice of one of the authors of this article, during a 4.5-year period and reported 3 adverse events (keratitis greater than grade 2). Each of these events resolved without loss of best-corrected visual acuity. This study showed that OrthoK is a very safe process for both children and adults and is effective in providing good vision correction.

Efficacy/retrospective analysis

Individual studies and meta-analyses

Individual studies and meta-analyses on myopia control with OrthoK have shown a 40% to 60% mean reduction in rate of refractive change compared with controls using spectacles to correct myopia [33–35]. It should be noted that studies reporting "mean reduction in rate of myopic progression" are describing the average for all subjects in the study. Within a study showing 50% mean reduction in myopia progression, some individuals may show 100% reduction in refractive change (no progression), whereas others may show 0% reduction (progression equal to that of the spectacle-wearing controls). Two studies reported results slightly differently [36,37]. These studies grouped the results in terms of the percentage of subjects who had little or no progression, moderate rate of progression, and fast progression. Both studies reported similar results with 60% of OrthoK wearers categorized as "slow progressors," 25% having "average" rate of myopia progression, and 15% "fast progressors," compares with spectacle wearers who showed rates of progression of 20% (slow), 60 (avg), and 20% (fast), respectively.

In a recent meta-analysis of 3 randomized controlled trials and 6 cohort studies, after 2 years of follow-up, OrthoK patients showed 0.27 mm less increase in axial length than the spectacle-wearing controls (weighted average change in 2 years of 0.36 mm in the OrthoK wearers vs 0.63 mm increase in the spectacle wearers) [38]. This equilibrates to a mean of 43% less axial length increase (study range of 24%–63%) versus controls (mean 43%) at 2 years. This same study also found that children of Asian ethnicity have less refractive increases with OrthoK than Caucasian children (about 0.10D less per year).

Quality of vision

Clarity of vision after removal of OrthoK lenses is very good. In the initial approval study for the Food and Drug Administration (FDA) [39], Paragon reported 57.4% of eyes achieved posttreatment unaided visual acuity of 20/20 and 88.5% achieved 20/40. More recent studies evaluating both objective and subjective ratings of visual acuity reported OrthoK patients having mean uncorrected visual acuity of 0.03 ± 0.07 logMAR (20/20-). In a cross-over study, OrthoK patients, on a validated questionnaire, rated their vision as equal to or better than with soft lenses after wearing OrthoK lenses versus soft lenses for 2 months each [40]. This subjective evaluation correlates well with the objective acuity of 0.06 logMAR (20/20-3) with OrthoK versus 0.04 (20/20-2) with the soft lenses. Overall, at the end of this study, 67.7% of the subjects chose to continue with OrthoK as their preferred method of correction.

Another study found unaided acuity of a group of OrthoK wearers to be −0.06 ± 0.12 logMAR (20/20 + 3) [41]. In this study, OrthoK wearers had a subjective level in this particular study of overall satisfaction with visual outcomes of 7.8 ± 1.8 (range, 3.5–10, on a 10-point scale). In both studies, a trend exists toward reduced level of overall quality of vision with higher level of baseline myopia. But both studies show OrthoK users have a high level of satisfaction with unaided vision and that individual variation occurs.

Theory of peripheral myopic defocus

The groundbreaking work on the effect of peripheral defocus on axial growth of the eye was done by Earl Smith [42,43]. He showed that ocular growth and refractive development are regulated by visual feedback associated with the eyes' effective refractive state, focus or defocus, of light peripheral to the macular area. Studies in humans demonstrate that myopic eyes show relative hyperopia in the periphery that hyperopic and emmetropic eyes do not, and children who develop myopia have more relative hyperopic peripheral defocus than emmetropic children 2 years before the onset of myopia. Children with peripheral hyperopic defocus are more likely to develop myopia. In addition, myopic children currently are corrected with standard spectacles that create significant hyperopic defocus. Therefore, peripheral hyperopia is likely the signal for increased eye growth. Light focusing posterior to the peripheral retina may act as a signal for increasing axial length and higher degree of myopia. Current research in spectacle design is investigating the creation of spectacle lenses to eliminate this hyperopic defocus (Fig. 5).

With OrthoK, the creation of an oblate shape of the cornea and the junction, where the oblate portion of the cornea returns to its original curvature, causes the image to clearly focus centrally at the fovea, while peripheral light focuses anterior to the peripheral retina (myopic defocus), and this results in an image profile focusing centrally at the fovea, while peripheral to the macula myopic defocus is created (see Fig. 5). This myopic defocus is believed to be the mechanism that slows myopia progression during OrthoK wear. Although these studies are quite convincing, studies exist that shows no effect of peripheral defocus on axial length increase, whereas other studies show a strong effect. Clinical research has demonstrated that peripheral myopic defocus created with OrthoK is the likely mechanism by which myopia progression is slowed with this process [42]. Other mechanisms occur that may also influence slowing of progression during OrthoK. One factor may be the change in lag of accommodation [44]. This change occurs because of the increase in positive spherical

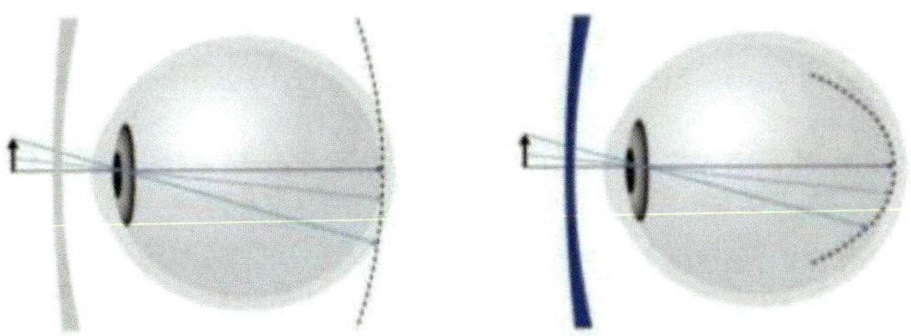

Fig. 5. A novel spectacle design to alter peripheral defocus. Traditional spectacle lens producing peripheral hyperopic defocus (*left*). Novel spectacle design creating peripheral myopic defocus (*right*).

aberration (more plus in the periphery) created after OrthoK and may be protective against progression of myopia. Another factor may relate to binocularity influencing myopic progression as OrthoK wearers show less esophoria and more exophoria, than single-vision soft lens wearers.

Myopia management with OrthoK—slowing of progression and refractive option

Currently, OrthoK lenses are designed and prescribed to correct myopic refractive error and provide good unaided visual acuity. A review of the literature on myopia control with OrthoK recently was published [45]. When prescribing OrthoK to correct refractive error, a secondary beneficial side effect of slowing myopia progression occurs [46]. Although OrthoK has a significant effect in slowing myopic progression, as described earlier, the results vary with individuals. Although some OrthoK patients show little or no myopic progression, some do continue to progress. Factors that may contribute to this variable effect include age of onset of myopia [22], age at start of OrthoK [36], increasing age, degree of baseline myopia, degree of baseline astigmatism, rate of progression before initiating OrthoK, pupil size, peripheral refractive profile (before and after OrthoK), retinal topography (shape), lens design, size of resulting treatment zone, and position of the treatment zone. These studies show that better myopia control (less myopic progression) positively is associated with older age of myopia onset, older age at start of OrthoK [13], higher degree of baseline myopia, larger pupil size [47], and smaller central treatment zone (more peripheral myopia induced by ring of steepening outside treatment zone). Even with these data, relative to peripheral refraction, the exact location or amount of peripheral myopic defocus that will result in the best control of myopic progression has not been determined. Future developments in testing peripheral refraction in combination with customized lens design may show even better myopia control with OrthoK.

Evaluation of the efficacy of various interventions to slow myopic progression has been performed by monitoring change in refraction (subjective or cycloplegic) and/or change in axial length. Many publications and researchers have stated that the gold standard for determining myopia control should be change in axial length [48]. But the changes in axial length do not always correlate directly with refractive changes. Certainly, slowing increases in axial length is the major reason to prescribe OrthoK, as longer axial length is associated with higher risk of serious ocular complications later in life. But, anecdotal reports exist of children who show axial length increases with no change in refraction and vice versa, children showing no change in axial length but with apparent refractive increases, which suggests that other growth-related factors occur that may influence these findings and that both measurements should be carefully monitored.

Quality of life

As with any medical treatment, patient-reported outcomes are an important measure of the acceptability and ultimate success of a treatment. OrthoK wearers report higher vision-related quality of life (VR-QOL) scores compared with spectacle and soft lenses wearers. The National Eye Institute Refractive Quality of Life (NEI-RQL 42) results showed higher "overall satisfaction with vision" in OrthoK wearers than in soft contact lens wearers [40]. Specific attributes that were significantly better with OrthoK were less activity limitations, symptoms (itching, burning, dryness), and dependence on correction.

A recent study reported significant psychological benefits of OrthoK [49]. Children using OrthoK showed more confidence, were more willing to try new things, were more active in participating in sports and recreational activities, and showed a trend toward increased outdoor activity time. Other effects reported here were self-esteem and overall improved VR-QOL. It already has been shown that children wearing contact lenses report better VR-QOL than those wearing spectacles. The added improvement in VR-QOL with OrthoK versus contact lenses worn during the day also has been demonstrated.

Of note is that the survey instruments used in these studies earlier are refractive measures that were not validated for use in OrthoK wearers. Now a new survey instrument has been validated for use with OrthoK wearers (and all forms of refractive correction) called the OrthoKeratology and Contact Lens Quality of Life Instrument [50]. Ongoing studies are evaluating OrthoK using this new questionnaire. The VR-QOL benefits of OrthoK will likely be even more impactful when considering the reduction in refractive and axial length increases.

Other considerations

Corneal and refractive changes with OrthoK are temporary. To maintain best vision, lenses should be worn every night for 7 to 8 hours while sleeping. Some patients report good vision even after skipping a night of wear. When lenses are worn regularly, most patients report consistently good vision during all their waking hours. If patients stop wearing OrthoK lenses, both refractive and topographic changes will return to baseline. Depending on the degree of baseline myopia, refraction should stabilize after 7 to 10 days while topography may take longer, 2 to 8 weeks, to completely stabilize.

No age restrictions exist for OrthoK. For young patients, the ideal age to start is when they are sufficiently motivated to wear lenses every night and when they are able to communicate in detail with parents and the practitioner about their vision and how their eyes/lenses feel. This could be as young as 5 years or as old as 18 years. Relative to management of myopic progression, starting at a younger age results in greater ultimate benefit in minimizing the child's eventual level of myopia as an adult.

Ongoing studies are investigating other factors that may affect development of myopia and myopia progression, which include choroidal thickness, hormonal factors, outdoor time, light exposure, and retinal/scleral shape [51–53].

CURRENT RELEVANCE/FUTURE INVESTIGATION

The benefit of prescribing OrthoK to myopic children is the limitation of axial length growth and the resulting reduction in the risk of ocular pathology associated with increased axial length. As described earlier, because of extensive study, we have learned much about the use of OrthoK. Summary of known attributes of OrthoK includes the following:

- Use of OrthoK in myopic children slows myopic progression 40% to 60% versus spectacles or traditional soft lenses.
- Unaided vision is good during all waking hours after regular wear of OrthoK lenses (OrthoK lenses are removed on waking in the morning).
- OrthoK is a safe process: the minimal risks are further minimized with compliance with lens care routines and regular follow-up.
- OrthoK is a temporary process that is 100% reversible.

Future study is needed to determine some of the unknowns involved in the development of myopia and myopia control with OrthoK.

Unknown issues include the following:

- What actually causes myopia to develop and progress? Although numerous factors have been associated with myopia development and progression, none have been isolated as causative. In addition, various patterns exist of myopia development and progression. Simply put, myopia and myopia progression are complex entities that vary from one patient to the next.
- As eye care professionals embrace the theory of peripheral defocus as the mechanism determining axial length growth or stability, it is still unknown as to the exact amount or the exact location of myopic defocus on the retina to provide optimal slowing of myopic progression.
- Why some patients show significant slowing or total arrest of myopic progression with OrthoK and others show continued progression?
- Can slowing of myopic progression be more effective by combining different modalities of intervention—behavioral, environmental, optical, or pharmaceutical?
- Can OrthoK be even more effective in slowing of myopic progression by customizing the design of the lenses for each patient?
- Is there an ideal age when OrthoK should be stopped (maybe no reason exists to stop as OrthoK is prescribed for adults)?
- Is there a rebound effect for those who do discontinue OrthoK wear?
- What is the effect of outdoor light, outdoor play, ultraviolet light, and other light sources on myopia progression?

SUMMARY

The importance of managing myopia and the progression of myopia have been demonstrated due to the long-term eye health risks associated with higher axial length. Studies show that OrthoK is effective in slowing increases in refractive error and axial length growth in children. OrthoK allows patients to enjoy good vision without need for vision correction during their waking hours. In addition, OrthoK provides excellent vision, improves vision-related quality of life, and is very safe. Since OrthoK gained FDA clearance in 2002 (in the United States) as an option to correct refractive error, it has become more popular with eye care practitioners and with patients, as they adapt quickly and enjoy the process. As described earlier, even without specific FDA clearance to slow myopic progression, most patients/parents state the reason they choose OrthoK is to slow increasing degree of myopia. Slowing myopic progression is of interest to eye care practitioners for reasons described earlier. A growing body of research shows OrthoK slows progression of myopia but that an individual's response is variable.

OrthoK may be prescribed for children or adults as an option to correct refractive error, as an alternative to spectacles and contact lenses worn during the day. As described earlier, wearers describe the excitement and freedom of being able to perform all their daily activities without the need for any vision-correcting device. In children, although OrthoK is prescribed to correct refractive error, extensive study has demonstrated a reduction in myopia progression. Current areas of interest for OrthoK in the future include the following:

- Individual custom-designed OrthoK lenses to improve on the efficacy of slowing myopic progression
- The use of OrthoK in combination with other modalities of myopia management

The practice of OrthoK is a unique specialty in contact lens–related eye care that requires practitioners to attain certification and specialty training. Proper fitting, detailed patient instruction on lens care and handling, as well as regular and careful follow-up are essential for long-term success and safety.

The process of OrthoK provides patients and practitioners an option to correct refractive error while slowing the rate of myopic progression. Future study may help further improve the effectiveness of OrthoK designs in slowing myopic progression.

References

[1] Holden BA, Jong M, Davis S, et al. Nearly 1 billion myopes at risk of myopia-related sight-threatening conditions by 2050—Time to act now. Clin Exp Optom 2015;98:491–3.

[2] Vitale S, Sperduto RD, Ferris FL III. Increased prevalence of myopia in the United States between 1971–1972 and 1999–2004. Arch Ophthalmol 2009;127:1632–9.

[3] Cho BJ, Shin JY, Yu HG. Complications of pathologic myopia. Eye Contact Lens 2016;42: 9–15.

[4] Saw SM, Gazzard G, Shih-Yen EC, et al. Myopia and associated pathological complications. Ophthalmic Physiol Opt 2005;25:381–91.

[5] Flitcroft DI. The complex interactions of retinal, optical and environmental factors in myopia aetiology. Prog Retin Eye Res 2012;31:622–60.

[6] Zadnik K, Sinnott LT, Cotter SA, et al, Collaborative Longitudinal Evaluation of Ethnicity and Refractive Error (CLEERE) Study Group. Prediction of juvenile-onset myopia. JAMA Ophthalmol 2015;133:683–9.

[7] Jones LA, Sinnott LT, Mutti DO, et al. Parental history of myopia, sports and outdoor activities, and future myopia. Invest Ophthalmol Vis Sci 2007;48:3524–32.

[8] Kurtz D, Hyman L, Gwiazda JE, et al, COMET Group. Role of parental myopia in the progression of myopia and its interaction with treatment in COMET children. Invest Ophthalmol Vis Sci 2007;48:562–70.

[9] Rose KA, Morgan IG, Ip J, et al. Outdoor activity reduces the prevalence of myopia in children. Ophthalmology 2008;115:1279–85.

[10] Dirani M, Tong L, Gazzard G, et al. Outdoor activity and myopia in Singapore teenage children. Br J Ophthalmol 2009;93:997–1000.

[11] Sherwin JC, Reacher MH, Keogh RH, et al. The association between time spent outdoors and myopia in children and adolescents. Ophthalmology 2012;119:2141–51.
[12] Mutti DO, Mitchell GL, Moeschberger ML, et al. Parental myopia, near work, school achievement, and children's refractive error. Invest Ophthalmol Vis Sci 2002;43:3633–40.
[13] Wang B, Naidu RK, Qu X. Factors related to axial length elongation and myopia progression in orthokeratology practice. PLoS One 2017;12(4):e0175913.
[14] Cho P, Cheung S-W. Retardation of myopia in orthokeratology (ROMIO) study: a 2-year randomized clinical trial. Invest Ophthalmol Vis Sci 2012;53:7077–85.
[15] Santodomingo-Rubido J, Villa-Collar C, Gilmarten B, et al. Long-term efficacy of orthokeratology contact lens wear in controlling the progression of childhood myopia. Curr Eye Res 2017; https://doi.org/10.1080/02713683.2016.1221979.
[16] Huang J, Wen D, Wang Q, et al. Efficacy comparison of 16 interventions for myopia control in children. Ophthalmology 2016;123:697–708.
[17] Koffler BH, Sears JJ. Myopia control in children through refractive therapy gas permeable contact lenses: is it for real? Am J Ophthalmol 2016;156:1076–81.
[18] Walline JJ, Lindsley K, Vedula SS, et al. Interventions to slow progression of myopia in children. Cochrane Database Syst Rev 2011;(12):CD004916.
[19] Lipson MJ. Long-term clinical outcomes for overnight corneal reshaping in children and adults. Eye Contact Lens 2008;34:94–9.
[20] Bullimore M, Sinott LT, Jones-Jordan LA. The incidence of microbial keratitis with overnight corneal reshaping lenses. Optom Vis Sci 2013;90:937–44.
[21] Wan L, Wei C-C, Chen CS, et al. The synergistic effects of orthokeratology and atropine in slowing the progression of myopia. J Clin Med 2018;7:259.
[22] Mutti DO, Hayes JR, Mitchell GL, et al. Refractive error, axial length, and relative peripheral refractive error before and after the onset of myopia. Invest Ophthalmol Vis Sci 2007;48: 2510–9.
[23] Zadnik K, Mutti DO, Friedman NE, et al. Initial cross-sectional results from the Orinda Longitudinal Study of Myopia. Optom Vis Sci 1993;70:750–8.
[24] Stone RA, Khurana TS. Gene profiling in experimental models of eye growth: clues to myopia pathogenesis. Vision Res 2010;50:2322–33.
[25] Young T. Molecular genetics of human myopia: an update. Optom Vis Sci 2009;86:E8–22.
[26] Lin Z, Vasudeven B, Mao GY, et al. The influence of near work on myopic refractive change in urban students in Beijing: a three-year follow-up report. Graefes Arch Clin Exp Ophthalmol 2016;254:2247–55.
[27] Wu P-C, Huang H-M, Yu H-J, et al. Epidemiology of myopia. Asia Pac J Ophthalmol (Phila) 2016;5:386–93.
[28] Tideman JWL, Polling JR, Hofman A, et al. Environmental factors explain socioeconomic prevalence differences in myopia in 6-year old children. Br J Ophthalmol 2017;1–5; https://doi.org/10.1136/bjophthalmol-2017-310292.
[29] Read SA, Collins MJ, Vincent SJ. Light exposure and physical activity in myopic and emmetropic children. Optom Vis Sci 2014;91:330–41.
[30] Koffler BK, Sears J, Wohl L, et al. Success rate of incorporating corneal refractive therapy into 3 different ophthalmology practices. Eye Contact Lens 2016;42:74–9.
[31] Bullimore M, Sinnott L, Jones-Jordan L. The risk of microbial keratitis with overnight corneal reshaping lenses. Optom Vis Sci 2013;90:937–44.
[32] Liu YM, Xie P. The safety of orthokeratology—a systematic review. Eye Contact Lens 2016;42:35–42.
[33] Wen D, Huang J, Chen H, et al. Efficacy and acceptability of orthokeratology for slowing myopic progression in children: a systematic review and meta-analysis. J Ophthalmol 2015; https://doi.org/10.1155/2015/360806.
[34] Si J-k, Tang K, Bi H-S, et al. Orthokeratology for myopia control: a meta-analysis. Optom Vis Sci 2015;92:252–7.

[35] Sun Y, Xu F, Ting Zhang ML, et al. Orthokeratology to control myopia progression: a meta-analysis. PLoS One 2015;10(4):e0124535.
[36] Cho P, Cheung S-W. Retardation of myopia in Orthokeratology (ROMIO) study: a 2- year randomized clinical trial. Invest Ophthalmol Vis Sci 2012;53:7077–85.
[37] Lipson MJ, Harris JK, Lather HD, et al. Axial length in orthokeratology patients: large case series. Adv Ophthalmol Vis Syst 2016;5(2):00154.
[38] Li S-M, Kang M-T, Wu S-S, et al. Efficacy, safety and acceptability of orthokeratology on slowing axial elongation in myopic children by meta-analysis. Curr Eye Res 2015;41: 600–8.
[39] Paragon CRT – FDA Approval Study, Premarket approval Application (PMA) Supplement Number: P870024/S43, June 2002. Available at: https://www.accessdata.fda.gov/cdrh_docs/pdf/P870024S043A.pdf. Accessed May 17, 2019.
[40] Lipson MJ, Sugar A, Musch DC. Overnight corneal reshaping versus soft disposable contact lenses: vision-related quality-of-life differences from a randomized clinical trial. Optom Vis Sci 2005;82:886–91.
[41] Hiraoka T, Okamoto C, Ishii Y, et al. Patient satisfaction and clinical outcomes after overnight orthokeratology. Optom Vis Sci 2009;86:875–82.
[42] Smith E, Campbell M, Irving E. Does peripheral retinal input explain the promising myopia control effects of corneal reshaping therapy (CRT or ortho-K) and multifocal soft contact lenses? Ophthalmic Physiol Opt 2013;33:379–84.
[43] Smith E. A case for peripheral optical treatment strategies for myopia. Optom Vis Sci 2011;88:1–16.
[44] Gifford K, Gifford P, Hendicott PL, et al. Near binocular visual function in young adult orthokeratology versus soft contact lens wearers. Cont Lens Anterior Eye 2017;40:184–9.
[45] Lipson MJ, Brooks MM, Koffler BK. The role of orthokeratology in myopia control: a review. Eye Contact Lens 2018;44:224–30.
[46] Lipson MJ, Sandall G. Myopia control: science or luck. Eye Contact Lens 2016;42:80–1.
[47] Chen Z, Niu L, Xue F, et al. Impact of pupil diameter on axial growth in orthokeratology. Optom Vis Sci 2012;89:1636–40.
[48] Cheung S-W, Cho P. Validity of axial length measurements for monitoring myopic progression in orthokeratology. Invest Ophthalmol Vis Sci 2013;54:1613–5.
[49] Zhao F, Zhao G, Zhao Z. Investigation of the effect of orthokeratology lenses on quality of life and behaviors of children. Eye Contact Lens 2018;44:335–8.
[50] McAlinden C, Lipson MJ. Orthokeratology and contact lens quality of life questionnaire (OCL-QoL). Eye Contact Lens 2018;44:279–85.
[51] Read SA. Ocular and environmental factors associated with eye growth in childhood. Optom Vis Sci 2016;93:1031–41.
[52] Gardner DJ, Walline JJ, Mutti DO. Choroidal thickness and peripheral myopic defocus during orthokeratology. Optom Vis Sci 2015;92:579–88.
[53] He M, Xiang F, Zeng Y, et al. Effect of time spent outdoors at school on the development of myopia among children in China a randomized clinical trial. JAMA 2015;314:1142–8.

Advances in Ophthalmology and Optometry 4 (2019) 89–100

ADVANCES IN OPHTHALMOLOGY AND OPTOMETRY

Adjustable Suture Strabismus Surgery in Children

Ahmed M. Kassem, MD[a,*], Richard Rivers, MD, PhD, MBA[b], David L. Guyton, MD[c]

[a]Pediatric Ophthalmology, Sanford Health, Sanford South University Medical Center, 1717 South University Drive, Fargo, ND 58103, USA; [b]The Johns Hopkins University, 400 North Broadway, Smith Building, Room 4041, Baltimore, MD 21287, USA; [c]The Johns Hopkins University, The Johns Hopkins Hospital, Wilmer 233, 600 North Wolfe Street, Baltimore, MD 21287-9028, USA

Keywords

• Anesthesia • Anesthetics • Oculomotor muscles • Propofol • Strabismus surgery • Suture techniques • Treatment outcome • Suture

Key points

- Adjustable sutures are rarely used in the pediatric age range.
- Children's cooperation with postoperative assessment was only very rarely reported to be a rate-limiting step in performing the adjustment procedure.
- Several techniques allow optional adjustment, obviating a second anesthetic when adjustment is not required.
- A single prospective randomized trial and several retrospective studies support the safety and feasibility of adjustable sutures in children in the postanesthesia care unit setting, and suggest an additional benefit compared with fixed sutures.
- Higher quality prospective studies are needed to prove the definitive advantage for using adjustable sutures in the pediatric age range in terms of improving the chances of successful alignment and reducing the reoperation rate.

INTRODUCTION

Adjustable suture strabismus surgery is a well-established technique among adult strabismus surgeons. It is particularly valuable in complex cases and reoperations in which the use of fixed sutures can be unpredictable. The use of adjustable sutures in the pediatric population is far less common, even among

Disclosure Statement: The authors have nothing to disclose.

*Corresponding author. *E-mail address:* kassema86@gmail.com

https://doi.org/10.1016/j.yaoo.2019.04.005
2452-1760/19/

strabismus surgeons who use adjustable sutures routinely in adults. Children are thought to be not cooperative enough for satisfactory assessment in the immediate postoperative period. Additionally, surgeons generally face resistance from anesthesia personnel and postanesthesia care unit (PACU) nursing teams because of the perceived complexity of the adjustment procedure in terms of cost, time, and stress on operating room (OR) and PACU resources. Also, there is emerging concern that a single anesthetic exposure is safe in the first 36 months of life but the effects of additional anesthesia on the developing child's brain is yet to be determined [1]. Added to that is the perception that the benefit of adjustable sutures in children is, at best, limited and does not justify the additional risk, cost, and time involved with the adjustment procedure. This article highlights the most commonly used adjustable suture techniques in the pediatric age group. Also, some tips that can facilitate the adoption of this procedure by strabismus surgeons and anesthesia teams are pointed out. Finally, the literature pertaining to the use of adjustable sutures in infants and children and the most commonly cited criticism is reviewed.

SIGNIFICANCE

Operative procedures

Several techniques have been described for performing adjustable suture techniques. Techniques pertaining to the pediatric age are highlighted in this article.

The bowtie

The bowtie technique was reported in the pediatric age group by Chan and colleagues [2]. They used the limbal approach to the surgery. This technique involved tying the muscle pole sutures into a bowtie over a strand of 6-0 silk after passing the suture ends through the original insertion. The 6-0 silk strand was then tied into a small loop to prevent displacement and loss. A so-called bucket handle of 6-0 Vicryl (Ethicon Sutures, Mercedes Medical, Lakewood Ranch, FL, USA) can be placed as a traction suture to allow globe manipulation during adjustment. The bowtie can be exposed to ease access during the adjustment process. During the adjustment, the bowtie is untied and the pole sutures tied to the desired adjustment, as in a nonadjustable hang-back technique. This requires both suture ends to be handled carefully to avoid unequal length of muscle sutures after retying. Adequate exposure is paramount. Importantly, this manipulation of loose sutures cannot be interrupted on anesthesiologist demand, which is a common occurrence during propofol-sedated adjustment in which excessive manipulation can stimulate the child excessively, requiring further manipulation be stopped and additional doses of propofol administered before the procedure can be safely completed without the need to take the child back to the OR [3].

The sliding noose

The sliding noose is perhaps the more commonly used technique in the pediatric age range. Several variations were introduced to the technique to make it more suitable for the pediatric age group. The basic technique involves securing the 2 pole sutures after passing them through the muscle stump with an overhand knot. A sliding noose is then fashioned around the pole sutures using a separate suture. This noose sliding up and down the pole sutures can be then used to increase or decrease the amount of recession [4]. The pole sutures are then tied against the sliding noose, and the sliding noose can be trimmed very short on the completion of the adjustment. Even if no adjustment is needed, an additional procedure is required postoperatively to tie the pole suture ends and trim the sliding noose. An adjustable resection involves an extra 1 to 3 mm of resection and hanging the muscle back by the same amount to allow advancement or recession [5].

One advantage of this technique is that it can be performed using a fornix or cul-de-sac incision with less postoperative discomfort and better healing. A Small Incision Muscle Hook (Katena, Denville, NJ, USA) was devised by Guyton [6] to minimize the conjunctival incision size, with subsequent reduction in postoperative inflammation and scarring. A sliding noose using a clove hitch with 3 slip knots was described by Deschler and colleagues [7]. Pulling sideways on this removable noose after adjustment removes the noose entirely and potentially reduces subsequent postoperative inflammation and discomfort.

Parsa and colleagues [8] and Awadein and colleagues [9] proposed the use of nonabsorbable sutures when large recessions of the inferior and medial rectus muscles are anticipated to reduce the incidence of slippage. They reported reduced incidence of overcorrections with this modification [8,9]. Such permanent sutures should be attached at least 4 mm posterior to the original muscle insertion to avoid later erosion of the suture ends and knot through the thin conjunctiva anteriorly.

Spielmann and Spielmann [10] proposed a semiadjustable method to reduce the risk of slippage of the inferior rectus muscle. They secured the corners of the muscle to the sclera using fixed interrupted sutures and secured the center of the muscle with a double-armed adjustable suture passing through the original insertion. This allows the advancement of the central muscle all the way up to the original insertion if desired postoperatively. A limitation of this technique is that it does not allow additional recession of the muscle farther than the 1 to 2 mm allowed by the sag in the central part of the muscle.

Several modifications to the adjustable noose have been proposed by Budning and colleagues [11], Nihalani and colleagues [5], and Engel and Rousta [12] that allow optional and possibly multiple adjustments to be made.

Both Budning and colleagues [11] and Nihalani and Hunter [5] described a new technique that keeps the sliding noose very short and a segment of only 6 to 7 mm in length above the sliding noose, such that the sliding noose and the pole sutures can be tucked under the conjunctiva and only exposed if adjustment is required. This also allows for multiple adjustments. Budning [11] reported being able to adjust a child 4 days after surgery and adults 6 days after surgery with adjustment limited by muscle attachment to the globe and suture absorption. Repeated adjustments are still limited by the need to put the child to sleep with every adjustment. Potential drawbacks include the potential for slippage of the muscle and the increased propensity to develop suture granulomas [5]. Because such optional adjustment procedures do not involve placement of a traction suture, and both the sliding noose and the pole sutures are kept short, more manipulation may be needed to locate the suture during the adjustment procedure. To avoid this, Tsai [13] reported the pull-string technique, which involves passing a thread of 6-0 Vicryl suture between the 2 arms of the pole sutures above the sliding noose. This pull-string suture can be taped to the skin. If no adjustment is required, 1 of the ends of the pull-string suture can be cut and the uncut thread can be pulled out to retrieve the whole thread. The investigator reported that neither the conjunctival closure nor the pole sutures were disturbed by this removal maneuver, and the removal maneuver required only 15 seconds.

Engel and Rousta [12] proposed another modification for optional adjustment that entails passing the ends of the muscle pole sutures through partial thickness scleral tunnels, thus keeping them buried under the conjunctiva. The adjustment process then required taking the child back to the OR to expose the buried pole sutures.

Hemihang-back technique for the lateral rectus muscle

Engel [14] and Engel and colleagues [15] reported a hemihang-back technique to be used in the adjustment of the lateral rectus muscle that does not involve using a sliding noose, which is a technique to possibly reduce conjunctival reactions and prevent vertical migration of the lateral rectus muscle during the healing process. The technique involves placing the initial scleral passes for the pole sutures in a position posterior to the original insertion but 2 to 3 mm anterior to the planned new insertion. This is followed by additional scleral passes and then bringing the extra suture up to the original insertion. The sutures are then tied, allowing the muscle to hang back 2 to 3 mm from the new insertion. If adjustment is needed, the knot at the original insertion is cut and the extra suture is unburied. The muscle can be advanced or recessed, and then the sutures are tied and the knot is trimmed, followed by conjunctival closure.

Ripcord technique and modifications

Coats [16] proposed a technique for optional suture adjustment that provides an all-or-none added 2-mm recession when a particular portion of the suture is cut, which behaves like a ripcord of a parachute. This was further modified by Hakim and colleagues [17] to a strengthened loop knot that can be released to produce additional 2 mm of recession. The inability to advance the muscle and the small amount of possible recession significantly limited the utility of this technique.

PREOPERATIVE AND POSTOPERATIVE CONSIDERATIONS

Preoperative assessment

As with every surgical procedure, the surgeon should have a thorough discussion about the adjustment procedure with the family, with every attempt made to involve the child in the decision-making. If the child is being considered for an awake adjustment, the cotton swab test, which involves observing the child's reaction to touching the nonanesthetized lateral conjunctiva with the tip of a piece of facial tissue or cotton swab, with the child looking away, should be used to assess the child's cooperation. Noting how the child reacts to eye drops in the clinic can give a guide to how he or she will behave during the adjustment procedure [15]. Awake adjustment can be attempted in some cooperative children as young as 7 years old based on the authors' experiences and previous studies [2,18,19].

ADJUSTMENT PROCEDURE

Choice of the timing for adjustment has varied in different studies, depending on the technique of adjustment used, the need for sedation or general anesthesia, and different PACU policies, from several hours to the first postoperative day. Kamal and colleagues [18] reported the time required for anesthesia to completely wear off so that the child could be reliably assessed as between 80 and 260 minutes, with an average of 156.5 minutes. The authors try to schedule adjustable cases earlier in the day and perform adjustment in the PACU 90 to 120 minutes postoperatively between subsequent cases [2,12,18,19].

Postoperative bedside assessment is ideally performed with prism and cover testing at a distance and near using a handheld muscle light for distance fixation and an accommodative target for near fixation, or at least using Krimsky measurement if the child is too young or uncooperative for the cover test. Adequate pain control for assessment can be achieved with topical anesthetic drops. It can be challenging at times to convince a fearful child to open his or her eyes and cooperate for alternate testing or Krimsky measurement, and it is not unusual for this to take up to 20 minutes to do so. Better cooperation can be achieved by asking the child to sit up with back unsupported and legs dangling over the edge of the bed. When all else fails in younger children, holding the child high up and feigning dropping the child on its face will typically elicit the reaction of the child's opening the eyes at least long enough to allow a brief assessment of alignment. The senior author (DLG) reported to have encountered only 4 children in his entire career who would not open their eyes for assessment of the alignment [15,18].

The target for adjustment, in the authors' experiences, is to aim in exotropia for single vision at near with esotropia of 3 to 6 prism diopter (PD) at distance, or double vision beyond 4 to 5 feet, and for esotropic patients to be left within 4 PD of orthotropia. We prefer to leave patients with hypertropia slightly undercorrected in straight-ahead gaze [18,19].

The adjustment process can be performed in the PACU or the OR, depending on the surgeon's and the anesthesiologist's comfort levels. It should be noted that propofol is a sedative hypnotic and does not provide adequate analgesia. Thus topical anesthesia should also be used and manipulation kept as minimal as possible. In awake adjustment, we have found the use of a lid speculum not to be necessary. Using it can further aggravate an uncomfortable child. An assistant can simply hold the lids open instead. The nonanesthetized lid margins should not be touched by the surgeon or the assistant during suture manipulation because this tends to cause further discomfort [2,3,19,21].

Our sterile adjustable suture kit typically consists of a lid speculum, 2 needle holders, tying forceps for holding the traction suture, Westcott scissors, and 2 pairs of 0.5 toothed forceps [19].

ANESTHESIA CONSIDERATIONS

Good coordination between the anesthesiologist and the strabismus surgeon is paramount for both phases of the adjustable surgery procedure to run seamlessly. The first goal is to allow both fast and adequate recovery from the OR anesthesia to permit good assessment of postoperative alignment. The second goal is to facilitate adjustment in the PACU with intravenous (IV) anesthesia only, without the need to return to the OR for adjustment.

Isoflurane and halothane are known to cause postoperative nausea, vomiting, and prolonged drowsiness, impeding timely assessment of postoperative alignment, and thus should not be used in these procedures [22,23]. The use of opioid analgesics should be kept to a minimum, especially in the postoperative period, to avoid excessive sedation and unwanted nausea and vomiting. Intraoperative ketorolac or rectal acetaminophen could be used instead to achieve adequate pain control [23–25].

Adjustment of children younger than the age of 10 years generally requires propofol IV anesthesia. IV propofol is associated with better recovery and less postoperative nausea and vomiting than the use of inhalational anesthetics. It can be administered in the PACU. Topical anesthetic drops should be used even with sedated adjustments to reduce the incidence of an oculocardiac reflex and reduce the total propofol dose needed to complete the adjustment [21,26,27].

None of the reviewed studies reported the occurrence of serious adverse events, such as apnea, hypotension, or bradycardia, during sedated or awake suture adjustments [12,18-21].

Phanphruk and colleagues [21] reported their experience with sedated suture adjustment in the PACU in 356 patients younger than the age of 18 years in a single center. No serious anesthesia events were reported. PACU stay was found to be a median of 132 minutes in those not needing adjustment compared with a median of 154 minutes in those adjusted without sedation and a median of 205 minutes in children requiring sedation for adjustment. Children undergoing nonadjustable bilateral medial rectus recessions at the same center spent an average of 90 minutes in the PACU. Median time from initial to final propofol dose was 7 minutes, and the median time the anesthesiologist spent at the bedside was 13 minutes (range 5–34 minutes). Median total propofol dose was 80 mg with 84% of patients undergoing sedated adjustment requiring more than a single bolus [28]. See later detailed discussion of the anesthesia protocol used for suture adjustment at the Wilmer Eye Institute of the Johns Hopkins Hospital, Baltimore, MD. The suture adjustment anesthesia protocol performed in Boston Children's Hospital has been published elsewhere [15].

On recovery from the general anesthesia in the OR, the surgeon needs the child to be as awake as possible so that the eye muscles are working under a normal state of consciousness. Children who are tired or sedated cooperate poorly and are not able to move their eyes in all directions as required for assessment by the surgeon.

Two anesthesia-related requirements exist for the successful adjustment of sutures in the PACU. During the initial surgery, avoid sedatives, such as midazolam, that may linger into the postoperative period. If such drug has been given, and the child does not adequately recover, a single dose of flumazenil in the PACU will increase the level of consciousness so that an effective postoperative assessment can proceed. Postoperative pain is not severe, therefore, a dose of IV ketorolac at the end of the OR procedure is usually sufficient for postoperative pain control. A single dose of nonsedating antiemetic is routinely administered to minimize the risk of postoperative nausea.

To minimize the chances of accidental termination of the IV, the authors recommend wrapping the IV with a cover of elastic, self-adhesive, bandage. Do not use any tension in the elastic, which might risk decreasing the blood flow distal to the bandage and making the limb very uncomfortable. It is only used as a cover to protect the IV catheter site.

As an extra precaution, start a second IV, with a heparin lock, in case the first IV fails or is accidently removed. Two IVs are recommended if the child is agitated or has postoperative delirium, he or she may accidently pull out the IV that was inserted under general anesthesia in the OR. Although this does seem like extra work, it might save the day in the end. If the IV is lost, and an awake insertion of a new IV seems inappropriate, then the only other option is another mask induction back in the OR, with all its usual barriers (Boxes 1 and 2).

Because the child has completely recovered from the prior anesthetic, this may be considered a new anesthesia encounter for billing, with all the appropriate base units. As such, this should be defined on the electronic medical record as a second surgical procedure in the new location.

Box 1: Preoperative and intraoperative planning

1. Avoid preoperative sedatives such as midazolam or antihistamines.
2. Secure the IV so it will outlast an arousing child, or awake child's mishandling. Alternatively start a second IV and cover it.
3. Use an antiemetic toward the end of the case.
4. Administer ketorolac toward the end of the case.

Box 2: Postanesthesia care unit planning

1. Maintaining spontaneous ventilation is the goal. Nonetheless, resuscitation equipment, including emergency airway supplies and medications, should be at hand.
2. Have adequate propofol on hand for a 30-minute case. Dose with intermittent boluses of propofol, depending on patient weight and responsiveness to the procedure. An initial dose of 1 mg/kg is typical. Pretreat with lidocaine to reduce the risk of pain during propofol injections.
3. Use doses of propofol that will maintain spontaneous ventilation through a green mask with 6 L/min oxygen.
4. Use end-tidal carbon dioxide ($EtCO_2$) sampling in the mask to assess and document adequate ventilation.
5. Use routine monitors such as electrocardiogram, blood pressure, oxygenation, and $EtCO_2$.
6. It is preferable to use device integration with an electronic medical record so time is spent caring for the patient instead of documenting the vital signs.

PRESENT RELEVANCE AND FUTURE AVENUES TO CONSIDER

To date, there is only a single prospective randomized study comparing the outcome of adjustable to nonadjustable strabismus surgery in children, and only a few retrospective comparative studies. An overwhelming number of the studies report success as within 10 PD of orthotropia and mostly analyze the horizontal component of the strabismus surgery. Most studies have excluded paralytic or restrictive strabismus and children undergoing surgery for compensatory head turn associated with nystagmus or Duane syndrome because of difficulty interpreting success in these conditions.

Kamal and colleagues [20] reported the only prospective randomized study comparing adjustable to nonadjustable strabismus surgery in a cohort of 60 subjects younger than 12 years of age. They compared success in the horizontal component of the strabismus only, after a follow-up period of 6 months, with success defined as alignment less than or equal to 8 PD at both distance and near. Adjustment was required in 33% of the subjects. The adjustable suture surgery group was more successful compared with the nonadjustable suture group (86.67% and 73.33%, respectively) but the difference was not statistically significant ($P = .197$). It should be noted that, although the overall adjustable and nonadjustable suture groups were equal in number, the proportions of esotropes and exotropes in the nonadjustable suture group versus nonadjustable suture group were not equal.

Kassem and colleagues [19] also reported the outcomes of the senior author's 19-year experience of using adjustable sutures in 521 children aged 15 years and younger in comparison with a historical group of 116 children who underwent nonadjustable suture strabismus surgery: 63% required adjustment and 85% had their sutures tied off with IV propofol anesthesia in the PACU. Success was defined as horizontal alignment less than or equal to 8 PD at the

3-month to 6-month follow-up visit. The overall success rate was significantly better in the adjustable suture group (77.7% vs 64.6%, $P \leq .03$). Success in esotropes and primary exotropes was found to be significantly greater in the adjustable suture group compared with the nonadjustable suture group. However, this could not be demonstrated in the entire exotropia group, the entire reoperation group, or reoperation subgroup, although the success in each adjustable suture group was always found to be greater than in the respective nonadjustable suture group: 15% of the adjustable suture group required reoperation compared with 21% of the nonadjustable suture group, and there were statistically significant lower cumulative rates of reoperation in the adjustable suture groups than in the nonadjustable suture group.

Dawson and colleagues [29] reported a similar overall success rate of 76% using a sliding noose adjustable suture technique in horizontal and vertical deviations in 45 children aged 10 to 15 years; 58% of the subjects had had previous operations, and subjects with restrictive and paralytic strabismus were included. Adjustments were performed under topical anesthesia and were needed in 67% of subjects. The reoperation rate was 11%.

Leffler and colleagues [30] reviewed a national insurance database for strabismus procedures performed in children 18 years old or younger between 2007 to 2013, comparing the reoperation rate between adjustable sutures and nonadjustable sutures. They identified 10,806 nonadjustable suture procedures compared with only 260 adjustable suture procedures. Reoperation rate was found to be higher in adjustable suture cases (9.6% vs 7.4%) but the difference was not statistically significant. The study is limited by the lack of preoperative and postoperative angles in both groups and by the possibility of incomplete claim data.

Chan and colleagues [2] reported the outcomes of adjustable suture surgery on horizontal deviations using awake adjustments on children aged 7 to 15 years using the bowtie technique. Adjustment was performed on the next day and was needed in 27% of the subjects: 60% had previous operations, and subjects with paralytic and restrictive strabismus were included. Success was defined as alignment within 10 PD of orthotropia at the final follow-up visit, with a mean follow-up of 13.3 months. The overall success rate was 74%. Fifteen percent of the subjects needed reoperations.

Surgeons using techniques allowing no further manipulation when no adjustment was needed reported lower adjustment rates, ranging from 14.6% to 54%. Success rates with such techniques continued to be comparable to traditional techniques, ranging from 72.6% to 88%. Reoperation rates ranged from 10% to 19% [3,12,23].

The overall results of the above-mentioned studies suggest a benefit of adjustable sutures compared with nonadjustable suture strabismus surgery in children. More importantly, these studies demonstrate an acceptable safety profile of the sedated adjustment protocol in PACU using propofol [5,18,19,21]. To be able to demonstrate a clear additional benefit of adjustable sutures, an ideal study should randomize all consenting participants, have at least 6 months of follow-up data, and include reoperation rates as an outcome measure [31].

SUMMARY

Despite the increase in OR and PACU time and subsequent higher initial cost associated with the use of adjustable sutures in the pediatric age range, these certainly have their place in the strabismus surgeon's armamentarium, whether used routinely in all children or in particularly challenging cases in which results cannot be predicted based on standard surgical tables alone.

Critics of adjustable sutures cite several reasons for not adopting the technique. There is a widespread conception that a child will not cooperate for assessment of alignment postoperatively. Although the authors agree that some children, especially at a younger age, can become difficult to assess in the immediate postoperative period, complete inability to assess a child was encountered only rarely, as was the case in other studies reviewed in this article.

Another concern is the safety of the adjustment procedure. No serious adverse events occurred associated with the use of propofol in sedated suture adjustments in the authors' experiences or in other studies describing the use of propofol in sedated suture adjustments [3,5,18,19,21]. Moreover, no reported deaths occurred in 49,836 IV propofol anesthesia encounters for procedures performed outside the OR [32].

Another criticism of adjustable sutures is the additional time required in both the OR and the PACU, and the added costs associated with additional OR time, PACU stay, and a second anesthetic procedure. Placement of adjustable sutures was reported to require an additional 3 to 5 minutes per muscle and 15 to 20 minutes for the adjustment process. Phanphruk and colleagues [21] reported that sedated adjustment prolonged the PACU stay by an additional 22 minutes if no adjustment was needed and an additional 50 minutes beyond that when an adjustment was performed. This highlights the need for a cost-benefit study to evaluate whether reduction in reoperation rate using adjustable suture surgery offsets the additional cost of additional OR and PACU time associated with the use of adjustable sutures.

Opponents of adjustable sutures in children also cite the lack of strong evidence supporting their use. Although a single prospective randomized study and several retrospective studies have shown improved outcomes with adjustable sutures, higher quality randomized controlled studies are needed to provide stronger evidence on the utility of this technique [18–20].

Another common perception is that adjustment could potentially disturb a good initial result. Mireskandari and colleagues [33] reported that subjects with alignment within the target range in the immediate postoperative period had statistically significant better outcomes regardless of whether adjustable sutures were used.

Strabismus surgeons are encouraged to familiarize themselves with adjustable suture techniques, particularly those that provide optional adjustment and thus avoid a second anesthetic when adjustment is not needed.

References

[1] Sun LS, Li G, Miller TL, et al. Association between a single general anesthesia exposure before age 36 months and neurocognitive outcomes in later childhood. JAMA 2016;315(21):2312–20.
[2] Chan TK, Rosenbaum AL, Hall L. The results of adjustable suture technique in paediatric strabismus surgery. Eye (Lond) 1999;13(Pt 4):567–70.
[3] Tsai CB. Adjustable suture strabismus surgery in pediatric patients using pull-string technique. Taiwan J Ophthalmol 2017;7:38–43.
[4] Jampolsky A. Current techniques of adjustable strabismus surgery. Am J Ophthalmol 1979;88(3 Pt 1):406–18.
[5] Nihalani BR, Whitman MC, Salgado CM, et al. Short tag noose technique for optional and late suture adjustment in strabismus surgery. Arch Ophthalmol 2009;127(12):1584–90.
[6] Guyton DL. A small-incision muscle hook for the Parks cul-de- sac approach for strabismus surgery. Binocul Vis Strabismus Q 2005;20(3):147–50.
[7] Deschler EK, Irsch K, Guyton KL, et al. A new, removable, sliding noose for adjustable-suture strabismus surgery. J AAPOS 2013;17(5):524–7.
[8] Parsa CF, Soltan-Sanjari M, Guyton DL. Non-absorbable suture should be used for adjustable inferior rectus muscle recessions. In: de Faber J, editor. Transactions 29th meeting European Strabismological Association, Izmir, Turkey. London: Taylor and Francis; 2005. p. 81–4.
[9] Awadein A, Marsh JD, Guyton DL. Nonabsorbable versus absorbable sutures in large, hang-back medial rectus muscle recessions. J AAPOS 2016;20(3):206–9.
[10] Spielmann A, Spielmann AC. Association of fixed suspensions of the capsulo-palpebral head of the inferior rectus with semi-adjustable recession of the inferior rectus muscle to minimize complications. In: Kaufmann H, editor. Transactions 21st meeting European Strabismological Association. Salzburg (Austria): Gahmig Druck; 1993. p. 175–80.
[11] Budning AS, Day C, Nguyen A. The short adjustable suture. Can J Ophthalmol 2010;45(4): 359–62.
[12] Engel JM, Rousta ST. Adjustable sutures in children using a modified technique. J AAPOS 2004;8(3):243–8.
[13] Tsai CB. Pull-string technique for recovering subconjunctival short-tag noose adjustable sutures. J AAPOS 2014;18(6):606–8.
[14] Engel JM. Adjustable sutures: an update. Curr Opin Ophthalmol 2012;23(5):373–6.
[15] Engel JM, Guyton DL, Hunter DG. Adjustable sutures in children. J AAPOS 2014;18(3): 278–84.
[16] Coats DK. Ripcord adjustable suture technique for use in strabismus surgery. Arch Ophthalmol 2001;119(9):1364–7.
[17] Hakim OM, El-Hag YG, Haikal MA. Releasable adjustable suture technique for children. J AAPOS 2005;9(4):386–90.
[18] Awadein A, Sharma M, Bazemore MG, et al. Adjustable suture strabismus surgery in infants and children. J AAPOS 2008;12(6):585–90.
[19] Kassem A, Xue G, Gandhi NB, et al. Adjustable suture strabismus surgery in infants and children: a 19-year experience. J AAPOS 2018;22(3):174–8.e1.
[20] Kamal AM, Abozeid D, Seif Y, et al. A comparative study of adjustable and non-adjustable sutures in primary horizontal muscle surgery in children. Eye (Lond) 2016;30(11): 1447–51.
[21] Phanphruk W, Alkharashi M, Bilge A, et al. Sedated suture adjustment in children undergoing adjustable suture strabismus surgery. J AAPOS 2017;21(3):196–200.
[22] Haynes GR, Bailey MK. Postoperative nausea and vomiting: review and clinical approaches. South Med J 1996;89(10):940–9.
[23] Nihalani BR, Hunter DG. Adjustable suture strabismus surgery. Eye (Lond) 2011;25(10): 1262–76.

[24] Padda GS, Cruz OA, Krock JL. Comparison of postoperative emesis, recovery profile, and analgesia in pediatric strabismus repair. Rectal acetaminophen versus intravenous fentanyl-droperidol. Ophthalmology 1997;104(3):419–24.
[25] Mendel HG, Guarnieri KM, Sundt LM, et al. The effects of ketorolac and fentanyl on post-operative vomiting and analgesic requirements in children undergoing strabismus surgery. Anesth Analg 1995;80(6):1129–33.
[26] Larsson S, Asgeirsson B, Magnusson J. Propofol-fentanyl anesthesia compared to thiopental-halothane with special reference to recovery and vomiting after pediatric strabismus surgery. Acta Anaesthesiol Scand 1992;36(2):182–6.
[27] Watcha MF, Simeon RM, White PF, et al. Effect of propofol on the incidence of postoperative vomiting after strabismus surgery in pediatric outpatients. Anesthesiology 1991;75(2):204–9.
[28] Wan MJ, Mantagos IS, Shah AS, et al. Comparison of botulinum toxin with surgery for the treatment of acute-onset comitant esotropia in children. Am J Ophthalmol 2017;176:33–9.
[29] Dawson E, Bentley C, Lee J. Adjustable squint surgery in children. Strabismus 2001;9(4):221–4.
[30] Leffler CT, Vaziri K, Schwartz SG, et al. Rates of reoperation and abnormal binocularity following strabismus surgery in children. Am J Ophthalmol 2016;162:159–66.e9.
[31] Hassan S, Haridas A, Sundaram V. Adjustable versus non-adjustable sutures for strabismus. Cochrane Database Syst Rev 2018;(3):CD004240.
[32] Cravero JP, Beach ML, Blike GT, et al. The incidence and nature of adverse events during pediatric sedation/anesthesia with propofol for procedures outside the operating room: a report from the Pediatric Sedation Research Consortium. Anesth Analg 2009;108(3):795–804.
[33] Mireskandari K, Schofield J, Cotesta M, et al. Achieving postoperative target range increases success of strabismus surgery in adults: a case for adjustable sutures? Br J Ophthalmol 2015;99(12):1697–701.

Section III: Ophthalmic Pathology & Ocular Oncology

Advances in Ophthalmology and Optometry 4 (2019) 101–128

ADVANCES IN OPHTHALMOLOGY AND OPTOMETRY

Biopsy Techniques in Ocular Oncology

Ashley Polski, BS[a], Sarina Amin, MD[a], Sagar Patel, MD[a], Jesse L. Berry, MD[a,b,*]

[a]Department of Ophthalmology, USC Roski Eye Institute, Keck School of Medicine of USC, 1450 San Pablo Street, Los Angeles, CA 90033, USA; [b]The Vision Center, Children's Hospital Los Angeles, 4650 Sunset Boulevard, Los Angeles, CA 90027, USA

Keywords

• Aspiration • Conjunctiva • Eyelid • Excisional biopsy • Incisional biopsy • Iris • Posterior segment • Tumor

Key points

- Ocular and periocular tumors comprise a diverse group of benign and malignant lesions in a variety of locations, including but not limited to the eyelid, conjunctiva/cornea, iris, ciliary body, and/or posterior segment.
- Appropriate surgical biopsy techniques facilitate the ability of surgeons to obtain samples of tumor tissue that can be examined histopathologically, which is considered the gold standard for diagnosis.
- The benefits and risks of biopsy techniques should be continually weighed and reevaluated as new, less invasive technologies in ocular oncology are developed.

INTRODUCTION

Ocular and periocular tumors comprise a wide and varied group of both benign and malignant lesions, located anywhere from the external lids to the retina and all ocular structures in between. Although new diagnostic and imaging techniques are continually developed that allow more detailed and less

Disclosure: The authors declare no conflicts of interest and have no financial interests to disclose. Dr J.L. Berry holds grants unrelated to the topic of this article from National Cancer Institute of the National Institute of Health Award Number K08CA232344, The Wright Foundation, The Knights Templar Eye Foundation, and the American Cancer Society #IRG-16-181-57.

*Corresponding author. Department of Ophthalmology, USC Roski Eye Institute, Keck School of Medicine of USC, University of Southern California, 1450 San Pablo Street, Los Angeles, CA 90033, USA. *E-mail address:* Jesse.Berry@med.usc.edu

https://doi.org/10.1016/j.yaoo.2019.04.006
2452-1760/19/

invasive characterizations of ocular lesions in ocular oncology, tumor biopsy, in which tissue is directly obtained for histopathologic analysis, remains the gold standard of diagnosis and management for many ocular lesions. This article discusses tumors of the eyelid, conjunctiva, iris, ciliary body, and posterior segment, and highlights the biopsy techniques that are most commonly used in their management.

EYELID LESIONS

Eyelid tumors represent 5% to 10% of all skin cancers and comprise a wide variety of both benign and malignant periocular conditions [1]. As with other skin tumors, periocular lesions are commonly, although not always, associated with exposure to ultraviolet radiation. Previous studies have shown only approximately 85% to 95% diagnostic accuracy in clinically distinguishing between benign versus malignant tumors; therefore, a surgical biopsy is critical for diagnosis [2].

Basal cell and squamous cell carcinoma

The most common malignant eyelid lesion is basal cell carcinoma (BCC; Fig. 1), comprising approximately 85% to 95% of all eyelid malignancies, followed by squamous cell carcinoma (SCC; 3.4%–12.6%) [3]. For BCC and SCC, the approach to biopsy for both diagnostic and therapeutic purposes is similar. Although both cancers generally can be successfully managed when treated early, SCC, compared with BCC, has the added risk of developing perineural spread and regional metastasis to lymph nodes, which can greatly increase the associated morbidity and mortality [4]. Thus, early identification

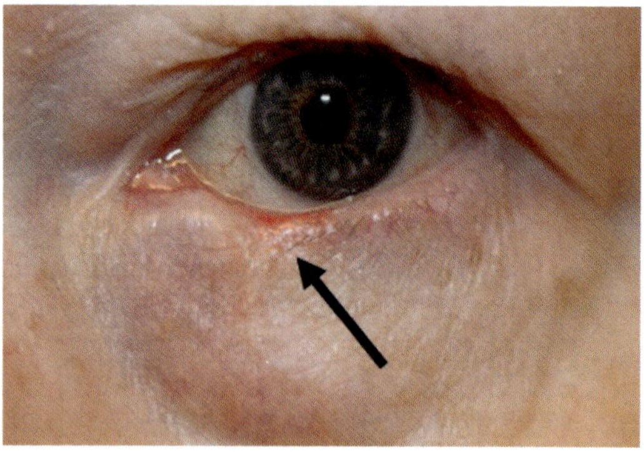

Fig. 1. Pearly cutaneous lesion with slightly rolled edges (*arrow*), later determined to be basal cell carcinoma via incisional biopsy, on the left lower eyelid, with accompanying madarosis and changes in lid architecture (ectropion). Incisional biopsy for diagnosis followed by full-thickness wedge resection or Mohs with subsequent reconstruction is indicated. (*Courtesy of* Jesse L. Berry, MD, USC Roski Eye Institute, University of Southern California, Los Angeles, CA.)

of such lesions via biopsy is an essential step in optimizing survival of these patients.

Incisional biopsy

Although some small, circumscribed lesions feasibly may be managed with excisional biopsy from the outset, less extensive biopsy techniques often are used first in order to guide planning for subsequent tumor removal and treatment. Incisional biopsy, which involves the surgical removal of a small portion of the tumor, is a simple and expedient method for diagnosing lid lesions. Of note, periocular lesions such as BCC and SCC often develop areas of central keratinization. Thus, incisional biopsies should be obtained from marginal areas of the tumor, with care taken to avoid both keratinization and any visible junction between tumor and noninvolved skin (so as to not disrupt the margin of the lesion). In general, incisional biopsy poses little risk to the patient and provides approximately 95% diagnostic accuracy [5].

Pentagonal wedge resection

Once the diagnosis of either BCC or SCC is made, complete tumor excision is the goal of treatment. Small BCCs or SCCs of either the upper or lower lid effectively can be managed with full-thickness pentagonal wedge resection. In this method, a surgical blade is used to make incisions in a symmetric pentagonal shape surrounding the lesion, with parallel vertical medial and lateral incisions made on either side of the tumor [6]. Incising in this manner, rather than in a triangular or V shape, helps to bolster structural integrity of the reconstructed lid and to minimize tension on the lid margin once closed [6,7]. Full-thickness incision is preferred because the lid is thin and malignant eyelid tumors may invade to the tarsus. Concurrent frozen-section control is often used so that margins may be microscopically examined for any residual tumor tissue. In most cases, sutures may then be used to achieve direct closure of the defect, although a description of Tenzel flap formation and other reconstructive procedures are outside the scope of this article.

Mohs excisional biopsy

For more extensive BCC and SCC of the eyelid, Mohs excision is considered the gold standard of effective and reliable management [4], especially in cases that show high-risk features such as recurrent disease or medial canthal location [8]. The purpose of Mohs surgery is to completely excise the lesion while maintaining control of both peripheral and deep resection margins, allowing mapping, identification, and removal of any microscopic tumor invasion while avoiding excision of excessive amounts of normal, noninvolved tissue. Typically, the visible margins of the tumor are outlined with ink before the procedure. Under local anesthesia, the tumor is excised with an approximately 3-mm (or less, depending on exact tumor location) margin of grossly normal tissue. Incisions are made with the knife beveled at a 45° angle to the surface of the skin, allowing a thin and flat tissue specimen. Once removed, the specimen is oriented appropriately to the defect using the ink markings, sectioned, and evaluated for any residual marginal tumor involvement. Any areas suspicious for tumor presence are noted and relayed to the surgeon in preparation for the next Mohs cycle. Overall, a complete cycle of excision, processing, and microscopic examination takes approximately 45 minutes [9].

Despite its reliability, Mohs surgery does present certain disadvantages. For example, increased wait time occurs in the operating room while intraoperative frozen sections are being completed, as well as potentially multiple rounds of Mohs surgery per case, all of which lead to increased cost for the procedure. In addition, the process may require the involvement of 2 physicians for the resection of the tumor and subsequent lid reconstruction postexcision, which can further add to procedure expense [4]. A cheaper alternative to frozen-section Mohs surgery is the use of formalin-fixed paraffin-embedded sections, or permanent-section evaluation, although this cost-effective approach may delay time to reconstruction [10]. Overall, the disadvantages of Mohs for eyelid BCC and SCC are generally outweighed by the unique ability of this tissue-sparing technique to achieve complete tumor excision while preserving the largest amount of uninvolved lid possible.

Melanoma

Melanoma of the eyelid accounts for less than 1% of all eyelid malignancies; although significantly rarer than either BCC or SCC, it has a much higher associated risk of metastasis and mortality. Precursor lesions that may transform to malignant melanoma include congenital nevi, dysplastic nevi, and lentigo maligna, all of which should be monitored closely by physicians over time [11]. Risk of metastasis and overall tumor prognosis is largely determined by the depth of microscopic tumor invasion (known as Breslow thickness), and thus surgical biopsy with histopathologic analysis is the gold standard for guiding both diagnosis and treatment.

Although partial incisional biopsy techniques entail the clear disadvantage of possibly underestimating the depth or breadth of tumor invasion, the specific biopsy type does not seem to significantly influence recurrence, metastasis, or overall outcome of the disease [12]. However, unlike for SCC and BCC, excisional biopsy is strongly preferred to incisional biopsy for diagnosing suspected melanoma because it is the most definitive method for elucidating the extent of tumor invasion, accurately staging the tumor, and providing potentially curative treatment [13].

Excisional biopsy

The central goal of excisional biopsy for suspected melanoma is the achievement of tumor-free margins, because surgical margin involvement leads to an increased risk of tumor recurrence and/or spread. Thus, excisional biopsy of melanomatous lesions is typically associated with wide surgical margins, significantly more so than with BCC or SCC [3,4]. Although dermatologic guidelines for melanoma removal generally recommend margins of at least 1 cm, such breadth can be difficult, even unachievable, for eyelid lesions. No formal consensus yet exists on exact margin requirements for periocular melanoma, but margins of at least 5 mm generally are considered acceptable for both managing disease and minimizing disfigurement, especially in cases of thin (<2-mm depth of invasion) melanoma [3,4]. If lesions present with higher-risk characteristics, such as greater than 2-mm thickness, ulceration, or mitotic figures, then 1-cm margins may be attempted as much as possible, accompanied with sentinel lymph node evaluation for potential metastatic disease [4,14].

In order to achieve margin control with excisional biopsy, Pavri and colleagues [13] suggest a permanent-section approach, because frozen sections, such as those used in Mohs surgery, have been shown to be inaccurate in distinguishing between normal versus malignant melanocytes. Although disease resolution following initial excisional biopsy is desirable, up to 30% of eyelid melanomas may require more than 1 excision in order to achieve adequate margin control [15]. Given the potential for severely metastatic and even fatal disease associated with melanoma, patients should be followed closely after wide surgical excision to monitor for any residual or recurrent tumor.

Sebaceous gland carcinoma

Sebaceous gland carcinoma represents approximately 0.6% to 10.2% of malignant eyelid tumors and most commonly presents in elderly women on the upper lid, where a high density of meibomian glands occur. Misdiagnosis frequently occurs, with sebaceous cell carcinoma often being mistaken for more common lesions such as BCC, SCC, or recurrent chalazion; loss of eyelashes in the region of the tumor is a diagnostic clue [3]. Given the risk of aggressive local extension and metastasis posed by sebaceous gland carcinomas, a diagnostic biopsy to confirm the identity of a suspected sebaceous cell lesion is paramount for guiding further surgical and management decisions.

Wedge and map biopsy

Before definitive management, the initial technique is full-thickness wedge biopsy, in which a wedge of the full thickness of the eyelid, including the anterior and posterior lamellae and the tumor tissue, is incised. This technique is the preferred method of diagnosis for sebaceous cell tumors of the eyelid, because more superficial biopsy methods may miss areas of local tumor invasion [4]. Sebaceous gland carcinomas also have the distinctive ability to develop pagetoid (intraepithelial) spread into not only large regions of periocular tissue but also into the contiguous epithelium of the palpebral and bulbar conjunctiva. In such cases of diffuse pagetoid spread, map biopsies are the most reliable and thorough method of histopathologic investigation and help to define the extent of disease. With this approach, 10 to 14 small, separate biopsies are taken from both the eyelid and conjunctiva (depending on the level of suspicion for conjunctival involvement), and each biopsied specimen is carefully labeled by biopsy site. The specimens are then submitted for permanent section to evaluate for sebaceous tumor involvement [16].

Excisional biopsy

Once histopathologic diagnosis of sebaceous gland carcinoma is established, definitive surgical management should be undertaken. The gold standard of treatment of malignant sebaceous lesions is complete, full-thickness excision with wide surgical margins and frozen-section control (Fig. 2). When feasible, surgical margins of at least 5 mm should be attempted for sebaceous gland carcinoma in order to minimize the risk of disease recurrence [3]. For conjunctival involvement, excision followed by topical chemotherapy, such as mitomycin C, may be indicated, but a surgical cure is always the goal [4,17]. Even following appropriate surgical therapy, up to 18% of cases show regional lymph node metastasis and up to 8% metastasize to more distant sites [17]. Thus, physicians

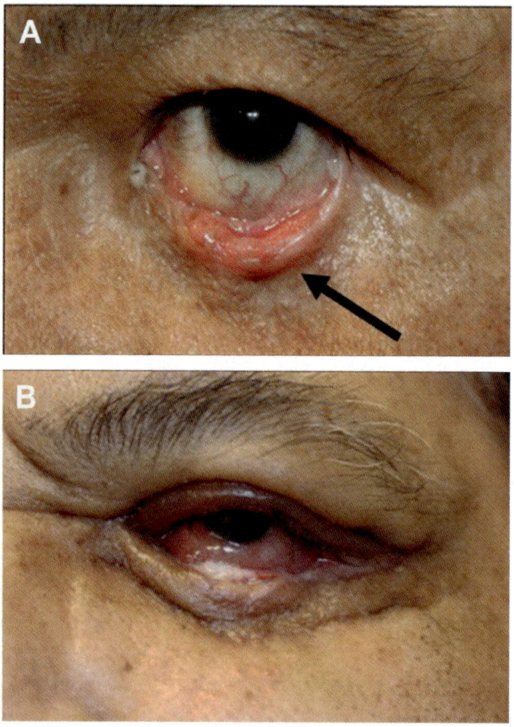

Fig. 2. (*A*) Multiple left lower eyelid nodules (*arrow*) clinically consistent with recurrent malignant disease in a patient with a history of sebaceous cell carcinoma that was previously treated with anterior orbitotomy, lower lid excision, and reconstruction with mucosal graft. (*B*) The same eye 1 month after full-thickness wedge excision and reconstruction of left lower eyelid for recurrent sebaceous cell carcinoma, with mild sloughing of mucosal graft but otherwise healing well. (*Courtesy of* Jesse L. Berry, MD, and Jessica Chang, MD, USC Roski Eye Institute, University of Southern California, Los Angeles, CA.)

should not hesitate to evaluate for potential lymph node involvement in cases of large, diffuse sebaceous gland carcinoma.

Merkel cell carcinoma

Merkel cell carcinoma (MCC) is a rare but potentially dangerous malignancy that can present in the elderly as a rapidly growing, violet-colored eyelid lesion with occasional telangiectasia and ulceration. Comprising less than 1% of all eyelid tumors, MCC has an aggressive growth that frequently spreads to preauricular and submandibular lymph nodes. However, despite its aggressive tendencies, many MCC lesions are either misdiagnosed or missed altogether given their resemblance to chalazia, keratoacanthomata, or BCCs [3]. Therefore, patients suspected to have possible MCC benefit from surgical biopsies in order to minimize delay in diagnosis and tumor spread.

Incisional biopsy

As with other aggressive tumor types, such as sebaceous cell carcinoma, the confirmatory diagnosis of MCC requires a full-thickness incisional biopsy (or excisional biopsy in cases of smaller, more confined nodules). Cytokeratin 20, as well as neuroendocrine markers such as chromogranin A, neuron-specific enolase, and synaptophysin, are specific markers of MCC that can be used on diagnostic biopsy samples [3].

Excisional biopsy

Following confirmatory biopsy and histopathologic diagnosis of MCC, the gold standard of management is wide local tumor excision with either frozen-section or permanent-section evaluation [4], although Mohs micrographic surgery also has been found to be an effective method of margin control for MCC [18]. Although 2.5-cm to 3-cm margins are generally preferred for cases of cutaneous MCC, 5-mm margins are allowable for achieving adequate local control [3,18]. Because nearly two-thirds of patients show regional lymph node metastases and one-third develop distant metastases within 1.5 years of initial diagnosis [3], all cases of MCC should be referred for sentinel lymph node biopsy in addition to their periocular management, regardless of tumor size [19].

In general, lesions of the eyelid require incisional biopsy for appropriate histopathologic confirmation followed by complete surgical excision with margin control, whenever possible.

CONJUNCTIVAL LESIONS

Conjunctival tumors include a range of benign, premalignant, and malignant lesions involving the bulbar and/or tarsal conjunctiva. Similar to lid lesions, conjunctival malignancies, such as ocular surface squamous neoplasia (OSSN) and melanoma, are often related to excessive solar radiation, with additional risk factors including immune deficiency (such as human immunodeficiency virus positivity), autoimmune conditions, xeroderma pigmentosum, and exposure to cigarette smoke [20]. Although innovations in imaging and topical chemotherapy have ushered in the possibility of both diagnosing and treating OSSN completely noninvasively [21–24], surgical biopsy remains a standard approach for managing tumors on the ocular surface.

Ocular surface squamous neoplasia

OSSN, comprising approximately 14% of conjunctival malignancies, includes a spectrum of squamous cell tumors, from dysplasia and carcinoma in situ to invasive SCC [20]. Such tumors are rare, with an incidence ranging from only 0.02 to 3.5 per 100,000, depending on geographic location. Nonetheless, OSSN remains the most prevalent conjunctival malignancy in adults and can lead to serious sequelae if untreated, including local invasion into intraocular or orbital spaces, involvement of regional lymph nodes in the head and neck, and even death [25]. Although more physicians are moving toward noninvasive management of OSSN lesions with topical chemotherapy [26], surgical excision with cryotherapy and possibly adjuvant topical chemotherapy is considered the current gold standard for both the diagnosis and treatment of OSSN.

Incisional biopsy

Incisional biopsy should be avoided whenever possible in cases of OSSN and conjunctival melanoma (further discussed later). However, although complete excision is ideal when approaching premalignant or malignant conjunctival lesions with surgical management, tumors with extensive ocular surface and/or lid involvement may not be fully resectable. In such cases, definitive histopathologic identification may be obtained with an incisional biopsy. For this technique, a full-thickness portion of the tumor is incised and then formalin fixed to allow for sectioning, staining, and microscopic analysis [27]. Although incisional biopsy may be limited in its ability to characterize the degree of tumor invasiveness, it may be helpful for characterizing otherwise unexcisable lesions in order to guide further management decisions.

No-touch excisional biopsy

For less extensive OSSN lesions, primary surgical management consists of excisional biopsy using the no-touch technique (Fig. 3). Described by Shields and colleagues [28] in 1997, the no-touch technique involves a conjunctival incision that typically respects a 3-mm to 4-mm margin of normal tissue around the epithelial lesion and has a primary goal of minimizing contact between surgical instruments and tumor cells in order not to cause tumor spread [25]. Direct manipulation of the tumor is avoided by using forceps to elevate the conjunctiva approximately 4 mm from the tumor edge, and scissors are then used to create a snip incision at this site. In the same manner, another incision in the conjunctiva is then made from the opposite side of the tumor. With these 2 incisions in place, scissors are used to complete the incision around the tumor, with care taken to handle only healthy, noninvolved tissue and never to directly manipulate the tumor.

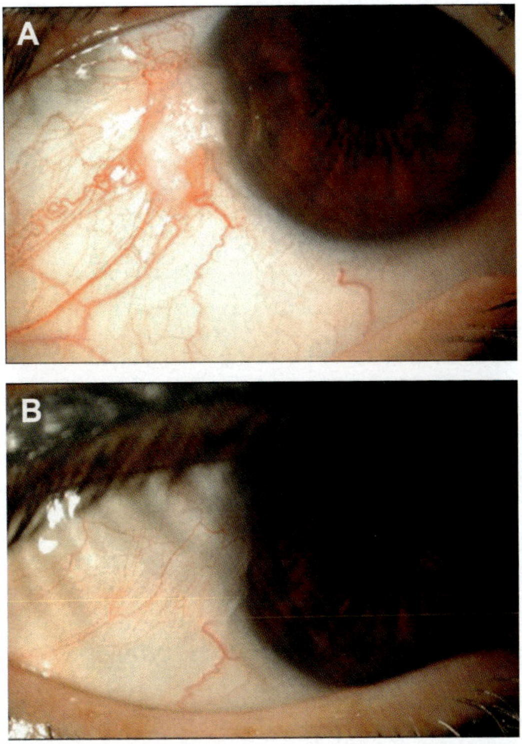

Fig. 3. (*A*) Temporal gelatinous mass at the corneal limbus with prominent sentinel-type vessels, concerning for OSSN. (*B*) The same eye 7 months after excisional biopsy (via the no-touch technique) and cryotherapy. Microscopic analysis confirmed the diagnosis of OSSN. There is mild pannus migration onto the corneal limbus in the location of the biopsy, without gross irregularity or signs of recurrence of OSSN. (*Courtesy of* Jesse L. Berry, MD, USC Roski Eye Institute, University of Southern California, Los Angeles, CA.)

If the sclera is involved clinically (eg, the tumor is not mobile and cannot be easily dissected from the sclera), a lamellar scleral flap is resected at the tumor base (2 mm posterior to the tumor margin) along with the lesion itself, while still avoiding direct contact between the surgical instruments and tumor. If scleral involvement extends to or abuts the cornea, dissection of the scleral flap should be done so as to avoid disruption of the Bowman membrane, which could lead to intraocular spread of the malignancy [28].

Once the conjunctival portion of the tumor is excised, double freeze-thaw cryotherapy is used at the surgical margins of the conjunctiva to reduce post-surgical tumor recurrence by eliminating any residual malignant cells. To perform cryotherapy, the exposed bulbar conjunctival margins are lifted gently with previously unused forceps, and a nitrous oxide cryoprobe tip is placed on the undersurface of the conjunctival edge (Fig. 4). The margin is frozen, allowed to thaw completely, and then refrozen at the same location [28]. Each

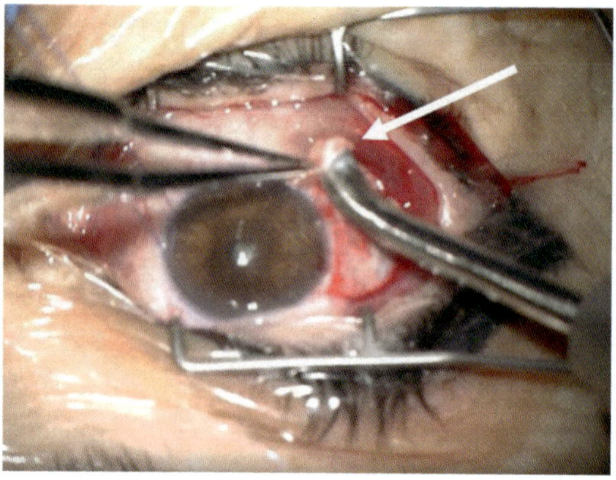

Fig. 4. Double freeze-thaw cryotherapy following no-touch excision of a conjunctival lesion. During this process, the bulbar conjunctival margin is lifted with forceps, and a nitrous oxide cryoprobe tip is placed under the conjunctival edge (*arrow*) to achieve freezing of tissue. This process (including 2 complete freeze/thaw cycles) is repeated along all exposed conjunctival margins in order to achieve adequate margin control. (*Courtesy of* Jesse L. Berry, MD, USC Roski Eye Institute, University of Southern California, Los Angeles, CA.)

nitrous oxide application lasts approximately 10 to 15 seconds or until an appropriate ice ball covers the conjunctival edge, and this double freeze-thaw technique is performed every 3 mm along the perimeter of the conjunctival margin. Cryotherapy for the sclera is generally avoided because it may lead to significant and devastating scleromalacia; however, some surgeons choose to apply it to the bare sclera following partial scleral flap removal if scleral involvement is suspected [29]. Other options for treating the sclera include absolute alcohol, which often is done even if overt tumor invasion is not seen, or subsequent plaque brachytherapy once scleral invasion has been confirmed [28]. Brachytherapy is the method of choice for the senior author of this article.

Because many OSSN lesions grow in a limbal location, abutting and even extending onto the corneal epithelium [30], definitive surgical treatment must include removal of the involved corneal epithelium. To accomplish this, a saturated cotton-tipped applicator is used to gently apply absolute alcohol onto the corneal surface approximately 2 mm from the visible tumor margin (Fig. 5A). The uninvolved corneal epithelium should be protected with viscoelastic. A surgical blade is then used to gently debride (bluntly) the affected epithelium taking great care to not penetrate the Bowman layer. Ideally the corneal epithelium is removed en bloc with the conjunctival tumor; however, it also can be placed on a cellulose sponge and submitted for microscopic analysis (Fig. 5B) [28].

Although Shields and colleagues [28] describe conjunctival wound closure with running or interrupted 6-0 or 7-0 absorbable sutures, certain surgical defects may be too large to close primarily. As an alternative, amniotic membrane placement may be used on the affected portion of the ocular surface in order to

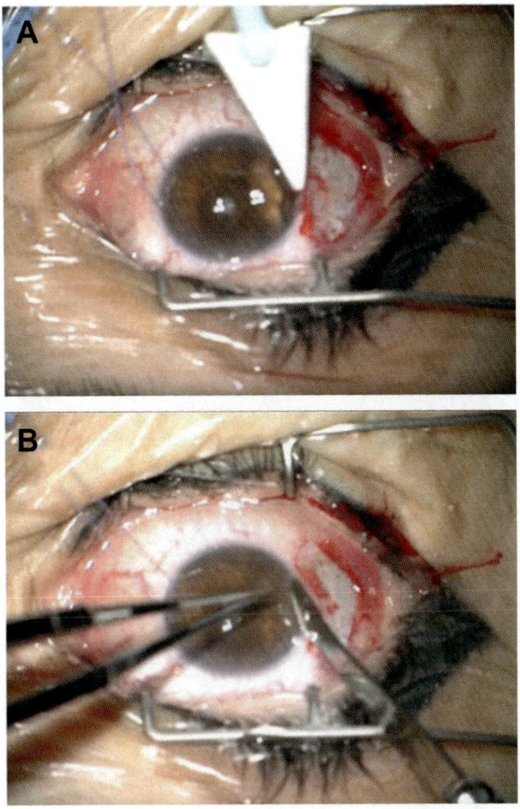

Fig. 5. (*A*) Saturated Weck-Cel sponge applicator applying absolute alcohol to the clinically involved corneal epithelium adjacent to the limbal tumor margin. The uninvolved corneal epithelium is protected with a viscoelastic agent. (*B*) Debridement of the affected corneal epithelium with a surgical scleral 57 blade following absolute alcohol application to the corneal surface. (*Courtesy of* Jesse L. Berry, MD, USC Roski Eye Institute, University of Southern California, Los Angeles, CA.)

minimize residual tissue defects and scarring and to facilitate more acceptable conjunctival reconstruction; the membrane can be anchored with interrupted sutures or fibrin glue [31,32].

Benign melanocytic lesions

In most cases, benign melanocytic tumors such as melanosis or conjunctival nevi do not require surgical excision unless concern for malignant conversion exists because of rapid clinical change. Such lesions are usually flat or minimally nodular, uninflamed, and nonvascularized [25]. Of the benign pigmented lesions on the ocular surface, primary acquired melanosis (PAM) is perhaps the most likely to require histopathologic investigation in order to rule out atypia [33]. Approximately 10% to 74% of conjunctival melanomas arise from PAM lesions with atypia [34], and up to 12% of clinically diagnosed PAM have been found to progress to melanoma over 10 years [33]. Because of this risk, generally it is recommended that all PAM lesions be surgically biopsied, especially if they are extensive, thickened, darkly colored, palpebral or corneal in location, or showing unusual vascularity [35]. Unilateral, non–limbal-based melanosis is more likely to be PAM than benign racial melanosis, and these lesions should be considered for biopsy [36]. A no-touch biopsy approach as previously described may be used to carefully excise melanocytic lesions and evaluate for the presence of atypical melanocytic cells (Fig. 6) [28]. If atypia is found, thus increasing the risk of progression to melanoma, then complete excision of all pigmented lesions should be done; if this is not possible, the entire ocular surface may be treated with topical mitomycin C [37].

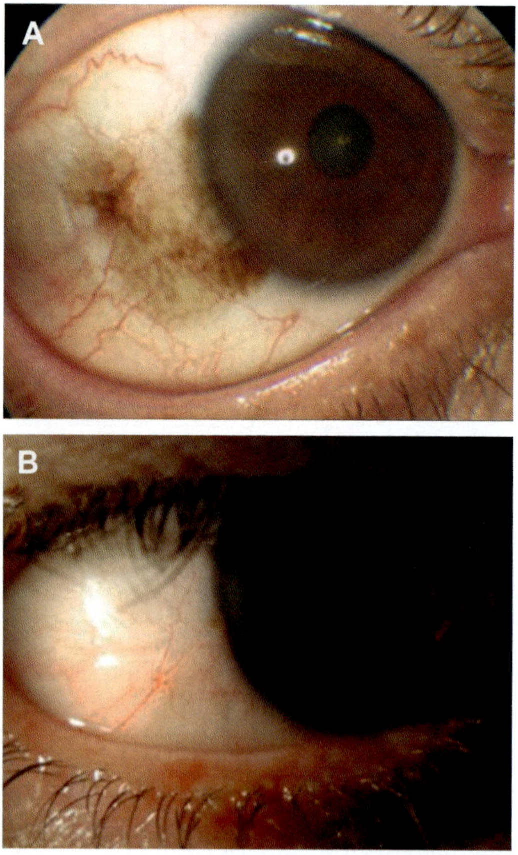

Fig. 6. (*A*) Right temporal conjunctival melanosis in 1 eye only displaying subtle growth concerning for PAM. (*B*) The same eye 11 months postexcision with cryotherapy for most prominent areas of melanosis, healing well with scant melanosis remaining. Histologic analysis of previously excised tissue showed PAM with atypia. No other pigmented lesions were seen and the patient has not recurred but is being followed closely. (*Courtesy of* Jesse L. Berry, MD, USC Roski Eye Institute, University of Southern California, Los Angeles, CA.)

Melanoma

Unlike with benign pigmented tumors, complete surgical excision is considered a therapeutic necessity in cases of malignant conjunctival melanoma, because untreated ocular surface melanoma has a high rate of metastasis and even death. The diagnosis and management of malignant melanocytic conjunctival lesions often is similar to that of OSSN, with nearly identical no-touch surgical excision methods and with increased surgical margins of 5 mm (Fig. 7) [28].

As with OSSN, incisional biopsy usually is not recommended for conjunctival melanoma, because partial tumor resection poses an increased risk for tumor seeding and metastasis [38,39]. En bloc tumor excision is the ideal approach to minimizing risk of metastasis, followed by cryotherapy and, if necessary, amniotic membrane placement. Following excision, adjuvant

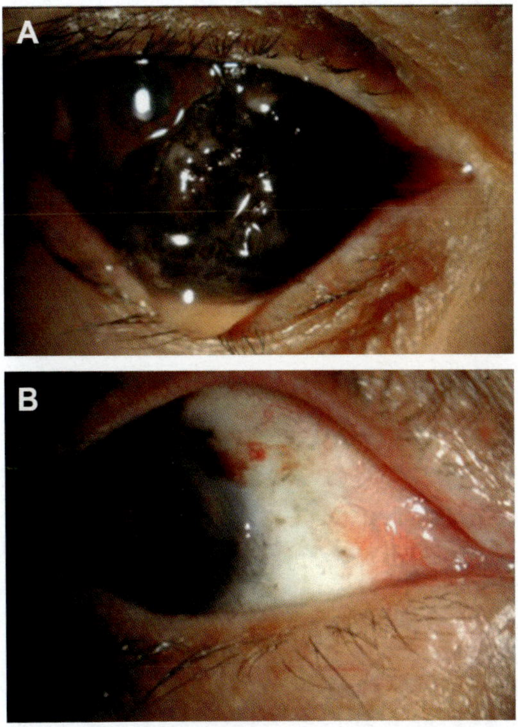

Fig. 7. (*A*) Large melanotic lesion involving the right nasal conjunctiva showing extensive nodularity and extension onto the cornea. Clinical diagnosis is a conjunctival melanoma that requires excisional biopsy via no-touch technique with 5-mm surgical margins. Incisional biopsy should be avoided. All pigmented area should be similarly excised (eg, if in the setting of diffuse primary acquired melanosis and excision is possible). (*B*) The same eye 2 months postexcision and reconstruction with an amniotic membrane. There is residual postoperative gray scleral pigmentation but no recurrent conjunctival melanosis. Histologic analysis showed malignant conjunctival melanoma; the patient remains free of disease. A sentinel lymph node biopsy was deferred. (*Courtesy of* Jonathan Song, MD, USC Roski Eye Institute, University of Southern California, Los Angeles, CA.)

brachytherapy and/or topical chemotherapy with mitomycin C may be used to reduce ocular morbidity and treat any residual melanocytic disease [39]. Some surgeons recommend sentinel lymph node biopsy as well for tumors greater than 2 mm, with ulceration, and/or a high mitotic rate [40].

IRIS LESIONS

Iris tumors include a spectrum of cystic and solid lesions that occur most commonly in middle-aged white adults. The differentiation between cystic and solid tumors is often apparent on slit-lamp examination alone, although ultrasonography biomicroscopy (UBM) or anterior segment optical coherence tomography may be used to confirm this as well as checking for posterior extension (UBM) [41]. Although most iris lesions are benign and require no further work-up or surgical management, intraocular biopsy is a useful approach in cases of diagnostic uncertainty, risk of malignancy or metastasis, or need for further grading and prognostic information.

Cystic iris lesions

Cystic lesions comprise approximately 21% of all iris tumors and may arise from either the iris pigment epithelium or the iris stroma (Fig. 8) [41]. Although iris pigment epithelium cysts are often quiescent and only rarely require surgical analysis or therapy, iris stromal cysts, although benign, have a propensity to enlarge within the anterior chamber, potentially leading to glaucoma with angle occlusion [42].

Fine-needle aspiration and sclerosis

In 2014, Shields and colleagues [42] investigated the use of microscope-guided needle aspiration followed by alcohol-induced sclerosis for iris stromal cysts.

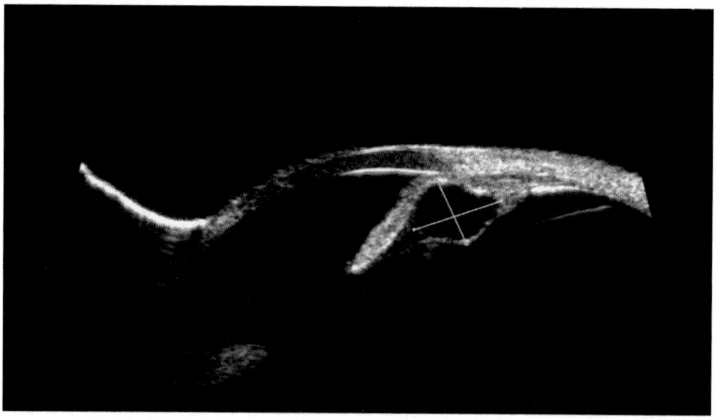

Fig. 8. Ellex ultrasound biomicroscopy image of the right eye, showing 2.65-mm by 1.98-mm iris stromal cyst with involvement of the ciliary body without ciliary body mass of thickening. There is narrowing of the angle in the region. This lesion was considered benign and was followed without clinical growth. (*Courtesy of* Jesse L. Berry, MD, USC Roski Eye Institute, University of Southern California, Los Angeles, CA.)

For this approach, a 30-gauge needle is inserted through the corneal limbus and directly into the cystic structure, avoiding entry of the needle into the aqueous. Microscopic visualization is used to guide aspiration until the cyst walls have nearly completely collapsed. Next, a second syringe is used to infuse the cyst with alcohol for 1 to 2 minutes before reaspirating the alcohol into the first syringe. The cycle is repeated until the cyst wall appears gray, taking great care not to rupture the cyst. At present, this method is considered a safe and effective approach to managing cysts of the iris stroma and preventing cyst recurrence.

Solid iris lesions

At 79%, solid tumors comprise most iris lesions and may be further categorized as either melanocytic or nonmelanocytic. Melanocytic tumors range from benign nevi to malignant melanoma, whereas nonmelanocytic tumors may consist of vascular growths, epithelial lesions, or even metastases originating from elsewhere in the body [41]. Although specific management varies depending on the identity and mortality risk of the tumor, solid iris lesions with uncertain diagnoses or that are suspicious for malignancy may be biopsied using similar techniques regardless of the tumor type.

Fine-needle aspiration biopsy

Fine-needle aspiration biopsy (FNAB) is a modality that uses 25-gauge to 30-gauge needles to obtain tissue samples for histopathologic analysis of iris lesions [43]. Although multiple specific approaches to FNAB exist, common indications for FNAB include tumor qualities such as lesion growth, seeding of the tumor on the iris or within the anterior chamber angle, hyphemas, malignancy, or suspected metastasis from an unknown location [44].

The direct-penetrating internal FNAB was described by Shields and colleagues [44]. A 25-gauge needle is attached to a 10-mL syringe and entered through the corneal limbus either temporally or inferiorly so as to avoid interference from the nose or eyebrow. The needle, bevel up, remains parallel to the surface of the iris and is inserted directly into the lesion. A gentle in-and-out sliding motion of the needle is performed in order to loosen cells within the tumor, and cells are then aspirated for at least 5 seconds with care being taken to not twist or rock the needle. Although aqueous leakage through the limbal entry site occasionally occurs and must be reconstituted with balanced salt solution [43], anterior chamber refilling or wound rehydration is only rarely required [44].

Although FNAB is a generally safe diagnostic procedure, requiring only local retrobulbar or peribulbar anesthesia, the procedure does have risks. Patients may (rarely) develop hyphema or blood clots within the anterior chamber [44], with a minor but present risk of tumor seeding [45]; both physicians and patients should be aware of such risks.

Additional aspiration techniques

Although FNAB is a reliable and less invasive technique of obtaining cells from iris tumors for microscopic investigation, alternative aspiration techniques exist that allow acquisition of larger tissue samples.

For example, the transcorneal fine-cannula aspiration technique produces tissue specimens of up to 1 to 1.5 mm in size that may be fixed and examined. Matthews and colleagues [46] described this method as a novel approach to sampling iris tumors. After application of topical anesthesia, a small incision using a straight 15° ophthalmic knife is made for corneal paracentesis 180° opposite the iris lesion of interest. Viscoelastic is introduced to prevent anterior chamber collapse, then a 25-gauge cannula, attached to a 2-mL syringe, is inserted into the anterior chamber. The bevel of the cannula is swept over the iris lesion, with negative pressure being applied to the syringe, until an adequate tumor sample is obtained. Similar to FNAB, no corneal sutures are required at the conclusion of this procedure.

Alternatively, the aspiration cutter technique combines aspects of FNAB and incisional biopsy to provide both tumor tissue and cells for microscopic examination [47]. To accomplish this, a microvitreoretinal blade is used to generate a 1-mm stab incision at the corneal limbus on the same side as the tumor. Once the anterior chamber is stabilized with sodium hyaluronate 1% or another viscoelastic substance, a 25-gauge vitrectomy probe is inserted through the incision and used to cut and aspirate portions of the iris lesion. Although this technique rarely leads to the development of postoperative hyphema, unlike FNAB, occasionally sutures are required for adequate corneal closure. The larger specimens obtained by this method facilitate accurate and definitive diagnosis of iris tumors.

Incisional biopsy techniques

If more than cytologic samples are desired for the identification of iris lesions, methods of incisional biopsy may be used to obtain tissue for fixing and examination.

The punch biopsy, described originally by Pe'er and colleagues [48], may be performed under local anesthesia using a Descemet membrane punch. Following clear corneal incision near the lesion and filling of the anterior chamber with viscoelastic, the punch is inserted through the incision and onto the iris tumor to obtain an approximately 1-mm diameter tumor sample. The tissue specimen may then be analyzed microscopically and stained for thorough histologic examination. Although not always necessary for the diagnosis of iris tumors, this method is particularly useful in cases for which FNAB was inconclusive.

Unlike the punch biopsy method, the Essen biopsy forceps technique typically requires 2 corneal incisions for successful sampling [49]. Although biopsy forceps grasp the lesion through 1 incision site, intraocular scissors are inserted through the second paracentesis site and dissect the tissue of interest. The tissue may then be enclosed within the forceps cavity and removed for fixation and analysis. Both corneal incisions are self-healing, usually without sutures, and only rarely do these techniques lead to temporary iris bleeding.

Given the friability of the iris and iris lesions, incisional biopsy is rarely done. Most commonly, these tumors are managed by FNAB followed by definitive excisional biopsy if needed (eg, in the setting of an iris melanoma). Some surgeons may proceed directly with excisional biopsy for iris melanoma [50].

Excisional biopsy techniques

Although the need for complete surgical removal of an iris lesion is rare, tumors that are posing a threat to vision by encroaching on either the pupillary margin or the trabecular meshwork, or a primary iris malignancy such as melanoma, may require surgical excisional biopsy.

Surgical iridectomy, performed under local anesthesia, is an ideal approach for managing small, peripheral iris melanomas (Fig. 9) [51]. Hood and colleagues [52] described a minimally invasive technique for excising tumors from the iris. In this method, 2 corneal incisions opposite the tumor site are made using a surgical blade; 1 incision is a 3-mm beveled clear corneal incision, and the second is a paracentesis incision approximately 4 clock-hours away from the first. Viscoelastic is introduced into the anterior chamber before

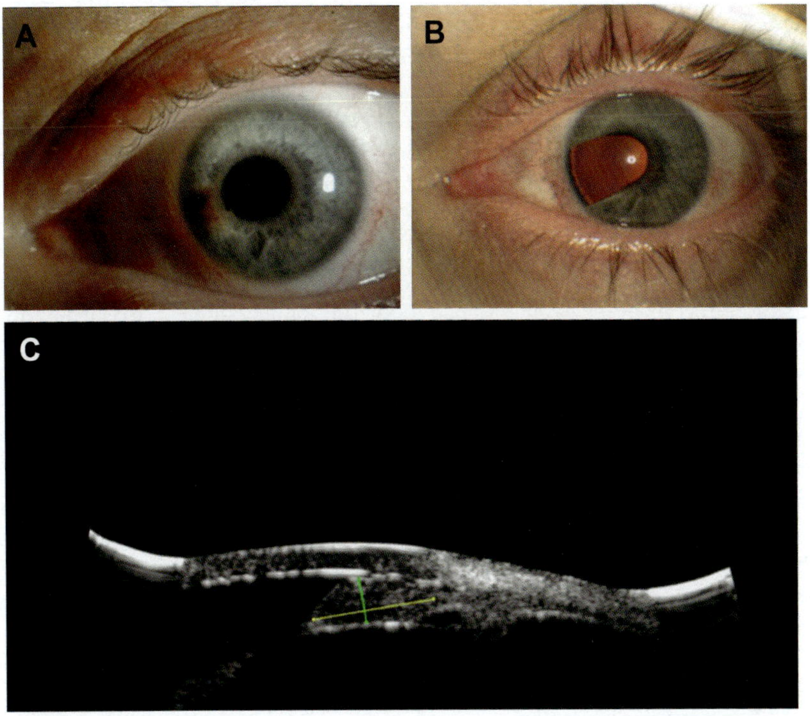

Fig. 9. (*A*) Slit-lamp image of a pigmented left nasal iris lesion that was elevated, amelanotic, and distorting the iris stroma concerning for malignant melanoma of the iris. (*B*) Slit-lamp image of the same eye 6 months after surgical iridectomy for treatment of iris melanoma, showing iris coloboma without evidence of disease recurrence. (*C*) Ellex ultrasound image of left nasal iris melanoma measuring 3.20 by 1.13 mm, before treatment with surgical iridectomy. (*Courtesy of* Jonathan W. Kim, MD, USC Roski Eye Institute, University of Southern California, Los Angeles, CA.)

tumor excision. Vitreous forceps and 25-gauge horizontal vitrectomy scissors are then entered through the corneal incisions and used to make radial cuts on either side of the iris tumor, allowing at least a 1-mm margin of unaffected tissue around the lesion [52,53]. Once the lesion is excised en bloc, the lesion is aspirated into viscoelastic-primed tubing with an attached syringe. After sodium hyaluronate washout, sutures may be used to achieve closure of both the iris and corneal wounds [52]. If iris suturing is not performed, the risk of postsurgical iris coloboma formation is increased, which may lead to both photophobia and unwanted cosmetic defect of the iris [51,52]. Less commonly, cataract development or progression may occur following iridectomy [51,54], although this complication is generally considered minor and manageable overall.

For iris melanoma that involves anterior portions of the ciliary body and angle, iridocyclectomy is the preferred treatment modality [51]. Performed under general anesthesia, this method involves the formation of a scleral flap for visualization of and access to the iris tumor. Conventional iridocyclectomy involves an anteroposterior approach to dissection following preoperative mydriasis with cyclopentolate and phenylephrine drops. Dissection occurs from the pupil margin inward in order to preserve the peripheral zonules [55]. However, Rospond-Kubiak and Damato [55] recommend an alternative posterior-anterior approach (termed cycloiridectomy) that involves preoperative miosis with pilocarpine followed by dissection from the iris root. Although no randomized trials have yet compared these approaches, Rospond-Kubiak and Damato [55] suggest that the novel approach may reduce the risk of large iris coloboma formation and more effectively conserve iris sphincter function.

Although considered largely effective for the management of iris melanoma with ciliary involvement, iridocyclectomy generally preserves superficial scleral layers, which may increase the risk of local tumor recurrence in cases that involve melanomatous invasion of the sclera. To reduce this risk, Naumann and Rummelt [56] suggest a block excision approach for removal of iris and ciliary body melanoma. Also known as full-thickness eyewall resection, this technique involves the complete, en bloc removal of adjacent iris, corneal and scleral layers in contact with the iris lesion, in addition to tumor excision. Alternatively, the use of plaque brachytherapy for iris melanoma has been shown to be highly effective in providing local tumor control and preventing recurrence with low complication rates [57,58]. This technique is the modality of choice for larger lesions that cannot be resected.

CILIARY BODY LESIONS

Ciliary body tumors include melanomas, melanocytomas, diktyoma, and metastatic tumors. The clinical presentation of these lesions varies and the combination of clinical examination in addition to noninvasive diagnostic studies (UBM) can suggest a specific diagnosis. The specific management varies depending on the classification of the tumor, and although clinical examination and imaging may suggest a specific diagnosis, many ciliary body tumors warrant a biopsy for diagnosis and further management. The biopsy techniques used to obtain tissue for ciliary body tumors are similar regardless of the tumor type.

Aspiration biopsy techniques

Fine-needle aspiration biopsy

A 3-mm partial-thickness lamellar scleral flap is dissected overlying the tumor. A 25-gauge short needle is attached to tubing and a biopsy gun and tangentially inserted through the scleral bed underlying the flap and into the choroid. Use of 27-gauge and 30-gauge needles has been described because of the lower potential for extraocular seeding but this is associated with more resistance and smaller tissue samples than are obtained with a 25-gauge needle. Once the sample is obtained, the scleral flap is then sutured back in position; cryotherapy or an absolute alcohol–soaked cotton-tipped applicator can be applied to the needle insertion site to reduce the potential for seeding if a plaque will not be placed immediately after [59].

Incisional biopsy techniques

Similar to the transscleral excisional biopsy technique described later, a partial-thickness scleral flap is created for the transscleral approach. A deep scleral incision is made and tumor samples are removed from the deep scleral bed using Essen forceps and Westcott scissors (Fig. 10). Diathermy is used to achieve hemostasis if needed. The scleral flap is then either glued or sutured back to its anatomic position, and the radioactive plaque is placed [60].

In the transvitreal approach, a standard 3-port pars plana vitrectomy is initiated with endoillumination provided by a chandelier or the infusion to allow for bimanual sampling of the tumor. Core vitrectomy is performed with

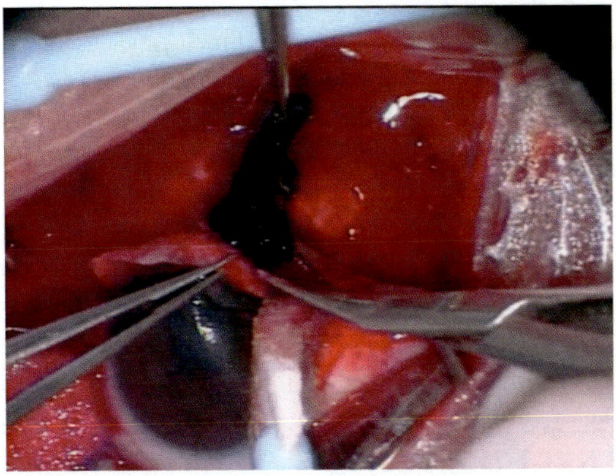

Fig. 10. Incisional biopsy for ciliary body tumor. A hinged partial-thickness lamellar scleral or corneoscleral flap is dissected with 4-mm margins around the tumor. The inner scleral fibers are then incised to expose uveal tissue and the mass. Tumor samples are removed from the deep scleral bed using Essen forceps and incised with Westcott scissors. Diathermy is used to achieve hemostasis. The scleral flap is sutured back to its anatomic position.

removal of the posterior hyaloid. The biopsy site is carefully chosen to avoid major vessels and to sample the tumor at its maximal height. Diathermy is applied to the incision site. Retinal incision of 1 mm × 1 mm is made using a diamond knife, during which time intraocular pressure is increased to achieve hemostasis. A 1 mm × 1 mm × 1 mm sample of tissue is then incised using the diamond knife and grasped with forceps, with the diamond knife in place to sever the base of the sample. The specimen is removed via the sclerotomy while infusion is off. Once the specimen is removed, infusion is reestablished and endolaser photocoagulation is applied to the biopsy retinotomy site. Air-fluid exchange is performed, and air is then replaced with isoexpansive sulfur hexafluoride gas [61].

Incisional biopsy allows for greater tissue sample than biopsy with fine-needle aspiration [59] and may provide better samples for thinner tumors [60]. In a series of 10 cases by Kvanta and colleagues [61] with the transvitreal approach, all cases had adequate samples for diagnosis and 30% of samples were benign lesions that were clinically suspected to be malignancies preoperatively. However, there was a high incidence of postoperative complications with the transvitreal approach described earlier, ranging from vitreous and subretinal hemorrhage to retinal detachment requiring repair with silicone oil tamponade; therefore, a staged approach with FNAB before incisional biopsy with vitrectomy was recommended [61,62]. Preoperative presence of retinal detachment also is associated with higher risk of retinal detachment progression postoperatively in the transvitreal approach [63]. Potential complications of the transscleral approach include perforation of the retina with consequent detachment, hemorrhage, endophthalmitis, buttonholing of the scleral flap, and potential damage to the radioactive plaque caused by excessive Histoacryl glue [60].

Excisional biopsy techniques

The transscleral approach involves partial lamellar sclerouvectomy and typically is reserved for smaller tumors or tumors in the ciliary body or peripheral choroid without associated retinal or vitreal seeding [64]. Smaller anterior choroidal or ciliary body tumors can be excised to avoid the potential complications of radiotherapy [60].

A hinged partial-thickness lamellar scleral or corneoscleral flap is dissected with 4-mm margins around the tumor. The inner scleral fibers then are incised to expose uveal tissue, and the tumor is removed in its entirety along with inner sclera. The scleral flap then is sutured back into position. The procedure can be combined with pars plana vitrectomy to aid in volume reduction and allow access to more posterior tumors, and silicone oil tamponade can be used in cases in which retinal breach occurs during biopsy [64].

The procedure is technically difficult and can be associated with a range of complications, including retinal prolapse, inability to remove the entire tumor because of posterior location, retinal breach leading to retinal detachment, vitreous hemorrhage, expulsive hemorrhage, and seeding [64]. Despite the complexity of the procedure and potential for complications, anterior tumors with well-defined margins are best suited for this type of biopsy, potentially avoiding radiotherapy [59].

POSTERIOR SEGMENT LESIONS

The most common malignant posterior segment lesions include choroidal metastases, melanoma, uveal lymphoma, primary intraocular/vitreoretinal lymphoma, and retinoblastoma (in children). In many cases of posterior segment tumors, clinical diagnosis in conjunction with noninvasive diagnostic imaging (fluorescein angiography, indocyanine angiography, optical coherence tomography, B-scan ultrasonography, computed tomography scans, and MRI) can establish the diagnosis with accuracy of up to 98% [65]. Biopsy is typically reserved for certain cases of diagnostic uncertainty in which conflicting or inconclusive results exist on noninvasive imaging or unusual clinical features with the potential for globe salvage. In the case of choroidal melanoma, a biopsy is routinely done not for diagnosis but to aid in prognosis by evaluating the molecular profile of the tumor, or sometimes for inclusion in clinical studies [62]. In general, the biopsy techniques used to obtain tissue from posterior segment lesions are similar regardless of specific tumor type. Note that it is contraindicated to biopsy retinoblastoma because it may lead to extraocular tumor spread, which significantly changes the prognosis for life for the child.

Approximately 10% of patients presenting with a choroidal mass have a history of systemic malignancy; however, up to 33% of patients with intraocular metastases have no known diagnosis of systemic malignancy [66]. In these cases, biopsy may play an important role in diagnosis, although, after systemic imaging, other lesions in the body may be more amenable to biopsy.

Aspiration biopsy techniques

Fine-needle aspiration biopsy

As with other anatomic sites, FNAB is an established technique for the identification of posterior segment tumors dating back to 1979, when the safety and reliability of the procedure was reported to be as high as 88% to 95% [67]. FNAB samples have adequate yield to aid in prognostic studies of melanoma. Small tumors less than 2.5 mm in height are typically associated with lower yields, so alternative methods for biopsy, or deferral of biopsy, should be considered [59,60].

The FNAB technique depends on the tumor size, tumor location, involved structures, and clarity of media. Preequatorial lesions typically are approached transsclerally, whereas postequatorial lesions are approached transvitreally. Transscleral approaches typically are performed before radioactive plaque placement or proton beam radiotherapy to provide fresh tissue for analysis [60]. Similar to the approach for ciliary body tumors, in the transscleral approach, a 3-mm partial-thickness lamellar scleral flap is dissected overlying the tumor. A 25-gauge short needle is attached to tubing and a biopsy gun and tangentially inserted through the scleral bed underlying the flap and into the choroid. Use of 27-gauge and 30-gauge needles has been described because of the lower potential for extraocular seeding but is associated with more resistance to aspiration and smaller tissue samples. Once the sample is obtained, cryotherapy or an absolute alcohol–soaked cotton-tipped applicator can be applied to the needle insertion site to reduce the potential for seeding if a plaque will not be placed immediately after. The scleral flap is then sutured back in position (Fig. 11) [60].

In the transvitreal approach, a 1.25 inch 27-gauge needle is inserted into the pars plana 3.5 to 4 mm posterior to the limbus in the meridian of the tumor. Under direct visualization with an indirect ophthalmoscope, the needle is placed through the overlying retina and into the tumor with care to avoid major vasculature (Fig. 12). Ocular oncologists generally prefer a 27-gauge needle for posterior lesions (less chance of penetrating the sclera), and a 25-gauge needle for anterior lesions biopsied via the transscleral route (because of better yield), but this is surgeon specific. If hemorrhage occurs, hemostasis can be achieved by applying gentle pressure with a cotton-tipped applicator on the ocular surface, or an injection of balanced salt solution to increase the intraocular pressure and tamponade the hemorrhage [59,68]. This technique can be modified to use an operating microscope and chandelier for intraocular illumination instead of the indirect ophthalmoscope, depending on the surgeon's preference. In cases with media opacity, most surgeons defer biopsy; however, FNAB can still be performed under ultrasonic guidance, although this should be done with extreme caution [69].

The transvitreal FNAB approach can be performed in conjunction with vitrectomy. A standard 3-port pars plana vitrectomy is initiated with core vitrectomy. Full separation of the hyaloid from the tumor biopsy site is recommended to prevent vitreous incarceration during biopsy. A long 25-gauge

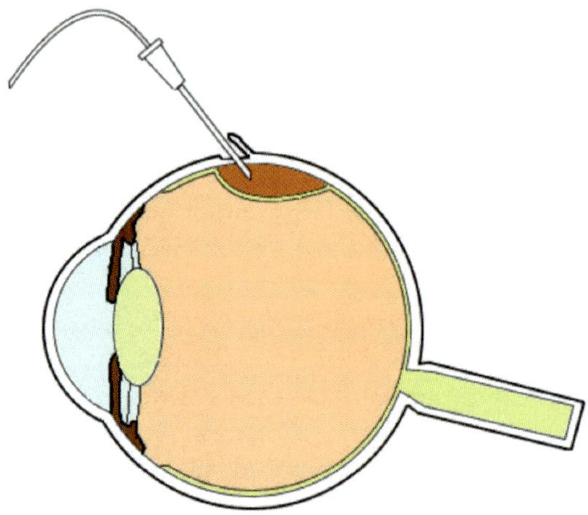

Fig. 11. Transscleral FNAB. A 25-gauge needle attached to a syringe via tubing is tangentially inserted into the scleral bed underlying the 3-mm partial-thickness lamellar scleral flap overlying the tumor.

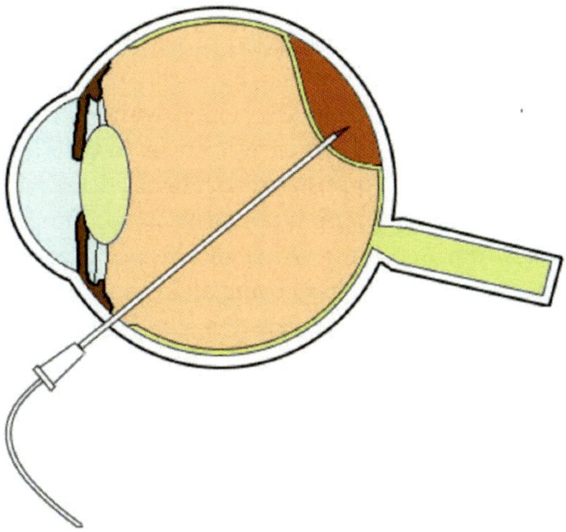

Fig. 12. Transvitreal FNAB. A 1.25 inch 25-gauge needle attached to a syringe via tubing is inserted into the pars plana 3.5 to 4 mm posterior to the limbus into the tumor via direct visualization with an indirect ophthalmoscope. In general, ocular oncologists prefer the 27-gauge for posterior (less chance of penetrating the sclera) and a short 25-gauge for transscleral (for better yield), but this is surgeon specific.

needle then is introduced through the port, and the intraocular pressure is increased just before insertion of the needle into the tumor. Once a tissue sample is obtained and hemostasis is established, the intraocular pressure is normalized [59].

Overall, FNAB of posterior segment tumors is well established and confers high diagnostic yield with low complication rate and low risk of tumor spread [67,70]. Adequate diagnostic yields have been reported in the range of 76% to 88% [68,71]. In 24% to 48% of cases, therapeutic plans have been altered by FNAB results [62]. Potential complications include inadequate biopsy sample, retinal detachment, vitreous hemorrhage, subretinal hemorrhage, endophthalmitis, and tumor seeding. No reported cases exist of local or systemic recurrence with use of 25-gauge or smaller needles [69]. FNAB in conjunction with vitrectomy can be complicated by cataract. Limitations of FNAB stem from the associated small sample size, which can confer false-negative results. False-negatives often are caused by low cellularity, and, therefore, a negative result should not definitely rule out the presence of intraocular malignancy [69]. FNAB yield can be improved by avoiding smaller-gauge needles, priming the syringe to avoid plunger retraction, and flushing the aspiration tubing for residual tissue sample [59,69].

Vitreous cutter aspiration biopsy

Use of vitreous cutter to aid in biopsy is an alternative to FNAB and may confer improved diagnostic yield of up to 97% [65]. In addition, the vitreous cutter provides more tissue than the standard FNAB approach, allowing for further testing such as immunohistochemistry and prognostic studies. Vitreous cutter sampling also allows for examination of paraffin-embedded tissue samples of many cohesive tumor cells rather than cell smears from FNAB [65].

Similar to the transvitreal FNAB in association with vitrectomy as described earlier, a standard 3-port pars plana vitrectomy is initiated with core vitrectomy, followed by induction of a posterior hyaloidal detachment. Full separation of the hyaloid from the tumor biopsy site is recommended to prevent vitreous incarceration during biopsy. After increase of intraocular pressure to achieve hemostasis, the retina is incised using an intraocular Sato knife to allow the head of the vitreous cutter to pass transretinally. Retinal vessels are avoided in choosing the biopsy site [60]. Once the vitreous cutter is placed into the tumor, sample is taken in 3 bites on high aspiration and low cut rate (Fig. 13). The vitreous cutter is then removed from the eye and residual tumor sample and fluid are aspirated from the tubing. Once a tissue sample is obtained and hemostasis is established, the intraocular pressure is normalized. In general, it is not necessary to apply cryotherapy or laser to the retinotomy site because the break usually is sealed by blood clot and there are strong retinal adhesions to the underlying mass, caused by degenerative changes that preclude the development of a retinal detachment [62,69].

According to a study by Bechrakis and colleagues [65] on 23 posterior intraocular tumors, only 1 case (4.3%) had inadequate sample for diagnosis because of loss of the sample in transport. The main complication noted in this series was vitreous hemorrhage; however, 1 patient developed multifocal intraocular metastases requiring enucleation. Additional complications are similar to those associated with standard vitrectomy: cataract, hemorrhage, endophthalmitis,

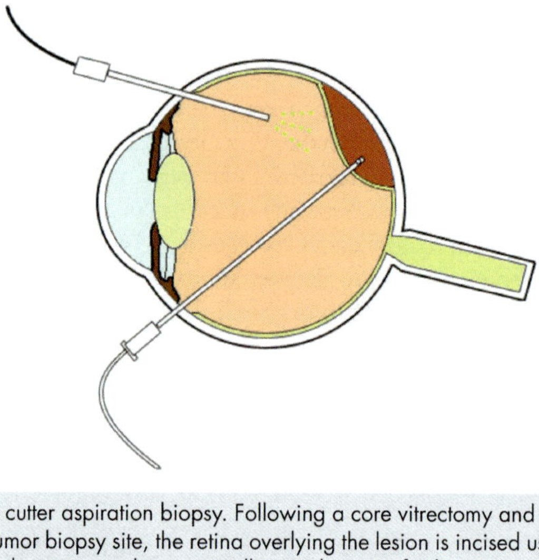

Fig. 13. Vitreous cutter aspiration biopsy. Following a core vitrectomy and separation of the hyaloid from the tumor biopsy site, the retina overlying the lesion is incised using a Sato knife. The vitreous cutter then is passed transretinally into the mass for biopsy.

retinal tear, or retinal detachment. A recent study using 27-gauge vitreous cutter suggested potential lower risk of complications with diagnostic yield comparable with larger-gauge vitrectomy systems [72].

Incisional biopsy techniques

Incisional biopsy has limited utility in the analysis of posterior segment tumors, but it does play a large role in the diagnosis of anterior segment lesions, as described earlier. Indications for incisional biopsy are limited to peripheral choroidal or ciliary body tumors [59], and are of particular use in thin tumors (<3 mm thick) [60].

Excisional biopsy techniques

Excisional biopsy for posterior segment tumors is rarely used. As described earlier, it can be a useful technique for tumors in the ciliary body or peripheral choroid without associated retinal or vitreal seeding [64].

Special considerations

Retinoblastoma

FNAB of suspected retinoblastoma is contraindicated because of potential for extraocular seeding of the tumor. Select cases in which clinical diagnosis cannot be established despite exhaustive noninvasive evaluation are potential candidates for FNAB; however, if the visual potential is low, it is preferred to simply enucleate the eye because the risk of tumor spread and the risk to the child's life in the setting of retinoblastoma is significant and not to be underestimated. A modified approach has been suggested in the literature to reduce the risk of seeding. The needle is passed through the peripheral cornea and iris and reaches the vitreous cavity via a transzonular approach to biopsy the suspicious lesion [69].

Intraocular lymphoma

Intraocular lymphoma can masquerade as uveitis, presenting a diagnostic challenge in cases of posterior uveitis refractory to steroid treatment, particularly in elderly patients. Vitreous biopsy is essential to diagnosis and is typically performed during core vitrectomy. Before initiating infusion, an undiluted vitreous specimen is obtained by aspiration from the vitreous cutter line into a syringe. Sample is obtained until the globe begins to involute because of lack of infusion. Vitrectomy can then be completed, and the sample is analyzed with flow cytometry and cytologic analysis [62]. It is critical that a conversation is had between the pathologist and surgeon if this diagnosis is suspected, given the challenges in managing this sample for histopathologic evaluation.

SUMMARY

In ocular oncology, surgical biopsy remains the gold standard of care for many lesions of the eyelid, ocular surface, iris, and posterior segment because of its unique ability to provide tissue samples for direct histopathologic analysis and thus bolster diagnostic certainty. Appropriate surgical technique is critical because it facilitates safely and effectively obtaining tissue for histopathologic evaluation in order to effect appropriate disease management.

References

[1] Cook BE, Bartley GB. Epidemiologic characteristics and clinical course of patients with malignant eyelid tumors in an incidence cohort in Olmsted County, Minnesota. Ophthalmology 1999;106(4):746–50.

[2] Deokule S, Child V, Tarin S, et al. Diagnostic accuracy of benign eyelid skin lesions in the minor operation theatre. Orbit 2003;22(4):235–8.

[3] Silverman N, Shinder R. What's new in eyelid tumors. Asia Pac J Ophthalmol (Phila) 2017;6(2):143–52.

[4] Allen RC. Surgical management of periocular cancers: high- and low-risk features drive treatment. Curr Oncol Rep 2017;19(9):57.

[5] Rice JC, Zaragoza P, Waheed K, et al. Efficacy of incisional vs punch biopsy in the histological diagnosis of periocular skin tumours. Eye (Lond) 2003;17(4):478–81.

[6] Garcia GA, Nguyen CV, Vo TA, et al. Lazy pentagonal wedge resection of eyelid margin lesions. JAMA Facial Plast Surg 2018;20(3):251–2.

[7] Divine RD, Anderson RL. Techniques in eyelid wound closure. Ophthalmic Surg 1982;13(4):283–7.

[8] Malhotra R, Huilgol SC, Huynh NT, et al. The Australian Mohs database, part II: periocular basal cell carcinoma outcome at 5-year follow-up. Ophthalmology 2004;111(4):631–6.

[9] Vuyk HD, Lohuis PJ. Mohs micrographic surgery for facial skin cancer. Clin Otolaryngol Allied Sci 2001;26(4):265–73.

[10] Morris DS, Elzaridi E, Clarke L, et al. Periocular basal cell carcinoma: 5-year outcome following Slow Mohs surgery with formalin-fixed paraffin-embedded sections and delayed closure. Br J Ophthalmol 2009;93(4):474–6.

[11] Sanchez R, Ivan D, Esmaeli B. Eyelid and periorbital cutaneous malignant melanoma. Int Ophthalmol Clin 2009;49(4):25–43.

[12] Mills JK, White I, Diggs B, et al. Effect of biopsy type on outcomes in the treatment of primary cutaneous melanoma. Am J Surg 2013;205(5):585–90.

[13] Pavri SN, Clune J, Ariyan S, et al. Malignant Melanoma: Beyond the Basics. Plast Reconstr Surg 2016;138(2):330e–40e.

[14] Pfeiffer ML, Ozgur OK, Myers JN, et al. Sentinel lymph node biopsy for ocular adnexal melanoma. Acta Ophthalmol 2017;95(4):e323–8.

[15] Yin VT, Warneke CL, Merritt HA, et al. Number of excisions required to obtain clear surgical margins and prognostic value of AJCC T category for patients with eyelid melanoma. Br J Ophthalmol 2014;98(12):1681–5.

[16] Shields JA, Saktanasate J, Lally SE, et al. Sebaceous carcinoma of the ocular region: the 2014 professor Winifred Mao lecture. Asia Pac J Ophthalmol (Phila) 2015;4(4):221–7.

[17] Shields JA, Demirci H, Marr BP, et al. Sebaceous carcinoma of the eyelids: personal experience with 60 cases. Ophthalmology 2004;111(12):2151–7.

[18] Peters GB, Meyer DR, Shields JA, et al. Management and prognosis of Merkel cell carcinoma of the eyelid. Ophthalmology 2001;108(9):1575–9.

[19] Campbell AA, Grob SR, Freitag SK. Controversies in sentinel lymph node biopsy for ocular neoplasms. Int Ophthalmol Clin 2015;55(4):73–9.

[20] Shields CL, Chien JL, Surakiatchanukul T, et al. Conjunctival tumors: review of clinical features, risks, biomarkers, and outcomes–the 2017 J. Donald M. Gass Lecture. Asia Pac J Ophthalmol (Phila) 2017;6(2):109–20.

[21] Kieval JZ, Karp CL, Abou Shousha M, et al. Ultra-high resolution optical coherence tomography for differentiation of ocular surface squamous neoplasia and pterygia. Ophthalmology 2012;119(3):481–6.

[22] Galor A, Karp CL, Chhabra S, et al. Topical interferon alpha 2b eye-drops for treatment of ocular surface squamous neoplasia: a dose comparison study. Br J Ophthalmol 2010;94(5):551–4.
[23] Hirst LW. Randomized controlled trial of topical mitomycin C for ocular surface squamous neoplasia. Ophthalmology 2007;114:976–82.
[24] Joag MG, Sise A, Murillo JC, et al. Topical 5-Fluorouracil 1% as primary treatment for ocular surface squamous neoplasia. Ophthalmology 2016;123(7):1442–8.
[25] Othman IS. Ocular surface tumors. Oman J Ophthalmol 2009;2(1):3–14.
[26] Adler E, Turner JR, Stone DU. Ocular surface squamous neoplasia: a survey of changes in the standard of care from 2003 to 2012. Cornea 2013;32(12):1558–61.
[27] Quhill H, Rundle PA, Mudhar HS. Conjunctival blue naevus in an anophthalmic socket. Ocul Oncol Pathol 2017;3(3):220–3.
[28] Shields JA, Shields CL, De Potter P. Surgical management of conjunctival tumors. The 1994 Lynn B. McMahan lecture. Arch Ophthalmol 1997;115(6):808–15.
[29] Honavar SG, Manjandavida FP. Tumors of the ocular surface: a review. Indian J Ophthalmol 2015;63(3):187–203.
[30] Lee GA, Hirst LW. Ocular surface squamous neoplasia. Surv Ophthalmol 1995;39(6): 429–50.
[31] Panda A, Kumar S, Kumar A, et al. Fibrin glue in ophthalmology. Indian J Ophthalmol 2009;57(5):371–9.
[32] Gündüz K, Uçakhan OO, Kanpolat A, et al. Nonpreserved human amniotic membrane transplantation for conjunctival reconstruction after excision of extensive ocular surface neoplasia. Eye (Lond) 2006;20(3):351–7.
[33] Harooni H, Schoenfield LR, Singh AD. Current appraisal of conjunctival melanocytic tumors: classification and treatment. Future Oncol 2011;7(3):435–46.
[34] Vora GK, Demirci H, Marr B, et al. Advances in the management of conjunctival melanoma. Surv Ophthalmol 2017;62(1):26–42.
[35] Gloor P, Alexandrakis G. Clinical characterization of primary acquired melanosis. Gaz Med Fr 1995;36(8):1721–9.
[36] Rodriguez-Sains RS. Pigmented conjunctival neoplasms. Orbit 2002;21(3):231–8.
[37] Finger PT, Czechonska G, Liarikos S. Topical mitomycin C chemotherapy for conjunctival melanoma and PAM with atypia. Br J Ophthalmol 1998;82(5):476–9.
[38] Shields JA, Shields CL, De Potter P. Surgical management of circumscribed conjunctival melanomas. Ophthalmic Plast Reconstr Surg 1998;14(3):208–15.
[39] Damato B, Coupland SE. Management of conjunctival melanoma. Expert Rev Anticancer Ther 2009;9(9):1227–39.
[40] Aziz HA, Gastman BR, Singh AD. Management of conjunctival melanoma: critical assessment of sentinel lymph node biopsy. Ocul Oncol Pathol 2015;1(4):266–73.
[41] Shields CL, Shields PW, Manalac J, et al. Review of cystic and solid tumors of the iris. Oman J Ophthalmol 2013;6(3):159–64.
[42] Shields CL, Arepalli S, Lally EB, et al. Iris stromal cyst management with absolute alcohol-induced sclerosis in 16 patients. JAMA Ophthalmol 2014;132(6):703–8.
[43] Gokhale R, Medina CA, Biscotti CV, et al. Diagnostic fine-needle aspiration biopsy for iris melanoma. Asia Pac J Ophthalmol (Phila) 2015;4(2):89–91.
[44] Shields CL, Manquez ME, Ehya H, et al. Fine-needle aspiration biopsy of iris tumors in 100 consecutive cases: technique and complications. Ophthalmology 2006;113(11):2080–6.
[45] Sellam A, Desjardins L, Barnhill R, et al. Fine needle aspiration biopsy in uveal melanoma: technique, complications, and outcomes. Am J Ophthalmol 2016;162:28–34.e1.
[46] Matthews BJ, Mudhar HS, Rennie IG. Trans-corneal fine cannula aspiration: Rycroft cannula aspiration technique for sampling iris tumours. Br J Ophthalmol 2012;96(3):329–31.
[47] Petousis V, Finger PT, Milman T. Anterior segment tumor biopsy using an aspiration cutter technique: clinical experience. Am J Ophthalmol 2011;152(5):771–5.e1.

[48] Pe'er J, Blumenthal EZ, Frenkel S. Punch biopsy of iris lesions: a novel technique for obtaining histology samples. Br J Ophthalmol 2007;91(5):660–2.
[49] Chronopoulos A, Kilic E, Joussen AM, et al. Small incision iris tumour biopsy using a cavernous sampling forceps. Br J Ophthalmol 2014;98(11):1539–42.
[50] Chong CF, Patel DV, Hadden PW, et al. Conservative biopsy excision and management of a large iris melanoma. Clin Exp Optom 2014;97(3):278–9.
[51] Klauber S, Jensen PK, Prause JU, et al. Surgical treatment of iris and ciliary body melanoma: follow-up of a 25-year series of patients. Acta Ophthalmol 2012;90(2):122–6.
[52] Hood CT, Schoenfield LR, Torres V, et al. Iris melanoma. Ophthalmology 2011;118(1):221–2.
[53] Lingam G. Options for management of intra ocular tumors. Indian J Ophthalmol 2015;63(3):204–10.
[54] Cardine S, Labetoulle M, Kirsch O, et al. Iris melanomas. A retrospective study of 11 patients treated by surgical excision. J Fr Ophtalmol 2003;26(1):31–7 [in French].
[55] Rospond-Kubiak I, Damato B. The surgical approach to the management of anterior uveal melanomas. Eye (Lond) 2014;28(6):741–7.
[56] Naumann GO, Rummelt V. Block excision of tumors of the anterior uvea. Report on 68 consecutive patients. Ophthalmology 1996;103(12):2017–27 [discussion: 27–8].
[57] Agraval U, Sobti M, Russell HC, et al. Use of Ruthenium-106 Brachytherapy for iris melanoma: the Scottish experience. Br J Ophthalmol 2018;102(1):74–8.
[58] Finger PT. Plaque radiation therapy for malignant melanoma of the iris and ciliary body. Am J Ophthalmol 2001;132(3):328–35.
[59] Rishi P, Dhami A, Biswas J. Biopsy techniques for intraocular tumors. Indian J Ophthalmol 2016;64(6):415–21.
[60] Damato B, Angi M, Coupland SE, et al. Miscellaneous uveal biopsy techniques. In: Singh AD, Damato BE, editors. Clinical ophthalmic oncology, chapter 4. Berlin: Springer-Verlag; 2014. p. 31–9.
[61] Kvanta A, Seregard S, Kopp ED, et al. Choroidal biopsies for intraocular tumors of indeterminate origin. Am J Ophthalmol 2005;140(6):1002–6.
[62] Eide N, Walaas L. Fine-needle aspiration biopsy and other biopsies in suspected intraocular malignant disease: a review. Acta Ophthalmol 2009;87(6):588–601.
[63] Seregard S, All-Ericsson C, Hjelmqvist L, et al. Diagnostic incisional biopsies in clinically indeterminate choroidal tumours. Eye (Lond) 2013;27(2):115–8.
[64] Shields JA, Shields CL, Shah P, et al. Partial lamellar sclerouvectomy for ciliary body and choroidal tumors. Ophthalmology 1991;98(6):971–83.
[65] Bechrakis NE, Foerster MH, Bornfeld N. Biopsy in indeterminate intraocular tumors. Ophthalmology 2002;109(2):235–42.
[66] Shields CL, Shields JA, Gross NE, et al. Survey of 520 eyes with uveal metastases. Ophthalmology 1997;104(8):1265–76.
[67] Singh AD, Biscotti CV. Fine needle aspiration biopsy of ophthalmic tumors. Saudi J Ophthalmol 2012;26(2):117–23.
[68] Shields JA, Shields CL, Ehya H, et al. Fine-needle aspiration biopsy of suspected intraocular tumors. The 1992 Urwick Lecture. Ophthalmology 1993;100(11):1677–84.
[69] Singh AD, Biscotti CV, Pelayes DE. Fine needle aspiration biopsy. In: Singh AD, Damato BE, editors. Clinical ophthalmic oncology, chapter 3. Berlin: Springer-Verlag; 2014. p. 17–30.
[70] Cohen VM, Dinakaran S, Parsons MA, et al. Transvitreal fine needle aspiration biopsy: the influence of intraocular lesion size on diagnostic biopsy result. Eye (Lond) 2001;15(Pt 2):143–7.
[71] Ausburger JJ, Schneider S, Ehya H. The role of transvitreal fine needle aspiration biopsy in small suspected choroidal melanomas. Invest Ophthalmol Vis Sci 1999;40:1287.
[72] Grewal DS, Cummings TJ, Mruthyunjaya P. Outcomes of 27-gauge vitrectomy-assisted choroidal and subretinal biopsy. Ophthalmic Surg Lasers Imaging Retina 2017;48(5):406–15.

Advances in Ophthalmology and Optometry 4 (2019) 129–145

ADVANCES IN OPHTHALMOLOGY AND OPTOMETRY

Specimen Processing for Ocular Tumors

Tips and Tricks from the Ocular Pathologist

Benjamin Kambiz Ghiam, MD[a], Alireza Ghaffarieh, MD[b], Anna J. Mathew, MD[b], Maria Sibug Saber, MD[b], Jesse L. Berry, MD[c,d,*]

[a]Oakland University, William Beaumont School of Medicine, Rochester, MI, USA; [b]Department of Pathology, Keck School of Medicine of USC, University of Southern California, 1450 San Pablo Street, Los Angeles, CA 90033, USA; [c]Department of Ophthalmology, USC Roski Eye Institute, Keck School of Medicine of USC, University of Southern California, 1450 San Pablo Street, Los Angeles, CA 90033, USA; [d]The Vision Center, Children's Hospital Los Angeles, 4650 Sunset Boulevard, Los Angeles, CA 90027, USA

Keywords

• Ocular tumors • Ophthalmic pathology • Specimen collection
• Specimen processing

Key points

- Proper diagnosis is critical in ocular oncology, which can be hampered by inadequate specimen collection.
- A collaborative dialog with the ocular pathologist is critical in the success of eye specimen handling.

Continued

INTRODUCTION

Despite abundant guidelines and recommendations published for ophthalmic pathologists regarding specimen handling and processing within the pathology laboratory, relatively little literature is available for guidance of specimen

Disclosure Statement: There are no financial conflicts of interest to disclose. Dr J.L. Berry holds grants unrelated to the topic of this article from the National Cancer Institute of the National Institute of Health Award, number K08CA232344; the Wright Foundation; the Knights Templar Eye Foundation; and the American Cancer Society, number IRG-16- 181-57.

*Corresponding author. Department of Ophthalmology, USC Roski Eye Institute, Keck School of Medicine of USC, University of Southern California, 1450 San Pablo Street, Los Angeles, CA 90033, USA. *E-mail address:* Jesse.Berry@med.usc.edu

https://doi.org/10.1016/j.yaoo.2019.04.007
2452-1760/19/

Continued

- Tips, tricks, techniques, and recommendations on specimen collection and handling are succinctly discussed for the busy surgeon and pathologist.
- Health care facility policy and procedure should be followed for the proper collection, labeling, and transportation of the specimen to the pathology department.

collection and handling for the ocular oncology surgeon. Following the surgical collection of a lesion specimen by the surgeon, adequate processing of the tissue by the pathologist largely depends on the information provided by the surgeon, the quality of the specimen submitted, and the container and fixative the specimen is submitted in. The improper submission of a specimen by a misinformed surgeon may result in an inadequate specimen that cannot be appropriately processed, leading to a delay in diagnosis and treatment, as well as possible additional procedures for the patient. Such a burden is often preventable with clear communication between the pathologist and surgeon regarding the adequate handling, timing, and submission of specimens. To optimize the specimen handoff, the authors describe general techniques and recommendations by pathologists on specimen collection and handling for the busy ocular oncology surgeon.

GENERAL RECOMMENDATIONS FOR TISSUE COLLECTION AND HANDLING

Effective and accurate communication is the most important element in the relationship between the ocular oncologist and the pathologist or pathology laboratory. For questions or concerns about proper specimen handling, it always is best to call the pathologist before the procedure. Information slips should always include date of birth, sex, race (if pertinent), laterality and location of the lesion, procedure performed, preoperative diagnosis, and postoperative diagnosis (if there is a change). The ophthalmologist's clinical impression is actually important to the pathologist because it may influence how the specimen is processed. Lesion is not a particularly helpful diagnosis, hence always list the suspected clinical diagnosis [1–3].

Generally, most specimens may be submitted to the pathology department fresh, in formalin (10%) (Fig. 1), or with a saline-moistened sponge or gauze. The specimen should be submitted as soon as possible, with clearly written instructions for any special testing. Unfixed specimens may be placed in a sterile container and kept moist with sterile saline or wrapped in saline-moistened sponges or gauze until the specimen can be properly placed in fixative (tissue should not be soaked in saline) [4]. If the specimen requires electron microscopy, 3% glutaraldehyde in 0.1 ml sodium cacodylate buffer is the fixative of choice [5]. Batching and submitting multiple specimens from different sites in the same container should never be done. There should be clear communication with the pathologist regarding the transfer of any unfixed specimens so

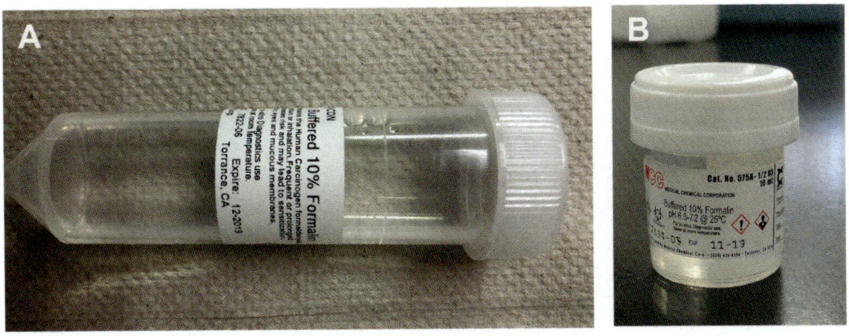

Fig. 1. Most specimens may be submitted to the pathology department fresh, or in a standard container (*A*) or jar (*B*) containing 10% formalin, or other specified medium (eg, Michel transport medium for direct immunofluorescence or glutaraldehyde if for electron microscopy) and submitted as soon as possible with clearly written instructions for any special testing.

there is no delay in their handling on delivery to the pathology laboratory (eg, on nights and weekends). See later discussion of specific recommendations, arranged anatomically, on specimen collection and processing for the ophthalmic surgeon.

ANTERIOR SEGMENT

When performing an aqueous tap for cytology, the pathology laboratory should be informed in advance to avoid delays in handling. The collected sample should be immediately delivered to the laboratory in a capped tuberculin syringe. During an anterior segment fine-needle aspiration biopsy (FNAB), the aspirated cells are located predominantly in the needle tip and should be flushed with a syringe into a small empty container using balanced salt solution (BSS). The collected sample is then sent for cytopathology processing and evaluation. Alternatively, the pathologist may join the surgeon in the operating room (OR) and the sample can be placed immediately onto a glass slide. This additionally allows for evaluation of the adequacy of the sample [6–8].

Focus points

- For aqueous tap specimens for cytology, inform the laboratory in advance and deliver the sample immediately.
- Use BSS to flush the FNAB specimen into a container, or collaborate with the pathologist in the OR to retrieve and evaluate the specimen directly.

CONJUNCTIVA AND CORNEA

Tumors of the conjunctiva and cornea comprise a large and varied spectrum of conditions. The most common ocular surface neoplasms are those of squamous origin. Others include lesions that arise from the melanocytes, including nevi, racial melanosis, primary acquired melanosis, and malignant melanoma [1,9]. A diagnostic biopsy is usually not necessary in cases of smaller tumors that appear benign. If a smaller tumor does require a biopsy, it is best to completely remove the lesion (excisional biopsy). In cases of larger lesions, it may be appropriate to remove a portion of the tumor (incisional biopsy) to obtain a histopathologic diagnosis before proceeding with therapy. Whenever possible, incisional biopsy should generally be avoided for conjunctival tumors, especially melanoma, because this can increase the risk for numerous tumor recurrences [10]. Occasionally, exfoliative cytology [11] and FNAB can provide useful information based on a few cells. The use of microscopically controlled excision (Mohs surgery) for some squamous lesions has been reported to ensure tumor-free margins, although this is rare [12].

Invasion of squamous cell carcinoma (SCC) and melanoma into the peripheral cornea may appear as a subtle, gray-surface opacity. For these cases, it is recommended that the surgeon note such corneal involvement before surgery because it often is less visible through the operating microscope than it is with slit-lamp biomicroscopy in the office [1].

For specimen submission of suspected squamous neoplasms of the ocular surface, the lesion should be placed flat, stromal side-down on non-adherent dressing or gauze pad such as Telfa paper (Covidien Products, Medtronic, Plymouth, MN, USA), specialized filter paper (Fig. 2), or thin cardboard (ie, that used to package sutures), and allowed to dry for 30 to 60 seconds before being placed in formalin fixative (so that its flat orientation is retained on the paper). Then the paper with specimen should be gently placed in a formalin jar; the paper also can be placed in a cassette (Fig. 3) and then placed in the jar. Taking at least 1 of these measure is essential because conjunctival biopsies tend to curl or ball up in fixative, making assessment of surgical margins difficult. It is ideal for the surgeon to mark 2 adjacent margins with different-colored sutures and to include a diagram depicting this orientation on the pathology requisition form. The status of the lateral and deep margins is important for prognosis [1,2,9,13].

The technique for excisional biopsy and specimen submission of primary acquired melanosis is similar to that previously described for squamous lesions. For suspected lymphoid lesions of the conjunctiva, an incisional biopsy may usually be performed in the office with topical or subconjunctival anesthetic; 4 to 5 mm of tissue generally is sufficient. The specimen should be submitted in formalin for routine hematoxylin-eosin (H&E) sections and immunohistochemistry. If possible, an additional 4 to 5 mm of tissue may be harvested and submitted in saline or special flow cytometry medium, on ice [1,9]. The pathology laboratory should be alerted before such fresh lesions are sent. See later discussion of further recommendations on the submission of lymphomatous lesions.

A wide range of corneal specimens can be submitted for histopathological analysis if involved by tumor. These include small biopsies, epithelial scrapings, and corneal membranes [14]. The cornea should be handled gently,

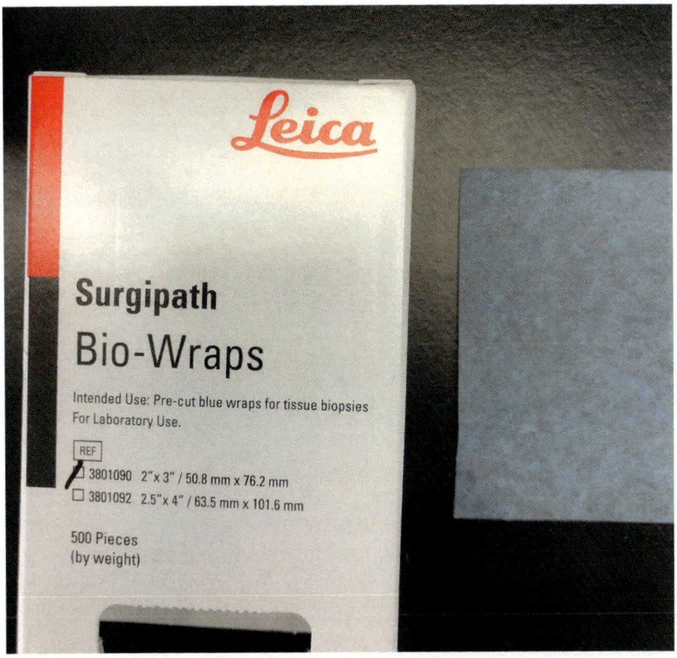

Fig. 2. Specimen submission of squamous neoplasms of the ocular surface, or other conjunctival lesions, should be placed flat, stromal side-down on specimen wrap paper, non-adherent dressing or gauze pad such as Telfa paper, filter paper, or thin cardboard (eg, that used to package sutures), and allowed to dry for 30 to 60 seconds. Then the paper with specimen should be gently placed in a formalin jar. This is essential because biopsies tend to curl or ball up in fixative, making assessment of surgical margins difficult.

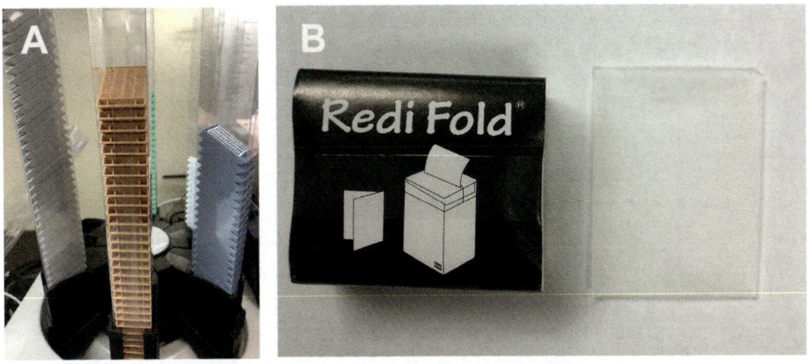

Fig. 3. Disposable plastic tissue cassettes (*A*) suitable for holding conjunctival tissue specimens. Small tissue specimens that may fall off the cassette during this process may be wrapped in the Redi-Fold (IMEB Inc., San Marcos, CA, USA) biopsy paper (*B*) and placed into the cassette.

with minimal trauma to the anterior and posterior surfaces. Corneal tissue is removed bluntly, often with the aid of absolute alcohol, so as not to perforate the cornea and facilitate intraocular spread of tumor. Small corneal biopsies do not require dissection and it is advised to submit all tissue for processing [5,14].

Focus points

- It can be difficult to see a tumor in the peripheral cornea when operating. Note these cases under the slit-lamp before operating.
- Conjunctival specimens will curl up, preventing adequate evaluation of the margins. The lesion should be placed flat on Telfa and allowed to dry before being placed in the formalin container. Mark 2 adjacent margins and include a diagram depicting this orientation for the pathologist.

EYELID

Basal cell carcinoma (BCC) is the most common malignant neoplasm of the eyelids, accounting for more than 90% of all eyelid malignancies [1]. The lower eyelid is most commonly involved, with the medial canthus being the second most common site of involvement. Although SCC may occur in the eyelids, it is 10 to 40 times less common than BCC [15]. Because most SCCs arise in solar-damaged skin, the lower eyelid is more frequently involved than the upper. After a diagnosis is confirmed with small incisional biopsy, complete excision with frozen section margin evaluation (conventional or Mohs microsurgery) is the treatment of choice. The overall 5-year recurrence rate is lower when using Mohs surgery than with conventional frozen sections [16–19]. When surgeons excise a full-thickness segment of the eyelid, a carefully performed gross examination (especially at the time of frozen section diagnosis) is critical. Meticulous specimen submission by the surgeon includes drawings of the excision site, with nasal and temporal margins labeled, or tagged with sutures or other markers [5,15]. A similar approach to specimen submission may be undertaken for melanoma of the eyelid (a much rarer tumor that accounts for <1% of all eyelid malignancies). However, it should be noted that there is no role for frozen margin control for melanoma, and permanent margin evaluation should be done.

Sebaceous carcinoma of the eyelid is less common than BCC or SCC, and more frequently affects the upper eyelid where there are a relatively greater number of meibomian glands [1,2]. Compared with wide local excision, Mohs micrographic surgery offers the potential of greater tissue conservation, and it may provide a lower recurrence rate [20,21]. The diagnosis of sebaceous carcinoma may be difficult both clinically and histopathologically. Even when examining tissue with optimal fixation and histologic preparation, these tumors may be mistaken for BCC or SCC. If a suspicion for a sebaceous carcinoma exists, this must be communicated with the pathologist and clearly listed as the suspected diagnosis so that the pathologist can generate frozen section slides for lipid stains to aid in the correct diagnosis. The demonstration of lipid within the cytoplasm of tumor cells by special stains, such as oil red O or Sudan black, is diagnostic, and must be performed on tissue before processing and paraffin embedding because these solvents dissolve the fat [22,23]. Additionally, sebaceous carcinoma may be multicentric in origin and may be missed by a single biopsy specimen. Also, 1 small biopsy specimen may not be adequate because inflamed areas within and surrounding the tumor may obscure the diagnosis. Therefore, multiple exploratory map biopsies are required for adequate evaluation [23]. Each separate small biopsy specimen must be placed in a separate small container or formalin. Care should be taken to label the location of each biopsy specimen in a drawing. Full-thickness eyelid biopsies are recommended in cases of suspected sebaceous carcinoma in which previous biopsy findings were negative. If there is extensive bulbar conjunctival involvement or if the orbit is involved, exenteration may be the treatment of choice [22].

Benign tumors can be removed by performing a simple skin ellipse (if not involving the lid margin), or a partial (usually cutaneous aspect only) or full-thickness (cutaneous, lid margin, and conjunctival aspect) lid resection [5]. When the clinical differential diagnosis is keratoacanthoma versus SCC, the lesion should be completely excised to permit optimal histologic examination of the lateral and deep margins of the tumor–host interface [1]. For actinic keratoses, the base of lesion must be examined histologically to determine whether invasive SCC is present; for this reason, shave biopsy not including the base of the lesion is contraindicated [1]. These specimen can be simply placed whole, in formalin, for evaluation.

Focus points

- When excising eyelid lesions, surgeons should provide a drawing of the excision site, with nasal and temporal margins labeled.
- If sebaceous carcinoma is suspected, inform the pathologist beforehand so appropriate stains can be used to aid in the diagnosis.

ENUCLEATION, EVISCERATION, AND EXENTERATION SPECIMENS

After enucleation, the globe should be placed into a large container (Fig. 4) with at least 60 mL of 10% neutral buffered formalin and transferred to the pathology laboratory where it will be allowed to fix for at least 24 hours before dissection. Formalin should not be injected into the globe or windows cut into the specimen for tumor collection before fixation unless this is discussed beforehand with the pathologist. If collection of a tumor specimen is done after enucleation, as is frequently done with retinoblastoma globes, a small incision is made in the sclera with a blade or a corneal keratome (the size of the keratome does not matter). This allows the surgeon to gently open the flap and dissect the tumor without placing unneeded pressure or suction on the intraocular contents [24,25]. This tumor sample is often sent separately for research

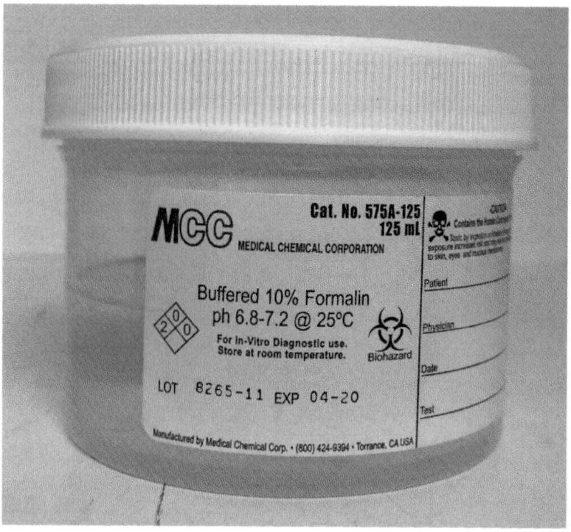

Fig. 4. Enucleated globes should be placed into a large container with at least 60 mL of 10% neutral buffered formalin and transferred to the pathology laboratory, where they will be allowed to fix for at least 24 hours before dissection.

protocols or other processing such as genetic evaluation. Before grossing the globe, enucleation specimens must be oriented by the pathologist, thus it is recommended to ensure identification of useful landmarks; the inferior oblique (IO) muscle serves as a great anatomic landmark. The IO muscle lacks a tendon; muscular fibers insert directly onto the sclera inferotemporally, with the nasal end of the IO muscle insertion lying close to the fovea. The superior oblique muscle inserts superiorly and temporally. It has a long tendon marked by parallel white bands, and serves as a landmark for the superior pole of the eye [2,26].

Ocular evisceration is a very rare procedure in ocular oncology. It never should be done if any suspicion of an intraocular tumor exists; imaging always should be done before evisceration to evaluate for tumor formation if there is no view to the posterior pole of the eye. After evisceration, the intraocular contents, including uvea, retina, and vitreous, are removed, including the entire cornea and a small rim of sclera. These specimens should be submitted whole in formalin fixative. Often, the anatomy of the eye is completely disorganized and much of the tissue is poorly recognizable. Most of the sclera is not removed. The pathologist will bisect the corneoscleral button and the intraocular contents [2].

Exenteration involves complete removal of the globe and all orbital contents that may be required in the setting of an advanced eyelid and/or orbital tumor wherein appropriate margins cannot otherwise be attained. In these cases, it is recommended to submit tissue from multiple surgical margins in separate containers. These separately submitted specimens represent the true surgical margin instead of the edges of the exenteration specimen [15,24]. These specimens require a greater volume of fixative and longer fixation because they are larger [24]. Before dissection by the pathologist, the external aspect of the surgical margins may be marked with India ink by the pathologist with special attention to any orientation details offered by the surgeon in respect to margins.

Focus points

- After enucleation, the globe should be placed in a large container with plenty of formalin (>60 mL); do not aspirate tumor from the globe because it distorts the intraocular anatomy.
- For exenteration specimens, submit tissue from multiple surgical margins in separate containers.

UVEA, RETINA, AND VITREOUS

Nevi and malignant melanomas arise in the iris, ciliary body, and choroid, and often are managed conservatively to avoid enucleation and preserve vision [26]. A melanoma can arise de novo or develop within a preexisting nevus, which may have been present for many years. For cases of iris melanoma, the extent of disease may not be appreciated by either the surgeon or the pathologist, thus careful orientation for clearance is important in iridectomy specimens. Clinical detection of small recurrences at the edge of the surgical coloboma can be delayed if the surgeon is not forewarned of the possibility [26,27]. Iridectomy specimens should generally be fixed in formalin because this will allow for adequate evaluation of the tumor specimen. If possible, it should be handled similar to conjunctival specimens and be placed on Telfa or specimen paper to prevent rolling.

If there is any suspicion of viral cause (eg, viral retinochoroiditis), a small piece of tissue should to be fixed in glutaraldehyde for transmission electron microscopy (whatever size is safely attainable is often sufficient). Additionally, in any suspected infectious cause associated with an iris lesion, the surgeon should submit material for microbiology (culture, polymerase chain reaction [PCR]–molecular testing) (Fig. 5) before placing the specimen in any fixative; the swab should not be used directly on the eye. Because these biopsies are quite small, they are best placed into sterile Eppendorf tubes (Fig. 6) containing formalin and not standard formalin pots or containers where the pathologist may have difficulty finding the specimen. For iridociliary body and (rarely) choroidal tumor local resection, the tissue should be submitted whole in formalin to the pathologist [5,26].

FNAB is an alternative method to obtain an iris tumor sample and may be used for diagnosing iris melanomas and to exclude common simulating conditions [28,29]. The risk for tumor seeding with transcorneal FNAB into either the adjacent iris or the anterior chamber is theoretic and considered to be extremely low [30]. Although only a small portion of patients require this diagnostic technique, it is important to consider that FNAB in the hands of a trained

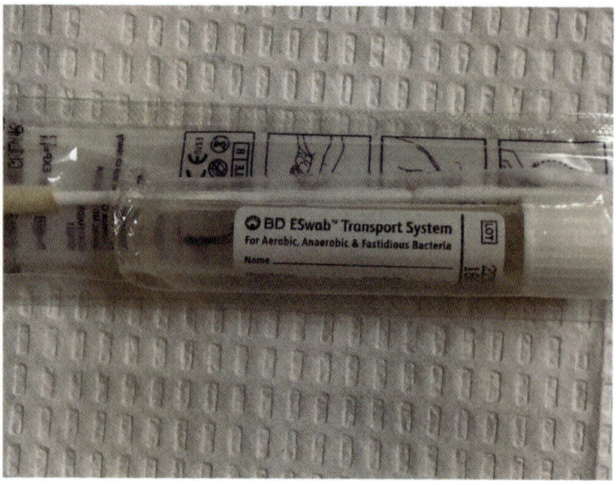

Fig. 5. Ensure that in any suspected infectious case, the surgeon submits material in designated microbiology containers for culture and/or PCR–molecular testing.

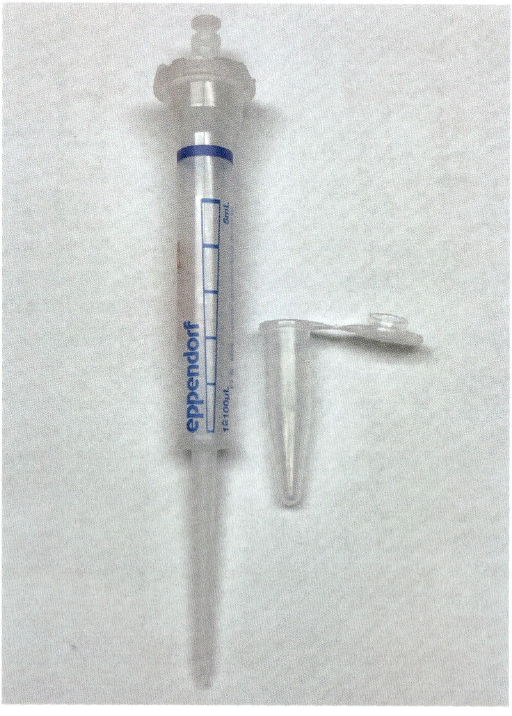

Fig. 6. Iridectomy biopsies are quite small and are best placed into sterile Eppendorf tubes (Eppendorf, Hamburg, Germany) containing formalin.

cytopathologist offers a definitive diagnosis [7]. See later discussion of recommendations on FNAB specimen handling.

If a lymphoid neoplasm (of the ocular adnexal tissues, uvea, or orbit) is suspected clinically, fresh unfixed tissue should be submitted for immunophenotypic assessment by flow cytometry to determine clonality. An adequate sample of fresh tissue is necessary; preferably of at least the volume of a green pea (4–5 mm). The specimen should be expeditiously delivered to the laboratory to avoid tissue degradation and be placed in a closed, moist container that contains a piece of gauze moistened with saline to prevent drying. The specimen should not be immersed in saline [2,31]. Additional tissue of similar volume should be separately submitted in formalin (eg, the entire specimen should not be submitted as a fresh specimen). The authors recommend that specimens not be submitted on Friday afternoons or after hours unless the surgeon can be assured the fresh tissue will be processed. If the sample must be collected after the flow cytometry laboratory has closed for the day, it is best to place it into a cell culture of 20 mL of Roswell Park Memorial Institute (RPMI) medium (Fig. 7) and then store in a refrigerator (4°C) overnight or over the weekend, for up to 5 days [32–34].

Although the diagnostic accuracy of FNAB for choroidal lesions is high when handled by a trained cytopathologist, the limited cellularity of some samples can compromise the diagnostic potential of ophthalmic aspirate samples. FNAB also is routinely used for prognostic evaluation with gene expression profiling or cytogenetic evaluation in combination with eye-conserving

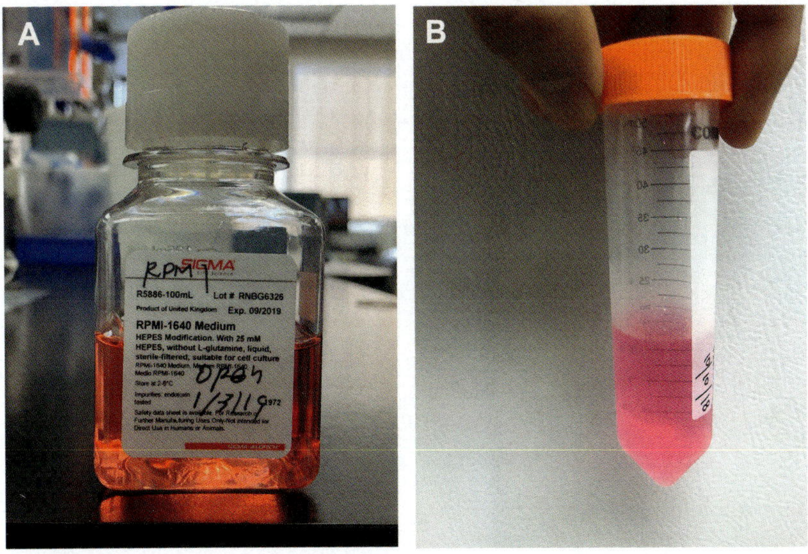

Fig. 7. RPMI medium (*A*) is a form of medium used in cell and tissue culture. Lymphomatous specimens that cannot be delivered to the laboratory expeditiously may be placed into a container with 20 mL of this medium (*B*) and stored at 4°C for up to 5 days.

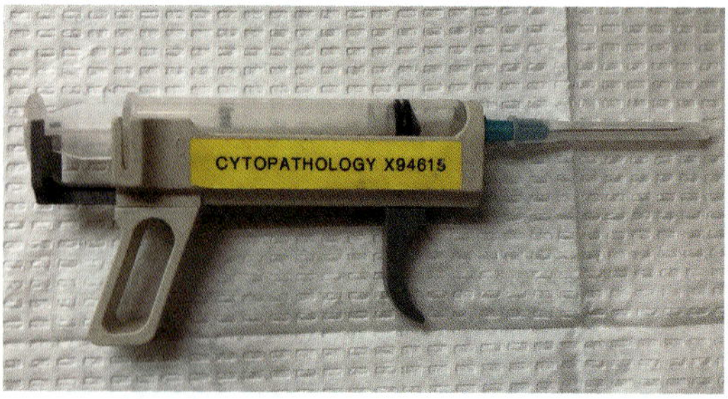

Fig. 8. In posterior segment FNABs, the needle is connected to a 5-mL syringe with a silastic tube on a tissue biopsy gun. The tissue material is aspirated from the needle and should be expeditiously sent for evaluation.

treatment such as plaque brachytherapy [7,8,35,36]. In posterior segment FNAB, the needle is connected to a 5-mL syringe with a silastic tube, often on a tissue biopsy gun (Fig. 8). (See Ashley Polski and colleagues' article, "Biopsy Techniques in Ocular Oncology," in this issue.) The tissue material is aspirated from the needle and immediately sent for cytopathologic examination and/or prognostic testing. Additionally, air-dried and/or alcohol-fixed smears may be prepared and sent to the pathology laboratory. It is acceptable to place the aspirated material into a methanol-based buffered preservative, such as Cytolyt (Hologic Inc., Marlborough, MA, USA), and submit it to the cytopathology laboratory for processing. As with FNAB in other anatomic sites of the eye, if a cytopathologist is available for rapid onsite evaluation, this can be done in the OR. In these instances, once the surgeon has aspirated the biopsy specimen from the tumor, the air-dried smears can be prepared by the pathologist, stained with Diff-Quik (Siemens, Munich, Germany) and directly evaluated and triaged accordingly (Fig. 9). Immunohistochemistry studies can be done

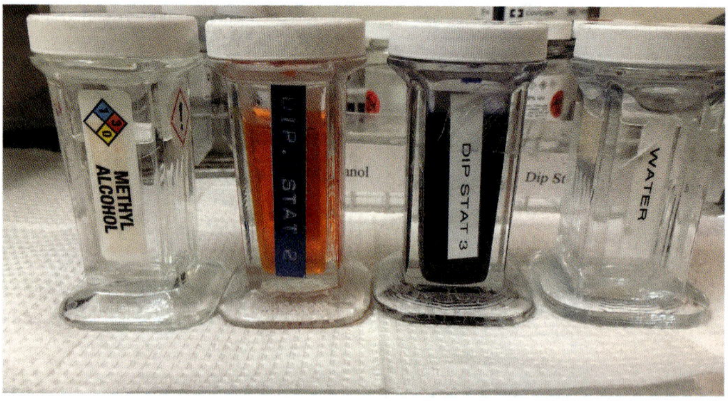

Fig. 9. Evaluation of FNAB samples may be performed in the OR using rapid onsite evaluation. Once the surgeon has aspirated the biopsy specimen from the tumor, the pathologist prepares the smears using the Diff-Quik solutions.

on these small samples for more precise classification and immunophenotyping of tumors [6,8]. The surgeon is encouraged to send some of the sample to microbiology for culture and PCR analysis if there is any suspicion of infection. Generally for melanoma (as previously discussed for iris tumors) this is not required; however, it may be for other retinochoroidal lesions if the diagnosis is not clear. In these instances, the authors encourage surgeons to send as much vitreous as is possible to safely aspirate in a capped tuberculin syringe or specimen container [5]. It should be noted that vitreous is not required for diagnostic evaluation of melanoma and other choroidal tumors, and aspiration of the vitreous should be avoided in these cases.

For vitrectomy specimens, surgeons are advised to submit as much vitreous as can be safely removed for complete analysis. The entire vitrectomy cassette or fluid collection bag should be submitted to aid in this. This should be done expeditiously because the contents are not fixed and the cells can degenerate rapidly. This is another instance in which the presurgical coordination with the pathologist is critical. If submission of the specimen needs to be delayed briefly, the entire cassette and sample can be placed in the refrigerator. Vitreous

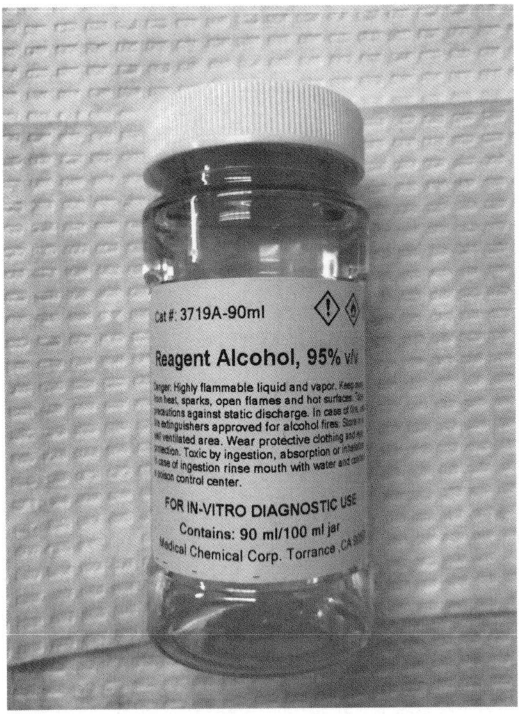

Fig. 10. Vitreous specimens obtained on the weekends, when the laboratory is closed, or when otherwise subject to delay, may be fixed by the surgeon by transferring the vitreous fluid into a container with an equal volume of 95% alcohol or 10% formalin. It is best to check with the laboratory as to which is their preferred fixative.

specimens obtained on the weekends, when the laboratory is closed, or when otherwise subject to delayed processing can be fixed by the surgeon by transferring the vitreous fluid into a container with an equal volume of neutral buffered formaldehyde or 95% alcohol (Fig. 10), if available. Alternative options include placing the vitreous specimen in culture medium (eg, bovine serum albumin) or in a mild cytofixative, such as herpes glutamic acid buffer-mediated organic solvent protection effect (HOPE) fixation or Cytolyt (Cytyc) for subsequent thin-prep slide preparation by the pathologist [2,37–39].

The diagnosis of primary intraocular lymphoma is made by cytologic analysis of vitrectomy specimens. Although ocular tissue can be obtained through vitreous aspiration; aqueous aspiration; external chorioretinal biopsy; or transvitreal, transretinal, or chorioretinal biopsy, a diagnostic vitrectomy is the preferred method and considered the gold standard [31,34,40,41]. Immunohistochemical study of cell markers, flow cytometry, or gene amplification studies (PCR) can be performed on vitreous specimens, though the standard method of diagnosis is cytology [1,42,43]. A standard 3-port pars plana vitrectomy is preferred for obtaining specimens for lymphoma evaluation; a complete core vitrectomy is recommended whenever possible. An initial core vitreous specimen of approximately 1 to 2 mL should be obtained at the start of the case. The specimen should be delivered fresh and/or in saline, or, if available, placed into a tube containing RPMI culture medium (20 mL) (see Fig. 7) to prevent cell death and taken immediately to an awaiting cytologist or pathologist for processing. Time is of the essence because lymphoma cells will rapidly degenerate [31,40,43,44].

Focus points

- If suspicion of infectious cause exists, submit material for microbiology (culture, PCR–molecular testing) before placing the specimen in any fixative.
- If lymphoma is suspected, fresh tissue should be placed in a closed container with a piece of saline-moistened gauze, and submitted expeditiously, preferably not on nights and weekends.
- For vitrectomy specimens, submit as much vitreous as can be safely removed. This should be done expeditiously, and in coordination with a pathologist who will rapidly evaluate the specimen.

SUMMARY

In summary, to optimize the surgeon-to-pathologist specimen handoff and minimize errors, clear communication between the surgeon and the pathology laboratory is a priority and should be considered a critical clinical step for any ocular oncologist before a biopsy is completed. Streamlining this process can eliminate substantial burdens, including a delay in diagnosis and treatment, as well as possible additional procedures for the patient. As techniques continue to evolve and as liquid biopsies and noninvasive diagnoses become more prevalent, these guidelines may change; however, a tenet unlikely to change in oncology is the clear mandate for open, active communication between the surgeon and pathologist.

References

[1] Rosa RH Jr. Basic and clinical science course (BCSC) section 4: ophthalmic pathology and intraocular tumors. San Francisco (CA): American Academy of Ophthalmology; 2014-2015. p. 3–326.
[2] Eagle RC Jr. Eye pathology: an atlas and text. Philadelphia: Lippincott Williams & Wilkins; 2016. p. 1–384. Available at: https://market.android.com/details?id.book-KxYRD-QAAQBAJ. Accessed May 9, 2019.
[3] Lott R, Tunnicliffe J, Sheppard E, et al. Pre-microscopic examination specimen handling guidelines in the surgical pathology laboratory. Northfield (IL): College of American Pathologists (CAP) and National Society for Histotechnology Published by HistoQIP; 2014. p. 1–49.
[4] Makary MA, Epstein J, Pronovost PJ, et al. Surgical specimen identification errors: a new measure of quality in surgical care. Surgery 2007;141(4):450–5.
[5] Ford AL, Mudhar HS, Farr R, et al. The ophthalmic pathology cut-up–part 2. Curr Diagn Pathol 2005;11(5):340–8.
[6] Rishi P, Dhami A, Biswas J. Biopsy techniques for intraocular tumors. Indian J Ophthalmol 2016;64(6):415–21.
[7] Augsburger JJ, Shields JA. Fine needle aspiration biopsy of solid intraocular tumors: indications, instrumentation and techniques. Ophthalmic Surg 1984;15(1):34–40. Available at: https://www.ncbi.nlm.nih.gov/pubmed/6700944.
[8] Singh AD, Biscotti CV. Fine needle aspiration biopsy of ophthalmic tumors. Saudi J Ophthalmol 2012;26(2):117–23.
[9] Shields CL, Shields JA. Tumors of the conjunctiva and cornea. Surv Ophthalmol 2004;49(1):3–24.
[10] Shields CL. Conjunctival melanoma: risk factors for recurrence, exenteration, metastasis, and death in 150 consecutive patients. Arch Ophthalmol 2000;118(11):1497.
[11] Spinak M, Friedman AH. Squamous cell carcinoma of the conjunctiva. Value of exfoliative cytology in diagnosis. Surv Ophthalmol 1977;21(4):351–5.
[12] Buuns DR, Tse DT, Folberg R. Microscopically controlled excision of conjunctival squamous cell carcinoma. Am J Ophthalmol 1994;117(1):97–102.
[13] Sudesh S, Rapuano CJ, Cohen EJ, et al. Surgical management of ocular surface squamous neoplasms: the experience from a cornea center. Cornea 2000;19(3):278–83. Available at: https://www.ncbi.nlm.nih.gov/pubmed/10832683.
[14] Bailey D. Tissue pathways for non-neoplastic ophthalmic pathology specimens. 2015. Available at: http://eyepath.org.uk/wp-content/uploads/2015/09/G141_TPOphthalmicPathology_Feb15.pdf. Accessed December 10, 2018.
[15] Chévez-Barrios P. Frozen section diagnosis and indications in ophthalmic pathology. Arch Pathol Lab Med 2005;129(12):1626–34.
[16] Mohs FE. Chemosurgery: microscopically controlled surgery for skin cancer. Springfield (IL): Charles C. Thomas Publisher; 1978. p. 378. Available at: https://books.google.com/books/about/Chemosurgery.html?hl.&id.CGZsAAAAMAAJ. Accessed May 9, 2019.
[17] Mohs FE. Micrographic surgery for the microscopically controlled excision of eyelid cancers. Arch Ophthalmol 1986;104(6):901–9. Available at: https://www.ncbi.nlm.nih.gov/pubmed/3718316.
[18] Mohs FE. Micrographic surgery for the microscopically controlled excision of eyelid cancer: history and development. Adv Ophthalmic Plast Reconstr Surg 1986;5:381–408. Available at: https://www.ncbi.nlm.nih.gov/pubmed/3331920.

[19] Conway RM. Surgery for primary basal cell carcinoma including the eyelid margins with intraoperative frozen section control: comparative interventional study with a minimum clinical follow up of 5 years. Br J Ophthalmol 2004;88(2):236–8.
[20] Dzubow LM. Sebaceous carcinoma of the eyelid: treatment with Mohs surgery. J Dermatol Surg Oncol 1985;11(1):40–4.
[21] Spencer JM, Nossa R, Tse DT, et al. Sebaceous carcinoma of the eyelid treated with Mohs micrographic surgery. J Am Acad Dermatol 2001;44(6):1004–9.
[22] Callahan EF, Appert DL, Roenigk RK, et al. Sebaceous carcinoma of the eyelid: a review of 14 cases. Dermatol Surg 2004;30(8):1164–8.
[23] Spencer WH. Ophthalmic pathology: an atlas and textbook. Philadelphia: Saunders; 1996. p. 3044. Available at: https://books.google.com/books/about/Ophthalmic_Pathology.html?hl=&id=lrhsAAAAMAAJ. Accessed May 9, 2019.
[24] Ford AL, Mudhar HS, Farr R, et al. The ophthalmic pathology cut-up—part 1: the enucleation and exenteration specimen. Curr Diagn Pathol 2005;11(4):284–90.
[25] Torczynski E. Preparation of ocular specimens for histopathologic examination. Ophthalmology 1981;88(12):1367–71. Available at: https://www.ncbi.nlm.nih.gov/pubmed/7033857.
[26] Lee WR. Examination of the Globe. Technical Aspects. In: Lee WR, editor. Ophthalmic histopathology. London, England: Springer; 2002. p. 1–33.
[27] Shields CL, Shields PW, Manalac J, et al. Review of cystic and solid tumors of the iris. Oman J Ophthalmol 2013;6(3):159–64.
[28] Gokhale R, Medina CA, Biscotti CV, et al. Diagnostic fine-needle aspiration biopsy for iris melanoma. Asia Pac J Ophthalmol (Phila) 2015;4(2):89–91.
[29] Grossniklaus HE. Fine-needle aspiration biopsy of the iris. Arch Ophthalmol 1992;110(7):969–76. Available at: https://www.ncbi.nlm.nih.gov/pubmed/1637283.
[30] Matthews BJ, Mudhar HS, Rennie IG. Trans-corneal fine cannula aspiration: Rycroft cannula aspiration technique for sampling iris tumours. Br J Ophthalmol 2012;96(3):329–31.
[31] Gonzales JA, Chan C-C. Biopsy techniques and yields in diagnosing primary intraocular lymphoma. Int Ophthalmol 2007;27(4):241–50.
[32] Coupland SE, Joussen A, Anastassiou G, et al. Diagnosis of a primary uveal extranodal marginal zone B-cell lymphoma by chorioretinal biopsy: case report. Graefes Arch Clin Exp Ophthalmol 2004;243(5):482–6.
[33] Aronow ME, Portell CA, Sweetenham JW, et al. Uveal lymphoma: clinical features, diagnostic studies, treatment selection, and outcomes. Ophthalmology 2014;121(1):334–41.
[34] Sen HN, Nida Sen H, Bodaghi B, et al. Primary intraocular lymphoma: diagnosis and differential diagnosis. Ocul Immunol Inflamm 2009;17(3):133–41.
[35] Singh AD, Dolan B, Biscotti CV. Future of ophthalmic fine needle aspiration biopsy. In: Vielh P, editor. Monographs in clinical cytology Vol. 21. Basel, Switzerland: Karger Publishers; 2011. p. 90–6.
[36] Ali MJ, Honavar SG, Vemuganti GK, et al. Fine needle aspiration biopsy of retinal tumors. In: Vielh P, editor. Monographs in clinical cytology Vol. 21. Basel, Switzerland: Karger Publishers; 2011. p. 72–81.
[37] Asencio-Duran M, Vallejo-Garcia JL, Pastora-Salvador N, et al. Vitreous diagnosis in neoplastic diseases. Mediators Inflamm 2012;2012:930704.
[38] Coupland SE. Vitreous biopsy: specimen preparation and interpretation. Monogr Clin Cytol 2012;21:61–71.
[39] Coupland SE, Perez-Canto A, Hummel M, et al. Assessment of HOPE fixation in vitrectomy specimens in patients with chronic bilateral uveitis (masquerade syndrome). Graefes Arch Clin Exp Ophthalmol 2005;243(9):847–52.
[40] Whitcup SM, de Smet MD, Rubin BI, et al. Intraocular lymphoma. Clinical and histopathologic diagnosis. Ophthalmology 1993;100(9):1399–406.

[41] Peterson K, Gordon KB, Heinemann MH, et al. The clinical spectrum of ocular lymphoma. Cancer 1993;72(3):843–9.
[42] Coupland SE, Hummel M, Müller H-H, et al. Molecular analysis of immunoglobulin genes in primary intraocular lymphoma. Invest Ophthalmol Vis Sci 2005;46(10): 3507–14.
[43] Levy-Clarke GA, Chan C-C, Nussenblatt RB. Diagnosis and management of primary intraocular lymphoma. Hematol Oncol Clin North Am 2005;19(4):739–49.
[44] Whitcup SM, Chan CC, Buggage RR, et al. Improving the diagnostic yield of vitrectomy for intraocular lymphoma. Arch Ophthalmol 2000;118(3):446. Available at: https://www.ncbi.nlm.nih.gov/pubmed/10721983.

Section IV: Cataract & Refractive Surgery

Advances in Ophthalmology and Optometry 4 (2019) 147–157

ADVANCES IN OPHTHALMOLOGY AND OPTOMETRY

The Flanged Intrascleral Intraocular Lens Fixation with Double-Needle Technique

The Yamane Technique

Madeleine Hasbrook, MD[a], David A. Crandall, MD[a,b,*]

[a]Department of Ophthalmology, Henry Ford Health System, 2799 West Grand Boulevard, Detroit, MI 48202, USA; [b]John Moran Eye Center, University of Utah, 65 Mario East Capecchi Drive, Salt Lake City, UT 84132, USA

Keywords

• Scleral-fixated intraocular lens • Yamane • Aphakia • Secondary intraocular lens

Key points

- Inadequate capsular support is a challenge both anterior and posterior segment surgeons encounter not infrequently. The flanged intrascleral intraocular lens fixation with double-needle technique is a novel approach to managing this.
- Several modifications have been made to increase the efficiency and ease of the surgery. With care taken during each step of the surgery, complications are low and visual outcomes high.
- The simplicity of the technique and readily available instruments make this surgery good for both first-world everyday surgery and surgical missions.

INTRODUCTION

Placement of an intraocular lens (IOL) in the capsular bag has long been considered the most reliable method for achieving optimal surgical outcomes, both refractive and anatomic. If during cataract extraction a break occurs in the posterior capsule, a sulcus-implanted 3-piece lens often is able to achieve the desired result [1]. For this most of the anterior capsule is required to be intact and sufficiently supported by the lens zonules. This support often is

The authors have nothing to disclose.

*Corresponding author. 2799 West Grand Boulevard, Detroit, MI 48202. *E-mail address:* Dcranda1@hfhs.org

https://doi.org/10.1016/j.yaoo.2019.04.008

absent in patients who have experienced ocular trauma, disorders of zonular weakness (eg, pseudoexfoliation, Ehlers-Danlos syndrome, Marfan syndrome, homocystinuria, hyperlysinemia, sulfite oxidase, retinitis pigmentosa, etc.), planned intracapsular cataract extraction, or suffered complications during cataract surgery, requiring the surgeons to have other techniques available in their surgical armament [2–6].

Currently, the surgical options for eyes that lack adequate capsular support include anterior chamber intraocular lenses (ACIOLs), iris-fixated intraocular lenses (IFIOLs), and scleral-fixated intraocular lenses (SFIOLs). ACIOLs classically had a poor reputation due to the high incidence of pseudophakic bullous keratopathy, chronic iritis, and pigment dispersion. This was in large part because of the original closed-loop design [7]. The arrival of ACIOLs with opened loops minimized these risks by decreasing contact with ocular tissue. This combined with the relatively reduced operating time, make ACIOLs attractive [8]. However, the commonly available PMMA ACIOLs do require large sclerocorneal incisions for insertion. IFIOLs lack some of the ease of surgical technique seen with ACIOLs and have pseudophacodonesis, pigment dispersion, chronic iritis, peripheral anterior synechia formation, and pupillary distortion as potential complications [9].

Multiple surgical techniques for SFIOLs have been developed to place IOLs in more anatomically correct position in the eye. These are placed in either the sulcus or the pars plana. SFIOLs can be secured with or without sutures, as well as with glue. Sutured SFIOLs tend to have good outcomes but have some inherent risks including suture breakage with lens dislocation and suture knot erosion with increased risk of endophthalmitis [10,11]. Some of these complications have been ameliorated with the switch to thicker sutures, such as polytetrafluoroethylene and burying suture under scleral flaps, in sclerotomies or in scleral pockets [12–14]. Other complications include lens dislocation, lens tilt, vitreous hemorrhage, and retinal detachment [15].

To avoid some of the potential pitfalls of sutures, several surgeons have found ways to perform sutureless scleral fixation, including using glue [15–18]. One of these techniques is the sutureless 27-gauge needle-guided intrascleral IOL implantation with lamellar scleral dissection described by Yamane and colleagues [19]. After 10-year follow-up in 35 eyes, no cases of retinal detachment, endophthalmitis, IOL dislocation, or vitreous hemorrhage occurred. The technique described in this article is Yamane's modification of his original technique.

The advantages of the flanged intrascleral IOL fixation with double-needle technique (a.k.a. the Yamane technique) lie in its simplicity and lack of specialized equipment. It avoids the potential risk of suture or glue-related complications. The smallest available gauge is used, which reduces the risk of postoperative hypotony. Peritomies and scleral flaps are not required. Although others have used small-gauged instruments to create sclerotomies, the Yamane technique was the first to secure the lens by merely fashioning a flange.

TECHNIQUE

The technique as first described by Yamane and colleagues began with a 25-gauge or 27-gauge pars plana vitrectomy under retrobulbar anesthesia. For subluxed crystalline lenses, phacoemulsification cataract was performed. Dislocated IOLs made of soft material were cut and removed through an approximately 3.0-mm sclerocorneal incision, whereas polymethyl methacrylate IOLs were removed through 6.00-mm sclerocorneal incisions. A 3-piece IOL was inserted into the anterior chamber using an injector. The trailing haptic was intentionally kept externally to prevent IOL from falling posteriorly into the vitreous cavity.

A tunneled sclerotomy 2 mm in length was made through conjunctiva 2 mm posterior to the surgical limbus (Fig. 1), angled posteriorly 15° following the angle of the haptics. Intraocular forceps through a conveniently placed paracentesis then were used to thread the leading haptic into the lumen of the needle. The second sclerotomy was made 180° away in similar fashion to the first but following the direction of the trailing haptic. The forceps again were used through the paracentesis to thread the trailing haptic into the needle lumen (Fig. 2). Once both haptics were secured, they were externalized by simultaneous removal of the needles. The tips of the haptics then were cauterized with a handheld low-temperature cautery to make a mushroom-shaped flange with a diameter of about 0.3 mm (Fig. 3). The flange of the haptics was pushed back into the scleral tunnels, effectively securing the lens in position. Finally, after miosis was induced, a peripheral iridotomy was performed with the vitrectomy cutter to prevent iris capture of the IOL [20].

CONSIDERATIONS FOR LENS CHOICE

The X-70 (Santen, Osaka, Japan) Tecnis ZA9003 (Abbott Medical Optics, Santa Ana, CA, USA), PN6A (Kowa, Tokyo, Japan), and MA60MA (Alcon

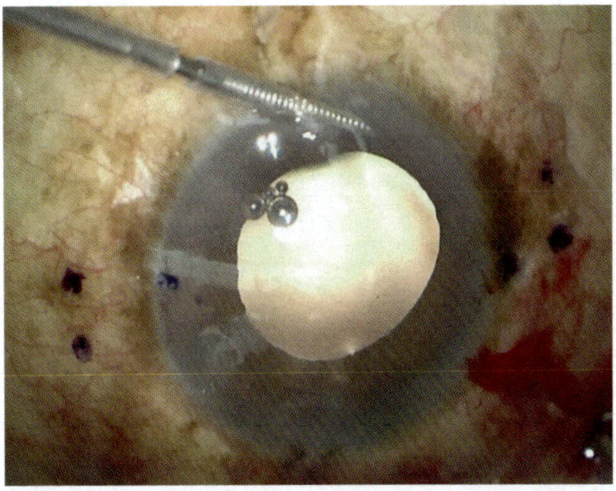

Fig. 1. Conjunctival markings for the needle passes 2 mm posterior to the limbus with guiding marks for the conjunctival and scleral entry point (more counterclockwise mark for each side) and the point for entry into the posterior chamber (more clockwise mark for each side).

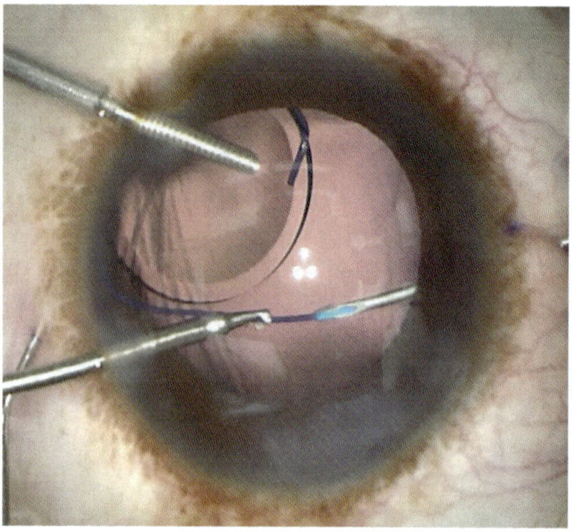

Fig. 2. Feeding the second haptic into the needle. Note significant displacement of the lens during the process, with the first haptic held in place within the needle to the left of the screen.

Laboratories, Inc, Fort Worth, TX, USA) were all the lenses used in the original Yamane technique paper. Although most 3-piece IOLs can be used in this technique, it is important to confirm that the haptic can be inserted into the needle being used (the diameter of the haptic must be smaller than the diameter of the needle lumen). Furthermore, one must ensure the flange can be created with heating element. A lower rate of iris capture did occur when IOLs with an optic diameter of 7 mm was used compared with an optic diameter of 6 mm (2.0% vs 14%) [20].

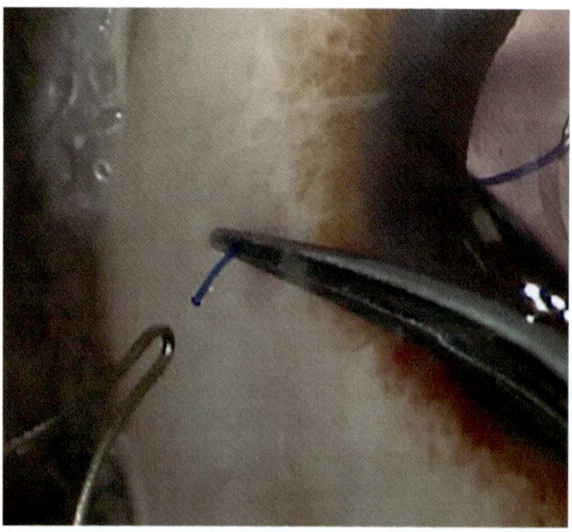

Fig. 3. Haptic bulb after cautery. The cautery should be brought near the haptic, but not make contact with it.

The material of the lens haptic may make a difference in the difficulty of the surgery. A few categories of material exist: poly(methylmethacrylate), polyimide (Elastimide), polypropylene (Prolene), and polyvinylidene fluoride (PVDF). Of these, PVDF is the more malleable and resists breaking better than the other listed options.

When learning the technique, it is recommended to use lenses with PVDF haptics, as these are very robust and are more tolerant to excess manipulation. Lenses with polyimide haptics are not recommended, as these become increasingly brittle and prone to breakage.

CONSIDERATION FOR NEEDLE CHOICE

The TSK ultrathin wall needle (Tochigi Seiko, Tochigi, Japan) was the needle used when the Yamane technique was originally described. The lumen of this needle is 0.2 mm versus a normal 30-gauge needle with an inner diameter of 0.14 mm. The haptic diameter of most available 3-piece IOLs range from 0.14 mm to 0.17 mm. Although the lumen of a 27-gauge needle would be sufficiently large enough to accommodate most haptics, the outer diameter is about 0.4 mm, which requires a larger flange [20].

OUTCOMES AND COMPARISON

Yamane reported a significant improvement in best-corrected visual acuity 36 months following surgery: logMAR 0.25 $\pm$ 0.49 before surgery to 0.04 $\pm$ 0.25 36 months following surgery. The angle of tilt of the IOL was measured by swept-source optical coherence tomography 3 months following surgery in both the vertical and horizontal positions. The reported mean lens tilt was $3.4^\circ \pm 2.5^\circ$ [20]. These outcomes show that this method provides excellent postoperative visual potential.

COMPLICATIONS

The overall complication rate reported by Yamane was low. Iris capture was by far the most common complication at 8%. In their analysis of this, they found no difference in lens tilt or IOL position between eyes with iris capture versus eyes without. The investigators, however, did find a difference in the mean patient age between the 2 groups; with younger patients (52.4 $\pm$ 11.4 years) demonstrating iris capture more frequently than older patients (68.5 $\pm$ 12.7 years; $P < .001$). The investigators felt younger patients had more movement to their iris inducing pupillary block, and while all patients received peripheral iridectomies at the time of surgery, some may have been ineffectively small. The iris capture was treated successfully with a mydriatic agent in 1 eye and 30-gauge needle in 7 eyes. In the 5 eyes in which the iris-capture recurred, a miotic agent was used for prophylaxis [20].

Other complications included vitreous hemorrhage (5%), elevation of intraocular pressure (IOP) (3%), postoperative hypotony (2%), transient corneal edema (1%), and cystoid macular edema (1%). Two of the eyes with elevated IOP experienced it postoperatively. The third eye developed pigment dispersion 18 months following surgery. Neither of the 2 eyes with hypotony had leaking from the 30-gauge sclerotomies, but rather had leaks from the vitrectomy sclerotomy or sclerocorneal wound. No incidence occurred of retinal detachment, endophthalmitis, or, most impressively, lens dislocation [20].

TIPS AND TROUBLESHOOTING

- The 30-gauge sclerotomy should be placed 90° away from the wound through which the IOL is inserted. This provides the optimal initial position of the leading haptic for threading into the needle.
- Using a toric marker and calipers to mark the conjunctiva aids in ensuring proper final position of the IOL, reducing tilt, or decentration. It also reduces risk of entering too posterior and puncturing the retina or too anterior and causing pigment dispersion or uveitis-glaucoma-hyphema (UGH) syndrome.
- Alternatively, intraoperative toric markers (eg, ORA, Callisto) can be used to insure the sclerotomies are 180° apart.
- Before inserting the needles, test the haptics within the needle lumens. Small size differences in the diameter of either the haptic or the needle lumen can be enough to prevent proper placement.
- The needle is bent with the bevel-up to easily engage the haptic. The bend in the needle should be long enough to be able to reach the haptic inside the eye, typically 5 to 6 mm from the end of the needle. Needles without bends tend to slide more inside the eye, potentially injuring intraocular structures, and are more difficult to keep at an appropriate angle, especially in patients with deep orbits. The needle is ideally bent less than 60°. Further bending can lead to the hub of the needle rolling forward and impeding the view.
- Have balanced salt solution fluid within the needle and syringe to avoid bubbles coming through the needle and impeding view.
- Before inserting the needles, loosen the connection between the needle and syringe to avoid excess manipulation removing the syringe.
- While making the tunnels and manipulating the lens in the eye, having continuous irrigation either through an anterior chamber maintainer or through a posterior infusion pressurizes the eye and reduces resistance.
- Both haptics should be within the needle lumens before attempting externalization. Externalizing the leading haptic before threading the trailing haptic will cause the IOL to rotate and make placement of the second haptic significantly more difficult.
- When removing the needles to externalize the haptics, be careful to remove along the original needle tracts. This is especially important if removing the haptics simultaneously as one of the haptics can easily become dislodged from the lumen of the needle and slip back into the eye.
- Only minimal cautery is required to create the flange. Too much cautery may shorten one haptic and cause lens decentration. Too little cautery would not produce the ideal 0.3 mm flange. Marking the haptics with a caliber may reduce likelihood of unequal haptic lengths. A tendency exists to make a larger than necessary flange when learning the technique, for fear that the haptics will slide into the sclera if the flange is too small.
- Be sure the conjunctiva is reapproximated and the flange is pushed in flush with the sclera to reduce risk of haptic exposure.
- Either superior or temporal surgeon approach is acceptable.

MODIFICATIONS

There have been several modifications to the Yamane technique in the short time since it was first reported.

- Trailing-haptic-first
  - The most difficult part of the procedure as originally described is securing the second haptic. Once the first haptic is fixated in the needle lumen, the second haptic is less mobile and often even out of view. Aggressive manipulation can cause deformation and even breakage of the haptics.
  - One modification has the surgeon make a paracentesis 180° away from the IOL incision and externalize the leading haptic through it with the aid of intraocular forceps (Fig. 4). The trailing haptic then is thread into the needle lumen with forceps [21].
  - This modification benefits most of the surgeons by allowing them to use their nondominant left hand first for placing the trailing haptic into the right needle while the leading haptic is safely outside the eye. Their right hand then can guide the second, more challenging haptic into the left needle.
- Externalizing one needle at a time.
  - Timing and skill are required to simultaneously remove both needles without dislodging one of the haptics or causing lens tilt.
  - After placing both haptics in the needle lumens, externalize one needle first, grasp the externalized haptic with tiers, and immediately cauterize the tip. Repeat for the second haptic.
  - It is important to ensure the haptics are firmly inserted in the needle lumens, so they are not dislodged during externalization.
- Inject leading haptic into needle lumen
  - Kim also described having the leading haptic directly into the needle lumen on the left with the aid of a surgical assistant.

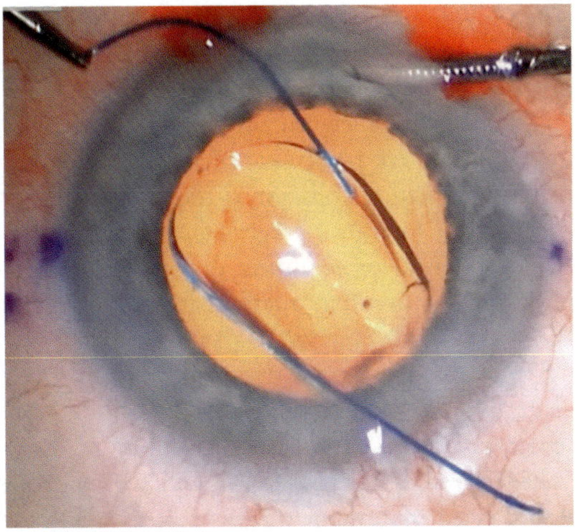

Fig. 4. Externalization of the leading haptic to place the trailing haptic first.

   - This reduces extra manipulation in the eye [22].
- Multiple companies are currently designing guides for correct placement of the needles.

CLINICAL SIGNIFICANCE

The Yamane technique is a simple yet effective way to correct aphakia and manage patients without adequate anterior capsular support. Once mastered, it can be performed relatively quickly through a standard cataract wound. Two thin-walled needles, high-temperature cautery, and intraocular forceps are the only nonstandard instruments required outside a cataract set. Furthermore, this technique has good potential for several particularly challenging surgical dilemmas.

No consensus exists for the optimal surgical management in aphakic children and children who lack capsular support. These cases often are managed with spectacles and aphakic contact lenses. In unilateral cases, however, anisometropia may make spectacles unreasonable; in addition, contact lenses may be intolerable for some patients. For this reason, some surgeons have explored SFIOLs. In one study 25 eyes with sutured SFIOL using 10 to 0 polypropylene sutures under scleral flaps were observed for 81.1 ± 46.2 months. Of these eyes 12 had greater than 1 Snellen line improvement, but 1 developed late endophthalmitis and late IOL dislocation due to breakage of polypropylene sutures after 7 to 10 years in 6 eyes (24%) [23]. Recently sutureless scleral tunnel IOL fixation, modified from a technique described by Prenner and colleagues [24], was performed in 10 eyes of 7 patients suffering from several lenticular disorders postoperative IOL subluxation, dislocation, decentration, iris capture, postoperative retinal detachment, corneal decompensation, endophthalmitis, or cystoid macular edema, although the maximum available follow-up was only 24 months for only 1 patient [25]. Theoretically the Yamane technique will provide a stable, long-term implant for these patients without risk of exposure or dislocation. Longitudinal studies are required.

The Yamane technique is beneficial in patients withglaucoma. Patient conditions that may lead to alternative placement of an IOL often have glaucoma as a comorbidity, including pseudoexfoliation syndrome, trauma, and vitrectomized eyes. For the glaucoma specialist, conjunctiva is sacred and should be preserved at all cost if a filtering or shunting procedure is required. With the Yamane technique there is minimal manipulation of the conjunctiva with only a 30-gauge needle wound. A glaucoma specialist easily can adjust his or surgical location, given that such a small area superiorly is taken. Furthermore, with the lens placed in a more anatomically correct position, a tube from a glaucoma drainage device easily can be placed in the anterior chamber, sulcus, or vitreous cavity, although the latter 2 still require a thorough vitrectomy. Finally, given the posterior placement of the lens, uveitis-glaucoma-hyphema syndrome, a severe complication in patients with already tenuous optic nerves, is much less likely to occur.

SUMMARY

The flanged intrascleral IOL fixation with double-needle technique (a.k.a. the Yamane technique) has not necessarily revolutionized SFIOLs but has simplified it significantly. Several techniques are available for SFIOLs, both sutured and sutureless techniques. Advantages and disadvantages exist to each technique. The Yamane technique allows for very efficient, safe lens placement with minimal special instrumentation. It can be performed primarily or with a dislocated three-piece lens that is already in the eye. This is a surgery that, in the right situations, can comfortably be performed by both anterior segment and posterior segment surgeons.

When performing this technique a few steps are required to be successful, several of which occur before even getting into the operating room. A few nonstandard pieces of equipment are required, including high-temperature cautery, anterior chamber irrigators, and thin-walled 30-gauge needles. Also, few surgical centers stock the Zeiss Lucia 3-piece lens, the best-suited lens for the procedure. It is important to be sure to have the necessary equipment along with backups in the operating room. Although simple, this surgical technique is precise, and substitutions may not lead to the desired outcome.

Unlike standard cataract extraction with phacoemulsification, the surgeon should consider having the patient discontinue any anticoagulation before surgery, if it is safe to do so. Although vitreous hemorrhage was rare in Yamane's original report, intraoperative vitreous hemorrhage during needle placement can complicate a straightforward surgery and even prevent the surgeon from completing the surgery. If hemorrhage does occur intraoperatively, elevating the intraocular pressure briefly may tamponade the hemorrhage. Remember it is always safer to live to fight another day if the view becomes too difficult to safely proceed.

Intraoperatively, the same care should be taken as with all microsurgery. A well-structured corneal wound helps maintain the anterior chamber while working inside the eye. A thorough anterior vitrectomy prevents traction on the hyaloids while manipulating the lens and needles posterior to the iris. Consistently measuring sclerotomy placement with calipers helps prevent lens tilt. Standardized surgical kits with equipment to aid in making perfectly angled sclerotomies currently are being designed, which will aid the surgeon in achieving reproducible outcomes. This along with surgeons continuing to share their experiences will make this innovative surgery more approachable and successful.

A very exciting benefit to the Yamane technique is in the area of outreach ophthalmology. In the outreach setting, options are limited in complicated cases with loss of capsule support or when intracapsular surgery has been performed. Either a patient will be left aphakic in a place with no resources for spectacle or contact lens correction or an anterior chamber lens will be placed; this potentially puts the patient at risk for long-term complications with limited resources and ability to correct them. It also requires the outreach team to have a consignment of anterior chamber lenses in addition to their regular lenses, which is especially difficult in remote settings. Outreach teams often are limited by space and weight for the equipment they can bring, so the range of sizes and powers of anterior chamber lenses will necessarily be limited, if available at all. The more remote the setting, the more severe these restrictions become. Before the Yamane technique, a three-piece lens could be placed in the capsular bag, in the sulcus, or fixated to the iris. With Yamane, now the 3-piece lens can be fixated to the sclera, which allows a team to travel with only a single type of lens, which simplifies planning and leaves space for other equipment or allows the team to offer care to patients in more remote areas.

References

[1] Dubey R, Birchall W, Grigg J. Improved refractive outcome for ciliary sulcus-implanted intraocular lenses. Ophthalmology 2012;119:261–5.
[2] Ascaso FJ, Huerva V, Grzybowski A. Epidemiology, etiology, and prevention of late IOL-capsular bag complex dislocation: review of the literature. J Ophthalmol 2015;2015:805706.
[3] Pascal D. Pathophysiology of zonular disease. Curr Opin Ophthalmol 2008;19:27–30.
[4] Hoffman RS, Snyder ME, Devgan U, et al. Management of the subluxated crystalline lens. J Cataract Refract Surg 2013;39:1904–15.
[5] Jehan FS, Mamalis N, Crandall AS. Spontaneous late dislocation of intraocular lens within the capsular bag in pseudoexfoliation patients. Ophthalmology 2001;108:1727–31.
[6] Zarbin M, Chu D, Por YM, et al. Diagnostic and surgical techniques of intraocular lens suspension in the absence of capsular/zonular support. Surv Ophthalmol 2005;50(5):429–62.
[7] Smith PW, Wong SK, Stark WJ, et al. Complications of semiflexible, closed-loop anterior chamber intraocular lenses. Arch Ophthalmol 1987;105(1):52–7.
[8] Wagoner MD, Cox TA, Ariyasu RG, et al. Ophthalmic technology assessment intraocular lens implantation in the absence of capsular support a report by the American Academy of Ophthalmology. Ophthalmology 2003;110:840–59.
[9] Michaeli A, Soiberman U, Loewenstein A. Outcome of iris fixation of subluxated intraocular lenses. Graefes Arch Clin Exp Ophthalmol 2012;250(9):1327–32.
[10] Zarbin M, Chu D, Por YM, et al. Techniques of intraocular lens suspension in the absence of capsular/zonular support. Surv Ophthalmol 2005;50(5):429–62.
[11] Heilskov T, Joondeph BC, Olsen KR, et al. Late endophthalmitis after transscleral fixation of a posterior chamber intraocular lens. Arch Ophthalmol 1989;107(10):1427.
[12] Mansukhani SA, Barkmeier AJ, Bakri SJ, et al. The risk of primary open-angle glaucoma following vitreoretinal surgery-a population-based study. Am J Ophthalmol 2018;193:143–55.
[13] Hoffman RS, Fine IH, Packer M. Scleral fixation without conjunctival dissection. J Cataract Refract Surg 2006;32(11):1907–12.
[14] Kir E, Kocaturk T, Dayanir V, et al. Prevention of suture exposure in transscleral intraocular lens fixation: an original technique. Can J Ophthalmol 2008;43(6):707–11.
[15] Stem MS, Todorich B, Woodward MA, et al. Scleral-fixated intraocular lenses: past and present. J Vitreoretin Dis 2017;1(2):144–52.
[16] Agarwal A, Kumar DA, Jacob S, et al. Fibrin glue-assisted sutureless posterior chamber intraocular lens implantation in eyes with deficient posterior capsules. J Cataract Refract Surg 2008;34(9):1433–8.
[17] Dajee KP, Abbey AM, Williams GA. Management of dislocated intraocular lenses in eyes with insufficient capsular support. Curr Opin Ophthalmol 2016;27(3):191–5.
[18] Todorich B, Stem MS, Kooragayala K, et al. Structural analysis and comprehensive surgical outcomes of the sutureless intrascleral fixation of secondary intraocular lenses in human eyes. Retina 2018;38(Suppl 1):S31–40.

[19] Yamane S, Inoue M, Arakawa A, et al. Sutureless 27-gauge needle-guided intrascleral intraocular lens implantation with lamellar scleral dissection. Ophthalmology 2014;121(1):61–6.

[20] Yamane S, Sato S, Maruyama-Inoue M, et al. Flanged intrascleral intraocular lens fixation with double-needle technique. Ophthalmology 2017;124:1136–42.

[21] Kim DB. Trailing-haptic-first modification of double-needle intrascleral haptic fixation technique. J Cataract Refract Surg 2018;44:424–8.

[22] Kim DB. The next big thing in scleral haptic fixation. Cataract and refractive surgery Today. 2017. Available at: https://crstoday.com/articles/2017-oct/the-next-big-thing-in-scleral-haptic-fixation/. Accessed May 24, 2019.

[23] Asadi R, Kheirkhah A. Long-term results of scleral fixation of posterior chamber intraocular lenses in children. Ophthalmology 2008;115(1):67–72.

[24] Prenner JL, Feiner L, Wheatley HM, et al. A novel approach for posterior chamber intraocular lens placement or rescue via a sutureless scleral fixation technique. Retina 2012;32(4):853–5.

[25] Walsh MK, Joshi M. Sutureless scleral tunnel intraocular lens fixation in the pediatric population. Retina 2014;34(4):807–11.

Advances in Ophthalmology and Optometry 4 (2019) 159–168

ADVANCES IN OPHTHALMOLOGY AND OPTOMETRY

Light-Adjustable Intraocular Lens

Kelly Williamson, MD

Drexel University College of Medicine, 219 N Broad Street 3rd Floor, Philadelphia, PA 19107, USA

Keywords

• Light-adjustable lens • Ultraviolet radiation • Cataract surgery • Emmetropia • Silicone macromers

Key points

- Refractive surprise after cataract surgery remains a top cause in patients requiring further invasive procedures postoperatively in order to achieve their visual goals.
- The RxSight Light Adjustable Lens uses silicone macromer technology and near-ultraviolet irradiation to noninvasively alter the shape of the intraocular lens (IOL) after implantation. This in turn results in predictable shifts in the refractive power of the lens.
- The Light-Adjustable Lens (LAL) has been shown to have good safety parameters and excellent outcomes in both animal models and in clinical use.
- The LAL can correct for small (up to about 2 diopters) residual myopia, hyperopia, and astigmatism and could even be adjusted to introduce multifocality or spherical aberration to IOLs after implantation.
- Certain limitations to the use of the LAL exist and may require consideration for future versions of the lens.

INTRODUCTION

Modern cataract surgery is a highly successful and safe procedure. As tools and techniques have been honed over the past few decades, surgeons have been able to focus more on achieving spectacle independence postoperatively. Improvements in the accuracy of intraocular lens (IOL) calculation formulae, biometry and intraoperative aberrometry, and IOL technology have allowed

The author has nothing to disclose.

E-mail address: kaw362@drexel.edu

https://doi.org/10.1016/j.yaoo.2019.04.009
2452-1760/19/

many surgeons to reach very high success rates for refractive targets. But despite a surgeon's best pre-, intra-, and postoperative efforts, still some patients have refractive outcomes different than predicted. For those patients, their options to achieve clear vision include spectacles or additional procedures, such as keratorefractive surgery or IOL addition or replacement. The recent approval of an IOL that can have its refractive power adjusted postoperatively introduces a new, noninvasive mechanism for correcting refractive surprise and achieving spectacle independence in patients without the financial and clinical burden of further surgical procedures. The Light Adjustable Lens (or LAL, RxSight, previously Calhoun Vision) is a silicone IOL that uses photosensitive molecule technology to adjust refractive power with the use of a near-ultraviolet (UV) light beam, which allows for refractive "touch-ups" to the IOL itself without modification of the cornea. The LAL was approved by the Food and Drug Administration (FDA) in the fall of 2017 [1]. Studies show that it can be a highly successful and safe tool to achieve emmetropia in cataract surgery patients. This article reviews the history, mechanism of action, safety, and clinical outcomes seen in the LAL and discusses potential uses and implications for cataract surgeons in the future.

History and mechanism of action

Several forms of modifiable IOL technologies have been suggested or prototyped over the past few years, as refractive accuracy has increased in priority for cataract surgeons. Multicomponent and mechanically adjustable IOLs have been suggested and some have even been implanted into patients with good results, but these technologies require a secondary surgical intraocular intervention to adjust the lens power. Intraocular lenses have been developed that can be noninvasively adjusted, such as a magnetically adjustable IOL and liquid crystal IOLs that can be adjusted using radiofrequency controllers, but the biocompatibility and appropriateness for intraocular use for these designs has yet to be fully evaluated [2,3]. The "holy grail" of modifiable IOL technology is a noninvasive, ideally repeatable or adjustable method by which to fine-tune the refractive power of the IOL after implantation. Both Alcon Laboratories, Inc, (Fort Worth, TX, USA) and Perfect Lens LLC (Aaren Scientific, Inc, Ontario, Canada) have developed IOLs that could be modified noninvasively with a femtosecond laser to change the refractive power of the lens. This technology holds significant promise, but it is still in the early stages of development and testing [2].

The RxSight (previously Calhoun Vision) LAL is the only modifiable IOL technology that has been FDA approved for commercial use in the United States. It also has been approved for use in the international community for about a decade. First conceptualized in 1996 by a team of researchers led by Daniel M. Schwartz, MD and Calhoun Vision, Inc, Pasadena, the LAL is a silicone IOL that can be adjusted using UV light after implantation into the eye. Silicone was the material of choice because of the ability of silicone molecules to diffuse in a polymer matrix at room temperature and because of the known biocompatibility of silicone, as it was already being used for implantable IOLs. The LAL uses a silicone matrix composed of polymer, resin, crosslinker, and platinum catalyst with photoreactive silicone macromers and UV absorbers conjugated therein. A benzoin-based photoinitiator is sensitive to light of 365 nm wavelength, which is in the near-UV spectrum. Irradiation of near-UV light to the silicone matrix results in photoactivation of the silicone macromers, which then polymerize. When the silicone macromers polymerize, macromers no longer exist at that part of the lens. This creates a diffusion gradient, resulting in diffusion of silicone macromers from nonirradiated portions of the lens into the irradiated zone. Over the course of 12 to 15 hours after irradiation, macromers diffuse into the irradiated zone and result in swelling of the lens at that site, thereby changing the refractive power of the lens. Irradiation of the central portion of an IOL results in central swelling of the lens, which increases the refractive power and corrects clinical hyperopia. Irradiation of the peripheral portion of the lens optic results in swelling of the periphery of the lens, making the IOL power more negative and correcting clinical myopia. Variations in size and location of the treatment zone and time of irradiation can result in correction of differing dioptric amounts of hyperopic or myopic correction. Irradiation in toric patterns can be used to correct for astigmatic error, and this technology has even been used to correct for higher-order aberrations and to introduce multifocality to the IOL. Once refractive correction is complete, a final "lock-in" procedure is required, which involves irradiation of the entire IOL optic to convert all silicone macromers into polymers, thereby preventing any further modifications to the shape and refractive power of the IOL [4].

As noted earlier, the IOL itself is a silicone foldable IOL that can be injected into the capsular bag similar to standard silicone IOLs on the market. It has a 6.0-mm optic with a posterior square edge and anterior round edge to minimize posterior capsular opacification. The 2 blue polymethyl methacrylate modified-C haptics result in an overall length of 13.0 mm. After insertion into the capsular bag in a standard fashion, patients are required to wear UV-blocking sunglasses for the initial 2 to 4 weeks postoperatively to prevent ambient irradiation of the IOL. After the eye has stabilized at 2 to 4 weeks, a refractive adjustment can be performed using a digital Light Delivery Device (LDD), which was developed in cooperation between Calhoun Vision and Carl Zeiss Meditec AG [2,4]. This is a slit lamp-mounted UV light delivery system that can irradiate the IOL in specific patterns to correct for myopic, hyperopic, and astigmatic refractive errors, reduce higher-order aberrations, and even introduce multifocality to the IOL [5,6]. One or more treatment sessions are applied to the IOL using this device based on refractive error of the eye at this time, sessions typically being under 120 seconds. After irradiation of the IOL to treat refractive error, the patient returns within 1 to 2 days. If the desired refractive outcomes are achieved, a "lock-in" treatment is then applied to the lens. As noted earlier, irradiation of the entire IOL optic during lock-in results in polymerization of all remaining macromers and stabilization of the refractive power of the lens [4].

During development, the lens underwent extensive testing to ensure biocompatibility and stability of the silicone matrix, both in the macromer and polymerized state, in vivo [4]. Studies in rabbit and cat eyes demonstrated no negative effects from the UV irradiation at the cornea or retina (these will be discussed later) [7–12]. The LAL and LDD were FDA approved for use in November of 2017 [1].

Safety of ultraviolet irradiation

A primary safety concern with the use of the LAL is that the postoperative adjustment and lock-in regimens require irradiation of the eye with UV light. Because of this, safety studies were performed in animal models before introduction to the market and in human eyes to determine the effect (if any) of this treatment on the radiation-sensitive tissues of the eye. Studies indicated that the irradiation required for adjustment and lock-in caused no significant toxicity to the eye and were appropriately safe for ocular administration. A newer model of the light-adjustable lens includes a 100-um silicone layer molded onto the posterior surface that contains a high concentration of UV-absorbing molecules in order to provide further protection to the retina from the irradiation required for adjustment and lock-in, but safety of direct UV irradiation to human eyes is still an important consideration [2,5].

The cornea is very sensitive to irradiation and is exposed to the highest doses of radiation from the LDD, so several safety studies have examined the effects on the structure and function of the cornea after LAL treatment and lock-in procedures. Studies during development of the lens evaluated changes in animal model corneas after irradiation at and above doses used with the LDD. Initial studies were done with rabbits with LALs implanted into the capsular bag. One group had irradiation performed with the LDD and a control group underwent lens implantation without radiation. On clinical and histopathologic analysis after implantation, no toxic effects from the lens or the irradiation were noted in the anterior or posterior segments of these rabbit eyes [4]. A similar study was done using cat eyes, because the ability of the endothelium in cats to recover from damage is more analogous to that seen in humans. In this study, cat eyes were irradiated with a UV light at a dose similar to that exposed to the human cornea during the lock-in procedure used with the LAL. The corneas were examined histopathologically at 1 day, 1 week, 1 month, and 3 months after irradiation and compared with eyes in a control group. A similar number of corneas in both the treatment and control groups were noted to have a few centrally located cells that showed signs of damage (staining with trypan blue), but these were felt to be due to folds in the corneas and on analysis were not found to be more prevalent in the treatment group compared with the control group [7].

A German group evaluated the effect of a maximal accepted level of near-UV treatment on human donor corneas and compared endothelial cell morphology and cell counts with human donor corneas that were exposed to white light only. Although this was a small study, no significant differences in cell count or morphology or the histologic presence of necrosis were observed between treatment and control corneas [8]. In 2011, the same group evaluated corneal changes in vivo in 122 eyes after surgery and LAL treatment and showed that change in corneal thickness and mean endothelial cell loss values at 1-year after surgery and treatment were similar to published data for phacoemulsification only [9]. A smaller study of 10 eyes from a group in Mexico also showed no difference in corneal endothelial health indicators 1 year after cataract surgery with LAL and near-UV treatment compared with those seen with standard phacoemulsification [10]. These studies, although small, demonstrate the safety of the levels of near-UV exposure required for adjustment and lock-in of the LAL for the corneal tissues.

UV light is known to cause damage to retinal cells, so it was important to evaluate potential retinal toxicity of the LAL treatment system. A study at the Moran Eye Institute compared the effects of near-UV treatment on the retinae of rabbits with one eye implanted with the LAL and the other eye implanted with a control IOL without a UV filter. The eyes were treated at up to 5 times the radiation level of the typical treatment dose and examined clinically and histopathologically for evidence of radiation damage. None of the eyes implanted with the LAL showed any clinical or histopathologic evidence of radiation damage to the retina, retinal pigment epithelium, or choroid. Three of the eyes in the control group showed areas of retinal and/or choroidal damage consistent with laser burn [11]. After introduction of the LAL to use in humans, a 2016 study was done to evaluate the effects of LAL treatment technology on macular structure and thickness. Macular optical coherence tomography was performed on patients preoperatively, postoperatively preadjustment, and at several time points up to 1 year after lock-in treatment. One hundred and twenty-five eyes were evaluated in the treatment group and compared with 104 eyes that underwent standard cataract surgery without LAL technology in the control group. The subjects were noted to have overall slight increase in the macular thickness in the initial postoperative weeks, but these returned to preoperative levels within 3 months of surgery. No structural changes in the retinal layers or retinal pigment epithelium were noted, and no increase in the risk of macular edema development occurred in the treatment group compared with the control [12].

Clinical outcomes and considerations

Clinical outcomes have been studied internationally over the past decade to demonstrate the accuracy and efficacy of the LAL and postoperative adjustments. Early small studies by Arturo Chayet's group in Mexico showed good accuracy when correcting residual myopia, hyperopia, and astigmatism. The myopia study evaluated 14 patients with residual myopic surprise of up to −1.5 diopters (D) after cataract surgery and implantation with the LAL. About 92.9% of these patients achieved a manifest refraction spherical equivalent (MRSE) of 0.25D or less at 1 day after lock-in procedure and 100% of patients achieved MRSE of 0.5D or less [13]. A similar study by the same group evaluated 14 patients with residual hyperopic refractive error up to +2.0D after implantation with an LAL. About 92.9% of eyes achieved MRSE within 0.25D of target at 1 day after lock-in and 100% of eyes were within 0.5D of target [14]. In both of these studies, the stability of refractive error was impressive–no significant change in manifest refraction spherical equivalent was observed over a 6-month follow-up in the hyperopia group and a 1-year follow-up in the myopia group. The mean rate of change in manifest refraction in both studies was 0.006D per month, which was stated to be 6 times more stable than current corneal refractive procedures [13,14]. Dr Chayet's group also evaluated 5 patients with postoperative astigmatic errors of 1.25 to 1.75D. MRSE for these patients after adjustment and lock-in remained within 0.25D of target for at least 9 months of follow-up, and all patients achieved uncorrected visual acuity of 20/25 or better [15]. A similar study by Lichtinger and colleagues evaluated 10 eyes with residual astigmatic error of 1.0 to 2.0D after implantation with an LAL and showed a final MRSE of −0.06 ± 0.25D at 1-year follow-up. This study also showed that the axis of cylinder correction was stable in 60% of eyes and showed less than 10° of rotation in 100% of eyes at 1 year [16]. Hengerer and colleagues evaluated the accuracy of the LAL in specific patient groups and found a high level of accuracy and stable manifest refractions in more than 90% of patients with both axial myopia and axial hyperopia. One eye in each study was noted to have a change in 0.325 to 0.38D over the course of 1-year postadjustment and lock-in, but all other eyes were noted to have a change in MRSE of less than 0.25D at the 12-month postoperative visit [17,18].

Larger studies have evaluated patients with a variety of residual refractive errors after implantation of the LAL and found similarly impressive results. Patients had residual refractive errors ranging from −1.98D to +2.3D after surgery requiring adjustment with the LDD. All studies achieved postadjustment manifest refractive errors of less than 0.5D in all patients, and postadjustment and lock-in mean MRSE ranged from 0.03 ± 0.17D to 0.15 ± 0.2D [19–23]. The largest of these studies followed 122 eyes over the course of 18 months and showed excellent final refractive results and stability over that time [22]. The FDA study that led to approval of the lens resulted in 91.6% of patients with 20/25 or better uncorrected visual acuity and 99.5% of patients with MRSE within 1D of goal after an average of 1.65 adjustments. Astigmatism results also were very good, with 82% of patients with less than or equal to 0.5D of astigmatism and 98.5% with less than or equal to 1.0D of astigmatism after adjustment and lock-in [23–25].

As mentioned previously, the LDD even can apply radiation to the IOL in arrays that can induce multifocality to the lens to allow for correction of presbyopia. Sandstedt and colleagues demonstrated the ability to reproducibly apply multifocal patterns to LALs in vitro with near add power ranging from +2 to +3.5D [26]. Hengerer's group also showed success in application of multifocal patterns to LAL, achieving improved near and intermediate vision in fifteen patients [27]. Villegas and colleagues applied arrays to simulate extended depth of focus and concurrently treated to reduce higher-order aberrations including spherical aberration and defocus [28]. Customized and premium refractive adjustments to the LAL show promise for minimizing not only postoperative refractive error but also visually significant higher-order aberrations that can be a drawback for some postkeratorefractive and multifocal IOL patients.

Concerns and future directions

Surgeons use several different methods preoperatively to try to achieve perfect refractive outcomes in cataract surgery. Newer-generation formulae and ray tracing, improved biometry, and intraoperative aberrometry have pushed the bar higher on preoperative evaluation and IOL selection. But refractive surprises still happen, particularly in patients with eyes at the extremes of axial length, with corneal pathology, or with prior keratorefractive surgery. Intraocular lens exchange for refractive surprise is one of the top causes of return to the operating room after cataract surgery, and surgeons anticipate the potential for more challenges as more postkeratorefractive surgery patients reach the age when they will need cataract surgery [3]. The LAL allows for an elegant and effective solution to noninvasively correct for refractive surprises that occur despite the surgeon's best preoperative efforts to select the ideal IOL.

Although not specifically approved for use in postrefractive surgery patients, a few reports have been published showing success in the use of the LAL in patients who have had previous LASIK or other keratorefractive procedures. A 2013 review in Canada of 34 eyes with a history of myopic keratorefractive surgery showed final MRSE within 0.25D of goal in 74% of eyes and within 0.5D of goal in 97% of eyes after adjustment and lock-in. Some patients in this study required up to 3 adjustment treatments, but ultimately the final refractive outcomes are promising [29]. Rocha and Mednick published a case report of a post-LASIK patient who suffered blunt trauma resulting in flap damage and a traumatic cataract in whom the use of a LAL allowed for a successful outcome in a complex clinical situation [30].

An important part of IOL power calculation for any IOL involves the development of optimized constants for that particular lens that is applicable across several different calculation formulae. A German study evaluated 125 eyes and developed optimized constants for the Hoffer Q, Holladay 1, and SRK/T formulae [31]. Increased use of this lens in clinical practice will allow for further evaluation and optimization of constants for newer-generation formulae in use. Optimized constants for preoperative calculations will hopefully reduce residual refractive error and, therefore, also reduce the need for postoperative adjustments.

Despite very promising results thus far, a few concerns and limitations to widespread use of the LAL remain. Successful use of this lens requires strict patient compliance with instructions to wear UV-blocking sunglasses in the 2 to 4 weeks before the adjustment and lock-in procedures. Lack of compliance with these recommendations could result in unintended refractive change in the lens; this is illustrated by a case presented by a group from Switzerland in which a patient did not adhere to UV sunglass protection in the week after her adjustment procedure (before lock-in) and was found to have a −3.25D induced refractive error with irregular elevation of the IOL noted at the slit lamp. This required explantation of the IOL and replacement with a standard monofocal lens [32]. Patient selection for the LAL would mandate ensuring that patients are capable of and willing to comply, with UV protection until the lens is "locked"; preoperative consent forms likely should be formatted to include this agreement. The number of postoperative visits required may be of concern for patients, as the adjustment and lock-in procedures require more visits than are typical for standard cataract surgery.

Another critical restriction in patient selection arises from the need for exposure of the entire 6.0-mm lens optic to UV irradiation for the lock-in procedure. This would restrict the use of this lens in patients who cannot achieve pharmacologic pupillary dilation to 6.0 mm or greater. Patients with pseudoexfoliation syndrome, prior alpha-blocker use, on chronic opiate therapy, or with physiologically small pupils should be carefully evaluated preoperatively to determine if they are candidates for the use of this lens [24]. The development of a contact lens that allows for irradiation beyond a small pupil has been discussed but would need to be tested before implementation [33]. Anterior capsular phimosis or opacification, if it occurred early enough in the healing process, could potentially limit the effectiveness of the lock-in procedure and result in unpredictable outcomes.

One unusual side effect noted in the FDA trial was that a small percentage of patients experienced color vision abnormalities or red-tinted vision (erythropsia) after the UV irradiation procedures. Up to 49% of patients reported erythropsia before the second lock-in treatment. This effect was not seen to be long-lasting in most of the patients, and only 0.5% of patients complained of erythropsia at a 6-month follow-up, but it would be important to mention this to patients undergoing the procedure. New tritan anomalies in color vision were noted in 1.8% of patients (7 cases) during the adjustment and lock-in period, but all but 2 of these ultimately resolved. This will be an important area to follow in long-term studies of safety and clinical outcomes [23,24].

Finally, there are some minor considerations surgically that could be addressed with future versions of the lens. The lens is a 3-piece silicone IOL, which means that it requires a 3-mm incision, which is larger than is used by most surgeons routinely. As a silicone lens, it can expand quicker in the eye than an acrylic IOL, which surgeons would have to make note of during the insertion process. These albeit minor adjustments should be taken into consideration by surgeons deciding whether to use the LAL. Finally, the cost of the lens may be prohibitive for some patients, which is no different from many premium cataract surgery options currently on the market. The cost of the LDD, however, may prohibit some physicians from offering this service at their own practice, which may result in patients being referred to an outside location for use of the LDD for adjustment and lock-in procedures [34].

SUMMARY

Modern cataract surgery is a field in which constant innovation drives the field closer to perfection year by year. Refractive accuracy, however, remains an area of unpredictability. Even with the use of intraoperative aberrometry and the newer-generation IOL calculation formulae, patients occasionally end up with a refractive error significantly different from their goal. The RxSight LAL allows surgeons to noninvasively adjust the lens itself after implantation, and clinical data in the series noted earlier show excellent outcomes. Although studies indicate that the level of UV radiation required for adjustment and lock-in are safe, long-term safety outcomes will be important to monitor. Concerns regarding patient compliance with UV-blocking sunglasses, pupillary dilation, and changes necessary to surgical technique are noted earlier and would be important for surgeons to consider in patient selection. Both the cost of the lens itself to the patient and that of the LDD for the practitioner are important considerations as well. But despite these concerns, the LAL is a truly unique introduction to the IOL field that may make the goal of perfect refractive outcomes much more attainable in the near future.

References

[1] U.S. Food and Drug Administration. FDA approves first implanted lens that can be adjusted after cataract surgery to improve vision without eyeglasses in some patients. 2017. Available at: https://www.fda.gov/newsevents/newsroom/pressannouncements/ucm586405.htm. Accessed February 22, 2019.

[2] Ford J, Werner L, Mamalis N. Adjustable intraocular lens power technology. J Cataract Refract Surg 2014;40:1205–23.

[3] Mamalis N. Adjustable intraocular lens technology. J Cataract Refract Surg 2014;40:1059–60.

[4] Schwartz DM. Light-adjustable lens. Trans Am Ophthalmol Soc 2003;101:417–36.

[5] Kohnen T. Light-adjustable intraocular lens technology. J Cataract Refract Surg 2011;37(12):2091.

[6] Schwartz DM, Sandstedt CA, Chang SH, et al. Light-adjustable lens: development of in vitro nomograms. Trans Am Ophthalmol Soc 2004;102:67–72.

[7] Werner L, Yeh O, Haymore J, et al. Corneal endothelial safety with the irradiation system for light-adjustable intraocular lenses. J Cataract Refract Surg 2007;33:873–8.

[8] Heinzelmann S, Hengerer F, Maier P, et al. Is there an endothelial cell toxicity of light-adjustable lens UVA irradiation on the human corneal endothelium? Eur J Ophthalmol 2012;22:S57–61.

[9] Hengerer FH, Dick HB, Buchwald S, et al. Evaluation of corneal endothelial cell loss and corneal thickness after cataract removal with light-adjustable intraocular lens implantation: 12-month follow-up. J Cataract Refract Surg 2011;37(12):2095–100.

[10] Lichtinger A, Sandstedt CA, Padilla K, et al. Corneal endothelial safety after ultraviolet light treatment of the light-adjustable intraocular lens. J Cataract Refract Surg 2011;37:324–7.

[11] Werner L, Chang W, Haymore J, et al. Retinal safety of the irradiation delivered to light-adjustable intraocular lenses evaluated in a rabbit model. J Cataract Refract Surg 2010;36:1392–7.

[12] Hengerer FH, Muller M, Dick HB, et al. Clinical evaluation of macular thickness changes in cataract surgery using a light-adjustable intraocular lens. J Refract Surg 2016;32(4):250–4.

[13] Chayet A, Sandstedt C, Chang S, et al. Correction of myopia after cataract surgery with a light-adjustable lens. Ophthalmology 2009;116(8):1432–5.

[14] Chayet A, Sandstedt CA, Chang SH, et al. Correction of residual hyperopia after cataract surgery using the light adjustable intraocular lens technology. Am J Ophthalmol 2009;147(3):392.

[15] Chayet A, Sandstedt C, Chang S, et al. Use of the light-adjustable lens to correct astigmatism after cataract surgery. Br J Ophthalmol 2010;94(6):690–2.

[16] Lichtinger A, Sandstedt CA, Schwartz DM, et al. Correction of astigmatism after cataract surgery using the light-adjustable lens: a 1-year follow-up pilot study. J Refract Surg 2011;27(9):639–42.

[17] Hengerer FH, Hutz WW, Dick HB, et al. Combined correction of sphere and astigmatism using the light-adjustable Intraocular lens in eyes with axial myopia. J Cataract Refract Surg 2011;37(2):317–23.

[18] Hengerer FH, Hutz WW, Dick HB, et al. Combined correction of axial hyperopia and astigmatism using the light adjustable intraocular lens. Ophthalmology 2011;118(7):1236–41.

[19] Villegas EA, Alcon E, Rubio E, et al. Refractive accuracy with light-adjustable intraocular lenses. J Cataract Refract Surg 2014;40(7):1075–84.

[20] Winkler von Mohrenfels CW, Salgado J, Khoramnia R, et al. Clinical results with the light adjustable intraocular lens after cataract surgery. J Refract Surg 2010;26(5):314–20.

[21] Hengerer FH, Conrad-Hengerer I, Buchner SE, et al. Evaluation of the calhoun vision UV light adjustable lens implanted following cataract removal. J Refract Surg 2010;26(10):716–21.

[22] Hengerer FH, Dick HB, Conrad-Hengerer I. Clinical evaluation of an ultraviolet light adjustable intraocular lens implanted after cataract removal: eighteen months follow-up. Ophthalmology 2011;118(12):2382–8.

[23] FDA.gov. LAL summary of safety and effectiveness. Available at: https://www.accessdata.fda.gov/cdrh_docs/pdf16/P160055B.pdf. Accessed March 8, 2019.

[24] Bethke W. RxLAL: say goodbye to postop surprise? Review of Ophthalmology 2018;12:15,66.

[25] Salgado JP, Khoramnia R, Schweiger B, et al. Six-month clinical results with the light adjustable lens. Klin Monbl Augenheilkd 2010;227(12):966–70.

[26] Sandstedt CA, Chang SH, Grubbs RH, et al. Light-adjustable lens: customizing correction for multifocality and higher-order aberrations. Trans Am Ophthalmol Soc 2006;104:29–39.

[27] Hengerer FH, Bocker J, Dick BH, et al. Light adjustable lens. New options for customized correction of presbyopia. Ophthalmologe 2012;109(7):676–82.

[28] Villegas EA, Alcon E, Mirabet S, et al. Extended depth of focus with induced spherical aberration in light-adjustable intraocular lenses. Am J Ophthalmol 2014;157(1):142–9.

[29] Brierly L. Refractive results after implantation of a light-adjustable intraocular lens in postrefractive surgery cataract patients. Ophthalmology 2013;120(10):1968–72.

[30] Rocha G, Mednick ZD. Light-adjustable intraocular lens in post-LASIK and post-traumatic cataract patient. J Cataract Refract Surg 2012;38(6):1101–4.

[31] Conrad-Hengerer I, Dick HB, Hutz WW, et al. Optimized constants for an ultraviolet light-adjustable intraocular lens. J Cataract Refract Surg 2011;37(12):2101.

[32] Hafezi F, Seiler T, Iseli HP. Light-adjustable lens complication. Ophthalmology 2010;117(4):848.

[33] Ronge LJ. Inside the Calhoun light-adjustable lens. American Academy of Ophthalmology EyeNet Magazine online. 2005. Available at: https://www.aao.org/eyenet/article/inside-calhoun-light-adjustable-lens. Accessed February 22 2019.

[34] Dalton M. An update on the Light Adjustable Lens. ASCRS EyeWorld online. 2015. Available at: https://www.eyeworld.org/article-an-update-on-the-light-adjustable-lens. Accessed February 22, 2019.

Section V: Vitreoretinal Disease

Advances in Ophthalmology and Optometry 4 (2019) 169–175

ADVANCES IN OPHTHALMOLOGY AND OPTOMETRY

Sterile Intraocular Inflammation After Intravitreal Injection—Diagnosis and Management

Jonathan P. Greenberg, MBBCh[a,*], Timothy J. Peiris, MD[a], Ronni M. Lieberman, MD[b,1]

[a]Department of Ophthalmology, Northwell Health, 600 Northern Boulevard Suite 214, Great Neck, New York, NY 11021, USA; [b]Icahn School of Medicine at Mount Sinai, 1 Gustave L. Levy Pl, New York, NY 10029, USA

Keywords

• Retina • Intravitreal injection • Infectious endophthalmitis
• Noninfectious endophthalmitis • Sterile intraocular inflammation

Key points

- Sterile inflammation has been reported with all intraocular antivascular endothelial growth factor medications, as well as with triamcinolone and ocriplasmin.
- Most cases present early with decreased visual acuity and intraocular inflammation, without injection, hypopyon, fibrin, or severe pain. Final visual acuity usually returns to baseline but remains decreased in a significant minority.
- Cases are either sporadic or clustered with potential mechanisms including patient-specific, medication-specific, and delivery-specific factors.

INTRODUCTION

Sterile intraocular inflammation is a known complication of therapeutic intravitreal injections. It is defined as any acute intraocular inflammation without infection that resolves without intravitreal antibiotics. Typical presentation is within a few days of injection with decreased vision and intraocular inflammation and classically without redness or severe pain. Cases generally are treated with topical steroids and most recover to baseline visual acuity (VA) after resolution of inflammation, which usually takes 2 to 12 weeks [1].

Disclosure Statement: The authors have nothing to disclose.

[1]Present address: 82-68 164th Street, Suite 452, Queens, NY 11432.

*Corresponding author. *E-mail address:* jonpgreenberg@gmail.com

https://doi.org/10.1016/j.yaoo.2019.04.010

Sterile inflammation has been reported with all antivascular endothelial growth factor (VEGF) medications (bevacizumab [Avastin] [2–7], ranibizumab [Lucentis] [8,9], aflibercept [Eylea] [8–14], pegaptanib [Macugen] [15], triamcinolone [Kenalog] [16–18], and ocriplasmin [JETREA] [19,20]. These events have occurred sporadically and in clusters, and variable incidences have been reported.

BEVACIZUMAB

Bevacizumab (Avastin) is a humanized monoclonal antibody binding vascular endothelial growth factor, originally developed to treat metastatic rectal and colon carcinoma.

Multiple case series in the literature have described noninfectious endophthalmitis after intravitreal administration of bevacizumab [2–7]. The Comparison of Age-related macular degeneration Treatment Trials reported no cases of sterile inflammation following bevacizumab administration, but incidence in other series ranges from 0.09% to 1.1% [2–7]. Patient characteristics, including sex, age, number of previous injections, and type and degree of pathology, have had little bearing on incidence of sterile inflammation after bevacizumab injection [21].

Clinical characteristics of this entity are similar across the various series. Patients usually presented within 1 to 7 days after injection with decrease in visual acuity and intraocular (anterior chamber [AC] and/or vitreous) inflammation [2–7]. Pain was common, but severe pain has not been commonly reported. Most cases resolved spontaneously and recovered baseline visual acuity without intravitreal antibiotics, although a significant minority did have a decrease in final visual acuity.

A large case series (63 patients) by Chong and colleagues [2] highlighted the most often seen presenting symptoms: blurred vision in 78% and AC and vitreous inflammation in 79% and 84%, respectively. Other notable but less common signs and symptoms include eye pain (46%), floaters (35%), hypopyon (13%), and fibrin (3%). When stratified into culture negative cases injected with antibiotics and those without antibiotic injection, pain was less common and no cases of hypopyon or fibrin occurred in the latter. Most studies include culture-negative cases injected with antibiotics; however, a proportion of these may be culture-negative infectious endophthalmitis. Chong and colleagues [2] found an average time to resolution of inflammation of 37 $\pm$ 5 days (range 3–159 days) and an average time to recovery of visual acuity of 53 $\pm$ 18 days (range 0–696 days). No statistically significant change occurred between visual acuity on day of presentation and that at last follow-up visit, a trend replicated in the literature [2].

Causes may include patient-specific, medication-specific, and delivery-specific factors. Contamination of the medication, such as from bacterial endotoxin, has been reported to cause clusters of inflammation. Wang and colleagues [3] reported that 69% (80/116) of eyes injected from 3 vials of endotoxin-contaminated bevacizumab in China developed intraocular inflammation. Another potential mechanism involves impurities introduced from the vehicle, such as silicone droplets coating the inside of the syringe, which may represent a TASS-like syndrome. Ness and colleagues [4] reported 10 cases of vitritis after intravitreal bevacizumab injection from various lots in one practice and implicated a particular syringe (Omnifix-F 1-mL tuberculin syringe), which was different from the syringes used for intravitreal injections of other drugs. Once the practice changed the brand of syringe, no further cases occurred from the same lot of drug.

RANIBIZUMAB

Ranibizumab (Lucentis) is a potent inhibitor of VEGF isoforms, with an affinity-matured antigen-binding fragment (Fab) based off of bevacizumab. Multiple studies have examined sterile inflammation after ranibizumab injection; and reported incidence ranges from 0.02% to 1.9% [1,8,9].

Williams and colleagues [8] evaluated 26,161 ranibizumab injections from 2006 to 2013 and found incidence of sterile inflammation to be 0.02% (6/26,161). Mean time to presentation was 2.7 days. The most common symptoms were blurred vision (5/6, 83%) and floaters (4/6, 66.7%). Two patients (2/6, 33.3%) complained of pain, and none had hypopyon. Median VA before injection was 20/40, at presentation was 20/80, and at final visit was 20/60. Daien and colleagues [9] investigated 54,776 intravitreal injections in treatment for naïve eyes with neovascular age-related macular degeneration over a 10-year period, using the Fight Retinal Blindness registry, and found an incidence of sterile inflammation with ranibizumab of 0.005% (3/54,776). This study also examined bevacizumab injections and found an incidence of 0.081% (8/9931) in this group. Of cases involving either ranibizumab or bevacizumab that completed greater than 12 months of follow-up, 25% lost greater than 2 lines of VA. Across both studies, the incidence of sterile inflammation after ranibizumab was found to be significantly lower than that of bevacizumab [8,9]. It is thought that ranibizumab does not elicit the proinflammatory effects of its predecessor by lacking the domain that activates complement-mediated toxicity and Fc receptors on immune cells [22].

AFLIBERCEPT

Shortly after aflibercept's approval in 2011, a cluster of 15 cases (13/15 from 3 lots) was reported [10]. Since this initial series, a total of 132 cases of sterile intraocular inflammation have been reported in the literature with an incidence of 0% to 0.55% [8–14]. Some cases were clustered but most were sporadic, and no reports thus far have been able to identify an inciting cause. Several hypotheses that exist are related to characteristics of the molecule itself as well as to production and handling of the medication [1,23,24]. Possible causes include patient-specific factors, such as a history of uveitis, and immunogenicity of drug itself, which could be increased by improper storage and handling. Contamination of the medication, such as from bacterial endotoxin, may cause clusters of inflammation. Another potential mechanism involves impurities introduced from the vehicle, such as silicone droplets coating the inside of the syringe, which may represent a TASS-like syndrome. The mechanism of aflibercept-related intraocular inflammation seems multifactorial, and the mechanism of action for single reports may be different from that of clustered cases.

Hahn and colleagues [11] reported the largest series to date of aflibercept-related sterile intraocular inflammation. Fifty-six cases from 12 practices were described, with events occurring between 12/2011 and 02/2014 [11]. Mean time to presentation was 3.5 days (range 0–30 days). Pain was present in 46% but severe in only 2% and 13% had conjunctival injection. Sixty-six percent were treated with topical steroids or observation alone. Mean time to resolution was 28.6 days (range 4–84 days), and 17% lost greater than or equal to 2 lines of final VA. No difference in visual outcome existed for topical therapy alone versus invasive procedures. The only factor associated with worse visual outcome was age greater than 80 years. Several subsequent reports of these events have occurred [8,9,12–14], all of which describe similar clinical presentations.

TRIAMCINOLONE

Triamcinolone is a synthetic glucocorticoid indicated in a variety of pathology, ranging from inflammatory conditions such as pseudophakic macular edema to neovascular processes such as proliferative retinopathy. Corticosteroids achieve their antiinflammatory effect through inhibition of leukotriene and prostaglandin synthesis; in addition, they exhibit stabilization of the blood-retinal barrier and reversal of capillary permeability [25].

Incidence of sterile inflammation following intravitreal triamcinolone administration has been found to range from 0.2% to 1.6% [16–18]. The largest series of this entity included 17 eyes from 17 patients [17]. Time to presentation ranged from 1 to 3 days, with all patients presenting with decreased vision. Five of the patients reported periorbital soreness and one reported photophobia. In contrast to sterile inflammation noted with other intravitreal agents, 11/17 (65%) of patients exhibited pseudohypopyon, defined as layering of triamcinolone crystals in the AC. Other clinical characteristics included vitreous haze and crystalline opacities in the vitreous and AC, believed to be secondary to dispersion of steroid crystals. Resolution of inflammation occurred after an average of 15.1 days (range 5–30 days).

Multiple hypotheses regarding the cause of triamcinolone-related sterile inflammation have been postulated. The preservative agent present in commercial triamcinolone, 0.99% benzyl alcohol, has been speculated to play a role. One report compared incidence of sterile inflammation between commercially available triamcinolone and preservative-free triamcinolone; the commercially available group was found to be more than 3 times as likely (1.9 vs 7.3%) to induce inflammation [26]. Other theories include contaminants in the drug suspension and mischaracterization of the pseudohypopyon as a cellular reaction. In addition, it has also been postulated that the vehicle used in intravitreal triamcinolone is toxic to the retina itself; however animal and human studies have failed to demonstrate this effect [25,26].

OCRIPLASMIN

Ocriplasmin is a proteolytic enzyme indicated for treatment of symptomatic vitreomacular adhesion. In phase 3 clinical trials, incidence of postinjection inflammation after intravitreal ocriplasmin versus vehicle alone was found to be 7.1% versus 3.7%, respectively [19]. The chemical composition of ocriplasmin is believed to contribute to its proinflammatory effects as it contains the active moiety of plasmin.

Han and Scott reported the first case of sterile inflammation after intravitreal ocriplasmin injection in 2015 [20]. Similar to other agents, onset of inflammation developed within 24 hours of injection and responded completely to topical steroids alone. Symptoms on presentation were decreased vision, pain, and photophobia. Within 48 hours, clinical response was noted, and inflammation was nearly completely resolved within 2 weeks.

DIFFERENTIATING INFECTIOUS AND NONINFECTIOUS ENDOPHTHALMITIS

Differentiating sterile inflammation from infectious endophthalmitis is critical as management and prognosis differ. The incidence of postinjection infectious endophthalmitis is roughly 1/5000 [27,28]. Infectious endophthalmitis generally presents with a greater decrease in VA–in the endophthalmitis vitrectomy study (EVS), 44% (185/420) presented with hand motion (HM) and 26% (110/420) with light perception (LP) vision [29]. On the other hand, HM vision is present only in the minority of cases of noninfectious endophthalmitis, and LP vision is rare. It is important, however, to note that the EVS described cases of infectious endophthalmitis postcataract extraction and not that after intravitreal injection. Infectious endophthalmitis classically presents after 3 to 5 days (mean 3.4 days [postinjection] [30]; median 6 days [after cataract surgery] [29]), whereas sterile inflammation tends to present a little sooner, often within 24 to 48 hours. However, significant overlap occurs in time to presentation. Pain often is present in sterile inflammation, although severe pain is uncommon–for example, severe pain was only present in 2% and 3.5% of cases in 2 series of aflibercept-related sterile inflammation [11,12]. In contrast, severe pain is common in infectious endophthalmitis, although pain is notably absent in roughly one-quarter of cases [29,31]. Other distinguishing features include differing frequencies of conjunctival injection (minority in sterile inflammation vs 82% in the EVS) [29] and hypopyon (minority in sterile inflammation [with exception of pseudohypopyon in triamcinolone] vs 85% in the EVS) [29]. Fibrin is found in less than 5% of cases of sterile inflammation, whereas it is more common but not always present in infectious endophthalmitis (33% of cases noted in one prior report) [31]. These distinctions indicate a generally more severe inflammatory response in infectious endophthalmitis. In addition, infectious endophthalmitis has a worse overall visual prognosis. One report found the 12-month VA in infectious and noninfectious endophthalmitis to be within 2 lines of baseline in 53% and 75% of eyes, respectively [9]. Importantly, infectious endophthalmitis often is culture negative–the EVS reported that 31% (129/420) of eyes had clinical findings consistent with infectious endophthalmitis but were culture negative [29]. In summary, factors that may suggest infectious rather than noninfectious endophthalmitis are later presentation, HM or worse vision, severe pain, conjunctival injection, hypopyon, and fibrin. Using these clinical guidelines, invasive procedures may be avoided in a certain subset of patients. However, both conditions have variable presentations with considerable overlap, and physicians should strongly consider administering intraocular antibiotics if infection is suspected.

SUMMARY

Sterile inflammation has been reported with all anti-VEGF medications as well as with triamcinolone and ocriplasmin. Most cases present early with decreased visual acuity and intraocular inflammation without injection, hypopyon, fibrin, or severe pain. Eyes respond to topical steroids with resolution occurring after a mean of roughly 1 month, although resolution may take several months. Visual acuity usually returns to baseline but remains decreased in a significant minority. Cases are either sporadic or clustered with potential mechanisms including patient-specific, medication-specific, and delivery-specific factors. Cautious evaluation and appropriate management are critical with any concern for infectious endophthalmitis, although increased awareness may reduce invasive procedures in select patients.

References

[1] Agrawal S, Joshi M, Christoforidis JB. Vitreous inflammation associated with intravitreal anti-VEGF pharmacotherapy. Mediators Inflamm 2013;2013:943409.

[2] Chong DY, Anand R, Williams PD, et al. Characterization of sterile intraocular inflammatory responses after intravitreal bevacizumab injection. Retina 2010;30(9):1432–40.

[3] Wang F, Yu S, Liu K, et al. Acute intraocular inflammation caused by endotoxin after intravitreal injection of counterfeit bevacizumab in Shanghai, China. Ophthalmology 2013;120(2):355–61.

[4] Ness T, Feltgen N, Agostini H. Toxic vitreitis outbreak after intravitreal injection. Retina 2010;30(2):332–8.

[5] Yamashiro K, Tsujikawa A, Miyamoto K, et al. Sterile endophthalmitis after intravitreal injection of bevacizumab obtained from a single batch. Retina 2010;30(3):485–90.

[6] Ricci F, Calabrese A, De Felici C, et al. A cluster of presumed, noninfectious endophthalmitis after intravitreal injection of bevacizumab: long-term follow-up. Digit J Ophthalmol 2016;22(2):41–5.

[7] Orozco-Hernández A, Ortega-Larrocea X, Sánchez-Bermúdez G, et al. Acute sterile endophthalmitis following intravitreal bevacizumab: case series. Clin Ophthalmol 2014;8:1793–9.

[8] Williams PD, Chong D, Fuller T, et al. Noninfectious vitritis after intravitreal injection of anti-VEFG agents: variations in rates and presentation by medication. Retina 2016;36(5):909–13.

[9] Daien V, Nguyen V, Essex RW, et al. Incidence and outcomes of infectious and noninfectious endophthalmitis after intravitreal injections for age-related macular degeneration. Ophthalmology 2018;125(1):66–74.

[10] Hahn P, Kim JE, Stinnett S, et al. Aflibercept-related sterile inflammation. Ophthalmology 2013;120(5):1100–1.

[11] Hahn P, Chung MM, Flynn HW Jr, et al. Postmarketing analysis of aflibercept-related sterile intraocular inflammation. JAMA Ophthalmol 2015;133(4):421–6.

[12] Fine HF, Roth DB, Shah SP, et al. Frequency and characteristics of intraocular inflammation after aflibercept injection. Retina 2015;35(4):681–6.

[13] Goldberg RA, Shah CP, Wiegand TW, et al. Noninfectious inflammation after intravitreal injection of aflibercept: clinical characteristics and visual outcomes. Am J Ophthalmol 2014;158(4):733–7.e1.

[14] Kim JY, You YS, Kwon OW, et al. Sterile inflammation after intravitreal injection of aflibercept in a Korean population. Korean J Ophthalmol 2015;29(5):325–30.

[15] Singerman LJ, Masonson H, Patel M, et al. Pegaptanib sodium for neovascular age-related macular degeneration: third-year safety results of the VEGF inhibition study in ocular neovascularisation (VISION) trial. Br J Ophthalmol 2008;92(12):1606–11.

[16] Roth DB, Chieh J, Spirn MJ, et al. Noninfectious endophthalmitis associated with intravitreal triamcinolone injection. Arch Ophthalmol 2003;121(9):1279–82.

[17] Yoon SJ, Rhee DY, Marx JL, et al. Anatomic and visual outcomes of noninfectious endophthalmitis after intravitreal triamcinolone. Am J Ophthalmol 2009;147(6):1031–6.

[18] Ahn SJ, Kim TW, Ahn J, et al. Associated factors and treatment outcome of presumed noninfectious endophthalmitis occurring after intravitreal triamcinolone acetonide injection. Graefes Arch Clin Exp Ophthalmol 2013;147(6):1031–6.

[19] JETREA® (ocriplasmin) Prescribing Information Available at: https://www.accessdata.fda.-gov/drugsatfda_docs/label/2016/125422s037lbl.pdf. Accessed December 8, 2018.

[20] Han IC, Scott AW. Sterile endophthalmitis after intravitreal ocriplasmin injection: report of a single case. Retin Cases Brief Rep 2015;9(3):242–4.

[21] Michels S, Rosenfeld PJ, Puliafito CA, et al. Systemic bevacizumab (Avastin) therapy for neovascular age-related macular degeneration twelve-week results of an uncontrolled open-label clinical study. Ophthalmology 2005;112(6):1035–47.

[22] Julien S, Biesemeier A, Taubitz T, et al. Different effects of intravitreally injected ranibizumab and aflibercept on retinal and choroidal tissues of monkey eyes. Br J Ophthalmol 2014;98(6):813–25.

[23] Palmer JM, Amoaku WM, Kamali F. Quality of bevacizumab compounded for intravitreal administration. Eye (Lond) 2013;27:1090–7.

[24] Liu L, Ammar DA, Ross LA, et al. Silicone oil microdroplets and protein aggregates in repackaged bevacizumab and ranibizumab: effects of long-term storage and product mishandling. Invest Ophthalmol Vis Sci 2011;22(52):1023–34.

[25] Lam A, Garg SJ, Spirn MJ, et al. Sterile endophthalmitis following intravitreal injection of preservative-free triamcinolone acetonide. Retin Cases Brief Rep 2008;2(3):228–30.

[26] Maia M, Farah ME, Belfort RN, et al. Effects of intravitreal triamcinolone acetonide injection with and without preservative. Br J Ophthalmol 2007;91(9):1122–4.

[27] Gregori NZ, Flynn HW, Schwartz SG, et al. Current infectious endophthalmitis rates after intravitreal injections of anti-vascular endothelial growth factor agents and outcomes of treatment. Ophthalmic Surg Lasers Imaging Retina 2015;46(6):643–8.

[28] Moshfeghi AA, Rosenfeld PJ, Flynn HW Jr, et al. Endophthalmitis after intravitreal vascular [corrected] endothelial growth factor antagonists: a six-year experience at a university referral center. Retina 2011;31(4):662–8.

[29] Endophthalmitis Vitrectomy Study Group. Results of the Endophthalmitis Vitrectomy Study. A randomized trial of immediate vitrectomy and of intravenous antibiotics for the treatment of postoperative bacterial endophthalmitis. Arch Ophthalmol 1995;113:1479–96.

[30] Shah CP, Garg SJ, Vander JF, et al. Outcomes and risk factors associated with endophthalmitis after intravitreal injection of anti-vascular endothelial growth factor agents. Ophthalmology 2011;118(10):2028–34.

[31] Mezad-Koursh D, Goldstein M, Heilwail G, et al. Clinical characteristics of endophthalmitis after an injection of intravitreal anti-vascular endothelial growth factor. Retina 2010;30(7):1051–7.

Advances in Ophthalmology and Optometry 4 (2019) 177–191

ADVANCES IN OPHTHALMOLOGY AND OPTOMETRY

Innovations in Secondary Intraocular Lens Placement

Peter J. Belin, MD[a,*], Sherief Raouf, MD[a], Ronni M. Lieberman, MD[b]

[a]Department of Ophthalmology, Hofstra Northwell School of Medicine, 600 Northern Boulevard #214, Great Neck, NY 11021, USA; [b]Department of Ophthalmology, Icahn School of Medicine at Mount Sinai, One Gustave L. Levy Place, New York, NY 10029, USA

Keywords

• Secondary IOL • ACIOL • Iris scleral fixated • Akreos • Envista • Yamane • Sutureless

Key points

- In cases in which capsular implantation of intraocular lenses (IOLs) is not feasible, there is a need for tenable alternatives.
- Anterior chamber IOLs have been a well-delineated option in such cases, albeit associated with high rates of known complications.
- More recent innovations in lens design and surgical technique have allowed ophthalmologists to achieve secondary IOL placement with more favorable outcome profiles.
- Among the techniques reviewed here are iris and scleral-fixated lenses, sutureless scleral fixation, and flanged IOL scleral fixation.

INTRODUCTION

In modern day cataract surgery, the lens is ideally placed in the capsular bag, which provides stable fixation at a position closest to the nodal point of the eye. In patients with trauma, complicated cataract surgery, or other conditions with insufficient capsular or zonular support, implantation into the capsular bag is not anatomically feasible. One option when the anterior capsule is intact is sulcus intraocular lenses (IOLs). However, they are placed close in proximity to

Disclosure Statement: The authors have nothing to disclose.

*Corresponding author. 50, 4th Avenue North #B10, Minneapolis, MN 55401, USA. *E-mail address:* petebelin@gmail.com

https://doi.org/10.1016/j.yaoo.2019.05.001
2452-1760/19/

the iris, allowing for contact between the 2 structures; this may lead to pigment dispersion, iris transillumination defects, dysphotopsias, and elevated intraocular pressure [1].

As an alternative when insufficient capsular support exists, placement more anterior in comparison to a lens within the capsular bag moves the implant farther from the nodal point of the eye and requires modification of the lens power. Insertion of an anterior chamber IOL (ACIOL) is another option in this patient population; however, it is associated with a relatively high rate of complications, including intermittent touch syndrome, iris chafing, inflammation, glaucoma, and corneal decompensation due to close proximity to the endothelium [2,3].

For these reasons, a functionally appealing option involves suturing the IOL to the sclera in the posterior chamber. Transscleral suturing of IOLs is a well-established and effective option in these patients [4–7]. To avoid contact with the iris, posterior segment surgeons may implant scleral-fixated posterior chamber IOLs (PCIOLs) farther back, up to 3 to 4 mm posterior to the limbus. This may avoid contact with the iris, and presumably place the implant in a position similar to that of one in the capsular bag. A variety of options exist for lens types to use, with some like the Akreos AO60 (Bausch & Lomb, Rochester, NY) being foldable and others such as the Envista lens (Bausch & Lomb) being more rigid, requiring a larger incision. As large incision surgery comes with risks of choroidal effusion, suprachoroidal hemorrhage, and wound rupture after trauma, it is desirable to minimize incision size. The type of sutures used over the years has progressed from the traditional polypropylene to more recently Gore-Tex sutures (off label) to maximize stability and minimize knot slippage, suture degradation, and conjunctival or scleral erosion. The methods of suture placement can be from inside the eye to the outside, ab interno, or outside to inside, ab externo. A number of innovative strategies have been used to reduce the risk of suture erosion, such as burying the knot within the sclerotomy, placing the suture within scleral flaps or pockets, gluing the haptic within a scleral tunnel, and creating a bulb at the haptic end with cautery to place within the scleral tunnel. To maximize lens stability and centration and decrease lens tilt, the number of points of fixation to sclera can vary between 2 and 4. Surgeons have combined these variables in several ways to enhance optical outcomes and reduce the risk for complications. Herein we review the more popular techniques, as well as newer advancements for secondary IOL placement.

Anterior chamber intraocular lenses

ACIOL implantation is an indicated alternative to capsular placement of lenses in eyes with poor capsular support and a normal iris anatomy. Early anterior chamber lens designs involved closed-loop haptics that were associated with high rates of complications stemming from physical contact of the lens to surrounding anatomy, such as uveitis glaucoma hyphema (UGH) syndrome and corneal decompensation [8]. For this reason, relative contraindications to ACIOL placement include corneal endothelial disease, iridocorneal-angle damage, or a shallow chamber.

Advances in lens design have provided safer alternatives. As a result, now the most commonly currently used ACIOLs use a flexible open-loop design, which is associated with fewer complications [9,10]. The open-loop haptic is typically designed with a footplate that provides a small and stable point of contact on the scleral spur within the anterior chamber angle. This prevents the capture of any iris tissue and disruptions of any existing iridectomies, if present [11]. Modern versions of the ACIOL commonly are positioned with less anterior vault, which minimizes corneal contact [12].

Anterior chamber lenses typically are placed through a temporal corneal or sclerocorneal incision. If vitreous is present in the anterior chamber as a result of complicated cataract surgery, an anterior vitrectomy is performed. Many surgeons use acetylcholine injection to induce miosis, followed by dispersive viscoelastic. A lens glide often is used to facilitate lens placement and to minimize the risk of abutting the iris during insertion by ensuring that the leading haptic stays anterior to the plane of the iris during placement [11].

Iris-fixated intraocular lenses

Iris fixation of IOLs has been a technique developed over the years as well. Both anterior and posterior chamber iris fixation of IOLs are used. Early designs of iris fixating IOLs were largely of 2 varieties: iris-clip lenses and iridocapsular lenses. Dr Binkhorst [13,14] of the Netherlands pioneered many of the early iris-supported IOLs that were designed with a 4-loop design to clip to the iris at the pupillary margin. These were associated with significant complications stemming from iris chafing and pupillary distortion, such as lens dislocation, pigment dispersion, uveitis, hemorrhage, and lens opacification [15]. Subsequent iterations of IOLs entailed modifications to the number and size of the IOL loops. In particular, the adoption of 2-loop iris-supported lenses produced a marked reduction in the incidence of many of the associated complications.

As the transition from intracapsular to extracapsular cataract extraction (ECCE) became more prevalent, the use of iridocapsular lenses became a feasible alternative. This type of lens was implanted into the anterior chamber with the posterior loops of the lens buried in the iridocapsular cleft. Subsequently, the lens optic was held in place by proliferating fibrous tissue that adhesed the lens capsule and the iris pigment epithelium [16,17]. This mechanism of function, however, did necessitate an iridectomy to facilitate aqueous humor outflow. Although these techniques are not currently used, because of clinical complications, the emphasis on IOL implantation, and ECCE was in many ways compelled by these innovations.

Separate from these outdated approaches, a technique still used for sutureless iris fixation can be achieved by the so-called "iris claw" fixation method (Fig. 1). This sutureless alternative involves the lens being secured into place

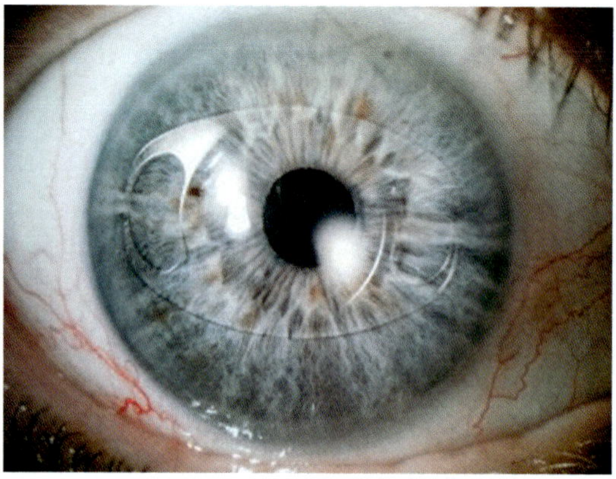

Fig. 1. Iris claw lens of the anterior chamber in an eye lacking capsular support. (*From* Touriño Peralba R, Lamas-Francis D, Sarandeses-Diez T, et al. Iris-claw intraocular lens for aphakia: Can location influence the final outcomes? J Cataract Refract Surg 2018;44(7):819; with permission.)

by pulling small sections of iris that are enclavated through specially designed IOL claws. The precise point of iris fixation is in the mid-periphery of the iris, which is nearly completely immobile during pupillary movements [15]. This affords the advantage of being centered over the pupil, even when the pupil itself is not centered in the anterior chamber, as is commonly the case in patients with high degrees of ametropia [17]. In addition, the fixation permits lens implantation with very good inhibition of lens movement, which renders the IOL amenable to astigmatism correction [18]. Implantation requires a 5.5-mm incision, an anterior chamber depth (ACD) $\geq$3 mm, 270° of iris tissue, and a 6-mm pupil; pupilloplasty can be performed if necessary. Iris claw lens use has been reported in phakic [19,20] and aphakic eyes [21]. Currently in the United States, the only iris claw IOL approved by the Food and Drug Administration is the Verisyse (Abbott Laboratories Inc, Abbott Park, IL) for phakic patients with moderate to high myopia [22]. The similar version for aphakic patients, the Artisan IOL (Ophtec, Boca Raton, FL) is not available in the United States [23].

This section has thus far treated iris fixation of anterior chamber lenses; however, there are inherent optical advantages to posterior chamber placement of IOLs. Posterior position is nearest to the optical nodal point of the eye and is farthest away from the corneal endothelium, which prevents the complications associated with endothelial decompensation.

Fixation of the haptic is typically achieved with sutures (commonly 9–0 or 10–0 polypropylene with long curved needle CTC-6 or CIF-4), which enter and exit the eye in the peripheral cornea [21]. The PCIOL is inserted and the haptics are placed into the ciliary sulcus before suturing. The suture is then guided with full-thickness passes through the midperipheral iris under the haptic and back through iris and peripheral cornea using the modified

McCannel knot [11,24] or a Siepser sliding knot [25]. The suture is then externalized through the paracentesis overlying the haptic using a Sinskey or Lester hook [26].

Scleral-fixated intraocular lenses

Fixation of the IOL with transscleral suture was first reported in patients status post-ICCE in 1986 [27–30]. Most broadly, the approach to sutured scleral fixation can be achieved either through an internal or external surgical incision. Common to both approaches is the eventual need to bury the knot required for fixation, so as to minimize the risk of conjunctival erosion or endophthalmitis [31,32]. Techniques also vary in the method of securing the haptic, the number of points of fixation required to lens stability, and the method to avoiding suture erosion [11]. An in-depth description of all surgical techniques and steps is beyond the scope of this article; a brief summary follows.

The seminal work by Malbran and colleagues [27] described a technique wherein a 10–0 polypropylene suture was used to the fix the haptics of an IOL to the sclera at a position 2 mm posterior to the limbus so as to give a final lens position in the ciliary sulcus. A needle was used to introduce suture loops at 3 and 9 o'clock. Through the corneal incision, the 2 loops of suture were then secured with a hitch to the lens haptic and then externalized. The lens was then placed in the eye, positioned posteriorly to the iris, and scleral sutures were tied. The technique entailed 2-point scleral fixation. Since then, surgeons have developed implantation techniques that use 3-point and 4-point fixation to increase lens stability [33,34]. Of course, the improved stability of the lens and diminished optic tilting is balanced against a greater number of scleral passes [35].

This method was refined to include the use of scleral flaps that functioned to cover suture knots [36–39]. A technique demonstrated by Lewis and colleagues [36] involved a suture being passed horizontally across the anterior chamber. The suture ends were docked in a straight needle and the middle of the suture was externalized through a corneal wound. This allows the suture to be cut (once externalized) and tied to the IOL haptic. The lens was then maneuvered into the eye and positioned with haptics resting in the ciliary sulcus. This technique is still used today, and study has demonstrated good results with low levels of IOL decentration on long-term follow-up [40].

In the early development of this technique, surgeons frequently sutured most PCIOLs via their haptic directly to the sclera. However, now many posterior IOLs are designed with eyelets that enable suture fixation [11,41]. Three commonly used PCIOLs are the Alcon CZ70BD, Akreos AO60, and the Bausch and Lomb Envista MX60. Moreover, 9–0 polypropylene (due to increased thickness) and 8–0 polytetrafluoroethylene (Gore-Tex; W.L. Gore & Associates, Newark, DE) sutures (due to their lack of degradation) are more commonly being used for improved long-term stability of scleral fixation as compared with 10–0 polypropylene [35,42]. In fact, several studies have documented no suture-related complications, such as lens dislocation, suture erosion, or suture breakage [43–45]. The CZ70BD lens is designed with only 2 eyelets for fixation, and as a result is thought be at risk for postoperative lens tilt [46]. The AO60 lens has 4 eyelets used for fixation, which is believed to improve the optical qualities of the lens in this regard [4]. In both IOLs, the lens position is adjusted by control of the tension of the fixating sutures. A notable drawback of the AO60 lens, is that it is made of hydrophilic acrylic material, which can opacify on intraocular gas exposure [47]. This is of particular concern in patients for whom the risk of future retinal detachment is elevated.

Akreos AO60

The Akreos AO60 IOL (Bausch & Lomb) has become one of the most popular secondary IOLs for both anterior and posterior segment surgeons. It is a hydrophilic acrylic IOL made of a single poly hydroxyethyl-methacrylate/ methyl methacrylate (HEMA/MMA) copolymer with a refractive index of 1.46. It is a single-piece equiconvex IOL consisting of 4 haptics with a 6.0-mm optic and 10.5-mm to 11.0-mm overall diameter [48]. Hydrophilic acrylics such as the AO60 have a range of qualities making them attractive options. With low refractive indices, hydrophilic acrylics may minimize problems with glare, reflections, and other unwanted dysphotopsias [49,50]. Their biocompatibility makes them a suitable option for long-term implantation and in patients with inflammatory conditions [51,52]. Studies also indicate better optical clarity and fewer discolorations or deposits found over time when compared with hydrophobic lenses [53]. The HEMA/MMA material of the Akreos AO60 is easily compressible and elastic, allowing the lens to be folded and injected through a small incision. In addition, hydrophilic acrylic lenses have been shown to demonstrate less damage during insertion secondary to fold marks or forceps damage when compared with silicone and other foldable acrylic IOLs [54,55]. These features and the 4 haptics with eyelets has made the AO60 a popular lens for scleral fixation with Gore-Tex sutures for the reasons mentioned previously.

Surgical technique

The surgical technique has been described in detail elsewhere in the literature [7]. First a vitrectomy is performed either via an anterior or pars plana approach to provide working space in the posterior chamber and avoid inducing vitreoretinal traction. The limbus is then marked at the 3 and 9 o'clock position, and then a partial peritomy is performed to expose bare sclera in these quadrants. Next, 2 sclerotomies are made 180° apart at a distance of 2 to 3 mm posterior to the limbus and 3 to 5 mm apart on either side (Fig. 2). Then 8–0 Gore-Tex suture with the needle removed is cut in half and each half is threaded through the adjacent eyelets on either side of the optic (Fig. 3). A 3.5-mm to 4.0-mm clear corneal incision is made, and the ends of the sutures are inserted through the incision and then externalized through the corresponding sclerotomies with microsurgical forceps. The lens is folded and inserted through the incision into the posterior chamber (Fig. 4). The IOL is centered by removing the suture slack and tying it down. The knots

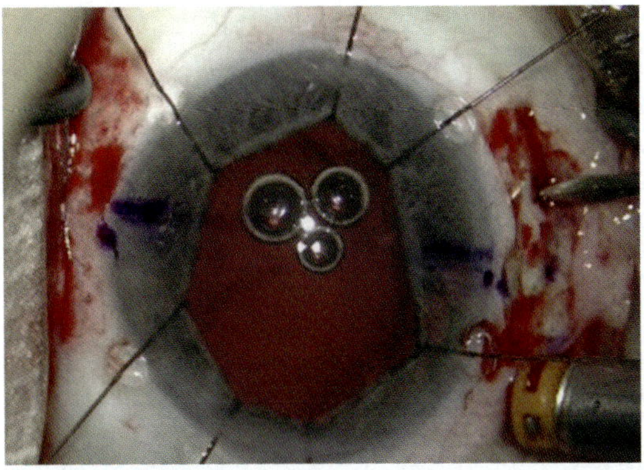

Fig. 2. Video still. Making 23-gauge sclerotomies 5.0 mm apart (and 3.0 mm posterior to limbus). (*From* Terveen DC, Fram NR, Ayres B, et al. Small-incision 4-point scleral suture fixation of a foldable hydrophilic acrylic intraocular lens in the absence of capsule support. J Cataract Refract Surg 2016;42(2):211–6; with permission.)

are trimmed and rotated into the sclerotomies, followed by closing the conjunctiva and corneal incision.

Outcomes

This procedure has been shown to effectively improve visual acuity in most patients, with low rates of complications. One study reported a mean postoperative visual acuity of 20/40, with 97% of patients having improved or unchanged visual acuity [7]. Complications reported in the literature in small series with low rates include transient ocular hypertension, hypotony, vitreous hemorrhage, hyphema, serous choroidal detachment, cystoid macular edema, and

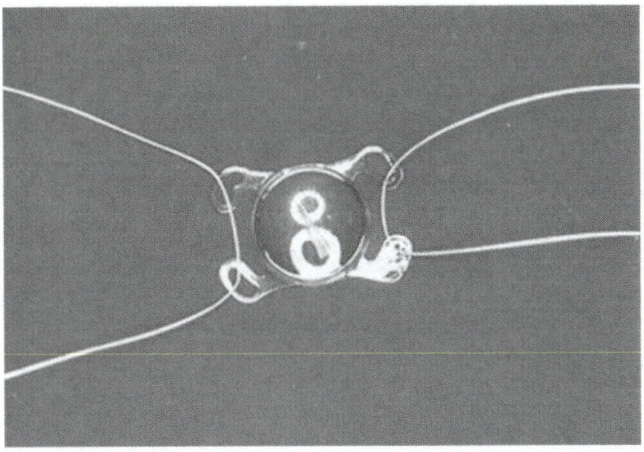

Fig. 3. The study IOL with eyelets threaded by polytetrafluoroethylene thread. (*From* Terveen DC, Fram NR, Ayres B, et al. Small-incision 4-point scleral suture fixation of a foldable hydrophilic acrylic intraocular lens in the absence of capsule support. J Cataract Refract Surg 2016;42(2):213; with permission.)

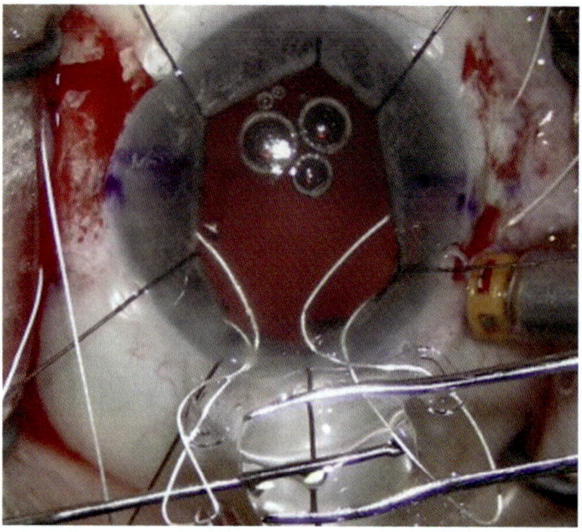

Fig. 4. Video still. Folding the Akreos AO60 IOL (with sutures placed through eyelets and brought through corneal incision and externalized through sclerotomies). (*From* Terveen DC, Fram NR, Ayres B, et al. Small-incision 4-point scleral suture fixation of a foldable hydrophilic acrylic intraocular lens in the absence of capsule support. J Cataract Refract Surg 2016;42(2):211–6; with permission.)

corneal edema [7,56]. It is possible that hypotony, the most common complication reported in one series (9.4%), may be less frequent with more surgeons using smaller 25-gauge or 27-gauge vitrectomy systems [56]. A recent retrospective study showed similar visual outcomes at 1 year between combined pars plana vitrectomy, ACIOL implantation, and combined pars plana vitrectomy, scleral-sutured AO60 IOL, with the only significant difference being higher rates of transient corneal edema in ACIOL group [43].

Envista MX60

The Envista MX60 (Bausch & Lomb, Rochester, NY) is an alternative IOL that has been used in scleral fixation techniques. The lens is one piece made of a hydrophobic PEG-HEMA (polyethylene glycol hydroxyethyl-methacrylate). The bridge between the haptic and optic is ring shaped, and as such several potential fixation sites exist for sutures (Fig. 5). Rho and colleagues [57] developed a technique for IOL scleral fixation that was similar to the one delineated previously for the Akreos lens, in that sclerotomies 3-mm posterior to the limbus were used.

Sutures are passed through one sclerotomy and out the other, such that 2 sutures enter and exit the eye 180° from one another in an ab externo technique. The sutures are pulled out of the eye at the midportion through a main wound equidistant between the 2 sclerotomies. The 2 sutures then are cut, such that 4 suture ends are present outside the main wound. At this point, the ends of the sutures are tied to the IOL. Some investigators have proposed straight forward suture fixation to the mid-haptic, and others have advocated

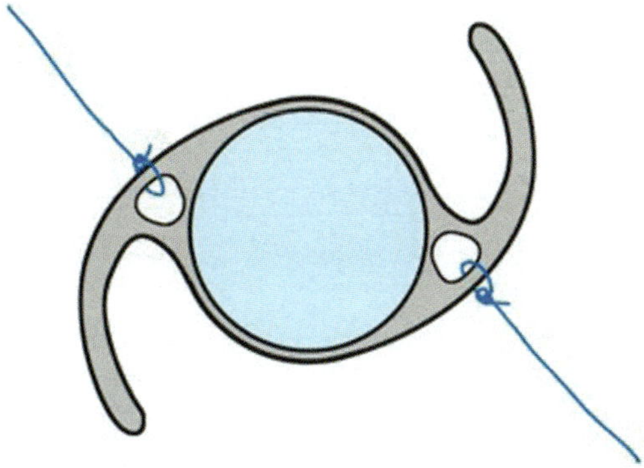

Fig. 5. Schematic of the Envista MX60 model IOL with loop haptic eyelets at the junction of the haptic and the optic. (*From* Yang JM, Yoon KC, Ji YS. Transscleral fixation of single-piece foldable acrylic lens with eyelets at the optic-haptic junction. Can J Ophthalmol 2015;50(5):368; with permission.)

for fixation through the ring in the bridge connecting the haptic and optic, with the advantage of the latter being less likelihood of suture slippage and lens tilt. The cut ends of the sutures can be tied to the ring bridge using a "European death knot," which is tied to both bridges before lens folding and insertion.

Patients treated with this method of scleral fixation of the IOL achieved significant improvements in best-corrected visual acuity (BCVA) with low rates of complications [57]. Given the hydrophobicity of the lens, the Envista represents an attractive alternative in secondary IOL implantation in patients with retinal detachment or at higher risk of requiring a future air or gas tamponade surgery.

Sutureless scleral fixation

Agarwal intraocular lens

In 2008, Agarwal and colleagues [58] described a novel technique of intrascleral haptic fixation of an IOL using fibrin glue. In this procedure, 2 partial-thickness limbal-based scleral flaps are created 180° apart from each other. A vitrectomy is performed to relieve vitreous traction of the retina as the IOL is manipulated. Two sclerotomies are made under the scleral flaps, and a scleral tunnel is prepared for introducing the IOL. The lens is passed through the tunnel, while a micro rhexis forceps passing through the adjacent sclerotomy is used to grasp the leading haptic, which is then pulled back through the sclerotomy and situated under the scleral flap. The trailing haptic (which has now been pulled back inside the eye), is similarly externalized through the contralateral sclerotomy. This has been termed the "handshake technique," in that the forceps passed through the opposite sclerotomy is ready to receive the haptic (Fig. 6). The haptics are then situated within each scleral bed and fibrin glue is injected beneath the scleral flaps for haptic fixation.

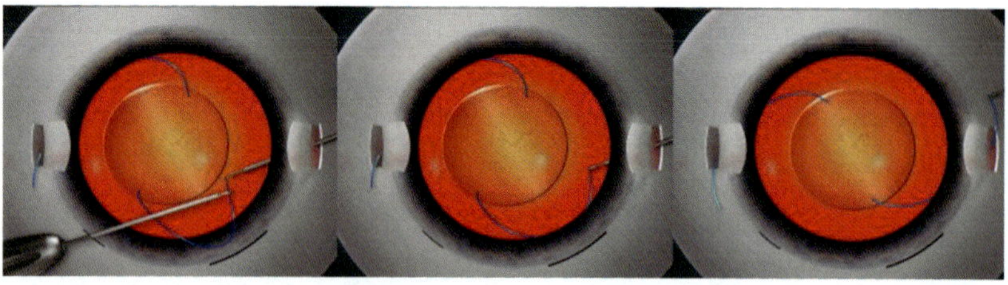

Fig. 6. The lens already having been passed into the AC via scleral tunnel, is manipulated by the "handing" of the haptic tip from one pair of forceps to another, which then secures it through the sclerotomy. (*From* Agarwal A, Jacob S, Kumar DA, et al. Handshake technique for glued intrascleral haptic fixation of a posterior chamber intraocular lens. J Cataract Refract Surg 2013;39(3):319; with permission.)

This technique was deemed of use in eyes that lacked posterior capsule support. Also, of note, the investigators did use the technique for the repositioning of already implanted, subluxated IOLs. In this case, the scleral flaps are created with the same technique, and the subluxated haptic was grasped and externalized beneath the scleral flap. Since then, modifications have occurred to the technique wherein the haptic tips were inserted through scleral tunnels, which provided more stability for the IOL [59].

A retrospective analysis of 735 eyes with glued IOLs demonstrated statistically significant improvements in BCVA at 1 and 3 years. The most common complications included IOL decentration (5.6% incidence), optic capture (2.4%), macular edema (4.8%), and endothelial cell loss [59]. Advocates of this technique have argued that externalization of a greater extent of the haptic would result in improved axial positioning and stability of the IOL. Although this technique may obviate the known risk complications of scleral fixation, such as suture breakage and erosion, long-term study is needed. Future retrospective studies will be able to elaborate the long-term stability of haptic fixation with fibrin glue.

Yamane technique

More recently, Yamane and colleagues [60] described a novel technique that entails haptic fixation to the sclera that does not require sutures or glue.

This was termed the flanged IOL fixation because it relied on a flange (created by the surgeon) at the end of the haptic for firm fixation [60]. The technique is similar to the sutureless technique described by Agarwal and colleagues [58] in that a vitrectomy is performed before lens insertion. A 3-piece IOL is introduced into the anterior chamber using an injector, while keeping the trailing haptic external. A sclerotomy was made using a 30-gauge needle, and the leading haptic, which is now in the anterior chamber, is threaded into the lumen of the needle with forceps. Viscoelastic is placed underneath the iris to provide adequate positioning of the optic, which has now traveled through the anterior chamber, through a dilated iris, and posterior to the iris plane. A second sclerotomy is then made 180° across from the first in a similar

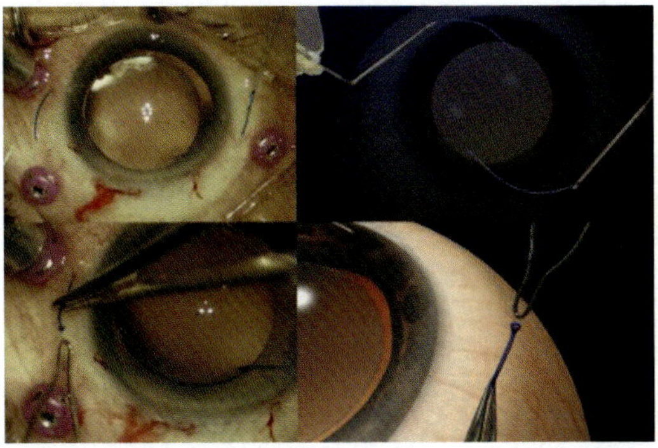

Fig. 7. The technique described by Yamane and colleagues [60] wherein the haptics are externalized with 2 needles (above) and subsequently the tips of the haptics are cauterized to create a flange that will fix the haptic within the sclera (below). (*From* Yamane S, Sato S, Maruyama-Inoue M, et al. Flanged intrascleral intraocular lens fixation with double-needle technique. Ophthalmology 2017;124(8):1138; with permission.)

fashion. The leading haptic is fed into this needle. At this point, both haptics have been fed into 30-gauge needle tips, which have been passed through sclerotomies on opposite sides. The haptic tips then are brought to the conjunctival surface, and cauterized to create a thermal deformity that acts as a flange to prevent the haptic from passing back inside the eye (Fig. 7).

The original investigators noted postoperative complications similar to those reported following transscleral IOL fixations, including iris capture of the optic, lens decentration, and cystoid macular edema. After a mean follow-up interval of 10 months in 35 eyes, the investigators had no cases of retinal detachment, endophthalmitis, IOL dislocation, or vitreous hemorrhage; however, ocular hypertension was present in 2 eyes and optic capture occurred in 3 eyes. One independent comparison study demonstrated transient intraocular pressure elevation to be the most common complication [61]. In addition, the investigators reported low incidence rates of mild decentration of the IOL and cystoid macular edema (CME), which were treated with refractive correction and local steroid therapy, respectively.

Other clinicians attempting the technique did report the advantages of a relatively short learning curve, as the procedure does not entail the use of sutures or glue adhesives, and often is a quicker procedure than other scleral-fixating surgeries [62].

SUMMARY

In the absence of capsular support, various options exist for secondary IOL implantation, including ACIOLs, iris-fixated IOLs, sulcus IOLs, and scleral-fixated IOLs, each with its own merits. No direct head-to-head prospective studies comparing these techniques exist to guide ophthalmologists; however, retrospective studies of postoperative outcomes of lens implantation are numerous, and significant attempts exist to summarize the known data to guide clinical decision making. In 2003, the American Academy of Ophthalmology (AAO) published a review of high-quality literature on the subject. The study concluded that no evidence existed to suggest the superiority of any of posterior iris-sutured, open-loop anterior chamber, or scleral-sutured IOLs over the other techniques in secondary lens implantation [1]. A more recently published study that compared the 3 methods in aphakic patients found no statistically significant difference in visual acuity, and similarly low complication rates of CME [63].

The improvements in visual acuity with all 3 techniques also are well-documented findings. The AAO review found that 95% of eyes with secondary iris-sutured PCIOLs achieved a postoperative BCVA within 1 line of the preoperative acuity. Unlike the older design of closed-loop ACIOL, the modern open-loop ACIOLs were in fact associated with comparable improvements in BCVA while achieving acceptable levels of complications (including the aforementioned corneal endothelial cell damage, secondary glaucoma, and CME) [1].

As many secondary ACIOLs are placed at the time of complicated cataract surgery, it is difficult to attribute postoperative pathology to the lens alone, as opposed to the confluent influence of other surgical events, such as capsule rupture or anterior vitrectomy. In this regard, outcome comparison of secondary open-loop ACIOLs placed after complicated versus uncomplicated cataract surgery is instructive. The AAO meta-analysis found that 90% of such lenses placed following uncomplicated cataract surgery achieved a BCVA within 1 line or better of the preoperative acuity, compared with 80% following a complicated cataract surgery.

Two separate large studies directly comparing ACIOLs with scleral-sutured lenses demonstrated no statistically significant differences in final BCVA [64,65]. In both studies, the investigators suggested that given the similar risk factor profiles, no sufficient evidence existed to favor one kind of lens approach over the other. This was the same conclusion reached by the review conducted with the AAO. Instead, it is reasonable for surgeon preference and relative comfort level to guide lens selection in secondary lens implantation in patients with poor capsular support.

Although many of the newer techniques reviewed previously aim to minimize complications, such as lens tilt or decentration, suture erosion, or breakage, iris chafe, UGH syndrome, and others, while maximizing visual and refractive outcomes, no long-term data exist. In the absence of large randomized prospective studies it will be difficult for any technique to be recommended over another with certainty. Yet, when considering which secondary lens to choose, it is important for surgeons to consider several factors, such as patient age, ocular comorbidities, and endothelial cell count. In addition, although placing an ACIOL is a relatively short and straightforward procedure, scleral-fixated PCIOLs tend to be longer and more technically challenging surgeries. In the end, if the procedure selected is one that the surgeon is comfortable doing well and the patient is monitored closely for complications, this will ensure the best possible outcomes.

References

[1] Wagoner MD, Cox TA, Ariyasu RG, et al. American Academy of Ophthalmology. Intraocular lens implantation in the absence of capsular support: a report by the American Academy of Ophthalmology. Ophthalmology 2003;110:840–59.
[2] Smith PW, Wong SK, Stark WJ, et al. Complications of semiflexible, closed-loop anterior chamber intraocular lenses. Arch Ophthalmol 1987;105:52–7.
[3] Chang DF, Masket S, Miller KM, et al. Complications of sulcus placement of single-piece acrylic intraocular lenses: recommendations for backup IOL implantation following posterior capsule rupture. J Cataract Refract Surg 2009;35(8):1445–58.
[4] Fass ON, Herman WK. Four-point suture scleral fixation of a hydrophilic acrylic IOL in aphakic eyes with insufficient capsule support. J Cataract Refract Surg 2010;36(6): 991–6.
[5] Oh H-S, Chu Y-K, Kwon O-W. Surgical technique for suture fixation of a single-piece hydrophilic acrylic intraocular lens in the absence of capsule support. J Cataract Refract Surg 2007;33(6):962–5.
[6] Khan MA, Gupta OP, Smith RG, et al. Scleral fixation of intraocular lenses using Gore-Tex suture: clinical outcomes and safety profile. Br J Ophthalmol 2016;100(5):638–43.
[7] Terveen DC, Fram NR, Ayres B, et al. Small-incision 4-point scleral suture fixation of a foldable hydrophilic acrylic intraocular lens in the absence of capsule support. J Cataract Refract Surg 2016;42(2):211–6.
[8] Dick HB, Augustin AJ. Lens implant selection with absence of capsular support. Curr Opin Ophthalmol 2001;12:47–57.
[9] Sawada I, Kimura W, Kimura I, et al. Long-term follow-up of primary anterior chamber intraocular lens implantation. J Cataract Refract Surg 1998;24:1515–20.
[10] Ellerton CR, Rattigan SM, Chapman FM, et al. Secondary implantation of open-loop, flexible, anterior chamber intraocular lenses. J Cataract Refract Surg 1996;22:951–4.
[11] Por YM, Lavin MJ. Techniques of intraocular lens suspension in the absence of capsular/zonular support. Surv Ophthalmol 2005;50:429–62.
[12] Apple DJ, Brems RN, Park RB, et al. Anterior chamber lenses. Part I: complications and pathology and a review of designs. J Cataract Refract Surg 1987;13:157–74.
[13] Binkhorst CD. Lens implants classified according to method of fixation. Br J Ophthalmol 1967;51:772–4.
[14] Binkhorst CD. About lens implantation. 2. Lens design and classification of lenses. Implant 1985;3:11–4.
[15] Yanoff M, Duker JS. Ophthalmology. Philadelphia: Elsevier Saunders; 2014.
[16] Manschot WA. Mechanism of fixation of two-loop iridocapsular lenses. Am J Ophthalmol 1978;85:465–8.
[17] Güell JL, Morral M, Kook D, et al. Phakic intraocular lenses part 1: historical overview, current models, selection criteria, and surgical techniques. J Cataract Refract Surg 2010;36: 1976–93.
[18] Baumeister M, Bühren J, Kohnen T. Position of angle-supported, iris-fixated, and ciliary sulcus-implanted myopic phakic intraocular lenses evaluated by Scheimpflug photography. Am J Ophthalmol 2004;138:723–31.
[19] Alió JL, Piñero DP, Sala E, et al. Intraocular stability of an angle-supported phakic intraocular lens with changes in pupil diameter. J Cataract Refract Surg 2010;36:1517–22.
[20] Fechner PU. Late loss of corneal endothelial density with refractive iris-claw IOLs. J Cataract Refract Surg 2010;36:352–3.
[21] Hirashima DE, Soriano ES, Meirelles RL, et al. Outcomes of iris-claw anterior chamber versus iris-fixated foldable intraocular lens in subluxated lens secondary to Marfan syndrome. Ophthalmology 2010;117(8):1479–85.
[22] Guell JL, Velasco F, Malecaze F, et al. Secondary Artisan-Verysise aphakic lens implantation. J Cataract Refract Surg 2005;31:2266–71.

[23] Tahzib NG, Nuijts RM, Wu WY, et al. Long-term study of Artisan phakic intraocular lens implantation for the correction of moderate to high myopia: ten-year follow-up results. Ophthalmology 2007;114:1133–42.
[24] Lorente R, de Rojas V, Vazquez de Parga P, et al. Management of late spontaneous in-the-bag intraocular lens dislocation: retrospective analysis of 45 cases. J Cataract Refract Surg 2010;36(8):1270–82.
[25] Chang DF. Siepser slipknot for McCannel iris-suture fixation of subluxated intraocular lenses. J Cataract Refract Surg 2004;30:1170–6.
[26] Ashraf MF, Stark WJ. McCannel sutures and secondary iris-fixated intraocular lenses. In: Azar DT, editor. Intraocular lenses in cataract and refractive surgery. Philadelphia: W.B. Saunders Company; 2001. p. 165–70.
[27] Malbran ES, Malbran E, Negri I. Lens guide suture for transport and fixation in secondary IOL implantation after intracapsular extraction. Int Ophthalmol 1986;9:151–60.
[28] Apple DJ, Price FW, Gwin T, et al. Sutured retropupillary posterior chamber intraocular lenses for exchange or secondary implantation. The 12th annual Binkhorst lecture, 1988. Ophthalmology 1989;96:1241–7.
[29] Zhang ZD, Shen LJ, Liu XQ, et al. Injection and suturing technique for scleral fixation foldable lens in the vitrectomized eye. Retina 2010;30(2):353–6.
[30] Gimbel HV, Brucks M, Dardzhikova AA, et al. Scleral fixation of a subluxated intraocular lens-capsular bag complex through a fibrotic continuous curvilinear capsulorhexis. J Cataract Refract Surg 2011;37(4):629–32.
[31] Hoffman RS, Fine IH, Packer M. Scleral fixation without conjunctival dissection. J Cataract Refract Surg 2006;32(11):1907–12.
[32] Lin CP, Tseng HY. Suture fixation technique for posterior chamber intraocular lenses. J Cataract Refract Surg 2004;30(7):1401–4.
[33] Oshika T. Transscleral suture fixation of a subluxated posterior chamber lens within the capsular bag. J Cataract Refract Surg 1997;23:1421–4.
[34] Rao SK, Gopal L, Fogla R, et al. Ab externo 4-point scleral fixation. J Cataract Refract Surg 2000;26:9–10.
[35] Stem MS, Todorich B, Woodward MA, et al. Scleral-fixated intraocular lenses: past and present. J Vitreoretin Dis 2017;1:144–52.
[36] Lewis JS. Ab externo sulcus fixation. Ophthalmic Surg 1991;22:692–5.
[37] Grigorian R, Chang J, Zarbin M, et al. A new technique for suture fixation of posterior chamber intraocular lenses that eliminates intraocular knots. Ophthalmology 2003;110:1349–56.
[38] Kumar M, Arora R, Sanga L, et al. Scleral-fixated intraocular lens implantation in unilateral aphakic children. Ophthalmology 1999;106:2184–9.
[39] Sharpe MR, Biglan AW, Gerontis CC. Scleral fixation of posterior chamber intraocular lenses in children. Ophthalmic Surg Lasers 1996;27:337–41.
[40] Cavallini GM, Volante V, De Maria M, et al. Long-term analysis of IOL stability of the Lewis technique for scleral fixation. Eur J Ophthalmol 2015;25:525–8.
[41] Holt DG, Young J, Stagg B, et al. Anterior chamber intraocular lens, sutured posterior chamber intraocular lens, or glued intraocular lens: where do we stand? Curr Opin Ophthalmol 2012;23:62–7.
[42] Price MO, Price FW Jr, Werner L, et al. Late dislocation of scleral-sutured posterior chamber intraocular lenses. J Cataract Refract Surg 2005;31(7):1320–6.
[43] Khan MA, Gupta OP, Pendi K, et al. Pars plana vitrectomy with anterior chamber versus Gore-Tex sutured posterior chamber intraocular lens placement: long-term outcomes. Retina 2019;39(5):860–6.
[44] Khan MA, Gerstenblith AT, Dollin ML, et al. Scleral fixation of posterior chamber intraocular lenses using Gore-Tex suture with concurrent 23-gauge pars plana vitrectomy. Retina 2014;34(7):1477–80.
[45] Parker DS, Price FW Jr. Suture fixation of a posterior chamber intraocular lens in anticoagulated patients. J Cataract Refract Surg 2003;29(5):949–54.

[46] Teichmann KD, Teichmann IA. The torque and tilt gamble. J Cataract Refract Surg 1997;23: 413–8.
[47] Cao D, Zhang H, Yang C, et al. Akreos Adapt AO Intraocular lens opacification after vitrectomy in a diabetic patient: a case report and review of the literature. BMC Ophthalmol 2016;16:82.
[48] Assouline M, Weber K, Welt R, et al. Akreos acrylic IOLs: clinical evidence continues to support biocompatibility and design features. North Clearwater (FL): Bausch & Lomb Incorporated internal memo; 2004.
[49] Davison JA. Positive and negative dysphotopsia in patients with acrylic intraocular lenses. J Cataract Refract Surg 2000;26(9):1346–55.
[50] Erie JC, Bandhauer MH. Intraocular lens surfaces and their relationship to postoperative glare. J Cataract Refract Surg 2003;29(2):336–41.
[51] Abela-Formanek C, Amon M, Schauersberger J, et al. Results of hydrophilic acrylic, hydrophobic acrylic, and silicone intraocular lenses in uveitic eyes with cataract: comparison to a control group. J Cataract Refract Surg 2002;28(7):1141–52.
[52] Schauersberger J, Kruger A, Abela C, et al. Course of postoperative inflammation after implantation of 4 types of foldable intraocular lenses. J Cataract Refract Surg 1999;25(8): 1116–20.
[53] Manuchehri K, Mohamed S, Cheung D, et al. Brown deposits in the optic of foldable intraocular lenses in patients with uveitis. Eye 2004;18(1):54–8.
[54] Mamalis N. Complication of foldable intraocular lenses requiring explantation or secondary intervention–2001 survey update. J Cataract Refract Surg 2002;28:2193–201.
[55] Schmidbauer JM, Peng Q, Apple DJ, et al. Rates and causes of intraoperative removal of foldable and rigid intraocular lenses: clinicopathological analysis of 100 cases. J Cataract Refract Surg 2002;28(7):1223–8.
[56] Patel NA, Shah P, Yannuzzi NA, et al. Clinical outcomes of 4-point scleral fixated 1-piece hydrophobic acrylic equiconvex intraocular lens using polytetrafluoroethylene suture. Clin Ophthalmol 2018;12:2145.
[57] Rho S, Song WK, Sung Y, et al. Scleral fixation technique using a hydrophobic foldable intraocular lens with ring-shaped connecting bridges. J Cataract Refract Surg 2015;41(2):262–7.
[58] Agarwal A, Kumar DA, Jacob S, et al. Fibrin glue–assisted sutureless posterior chamber intraocular lens implantation in eyes with deficient posterior capsules. J Cataract Refract Surg 2008;34(9):1433–8.
[59] Kumar DA, Agarwal A, Agarwal A, et al. Glued intraocular lens implantation for eyes with defective capsules: a retrospective analysis of anatomical and functional outcome. Saudi J Ophthalmol 2011;25:245–54.
[60] Yamane S, Sato S, Maruyama-Inoue M, et al. Flanged intrascleral intraocular lens fixation with double-needle technique. Ophthalmology 2017;124:1136–42.
[61] Kelkar A, Kelkar J, Kothari A, et al. Comparison of two modified sutureless techniques of scleral fixation of intraocular lens. Ophthalmic Surg Lasers Imaging Retina 2018;49(10):e129–34.
[62] Kelkar A, Fogla R, Kothari A, et al. Sutureless 27-gauge needle-assisted transconjunctival intrascleral intraocular lens fixation: initial experience. Indian J Ophthalmol 2017;65:1450–3.
[63] Hazar L, Kara N, Bozkurt E, et al. Intraocular lens implantation procedures in aphakic eyes with insufficient capsular support associated with previous cataract surgery. J Refract Surg 2013;29:685–91.
[64] Donaldson KE, Gorscak JJ, Budenz DL, et al. Anterior chamber and sutured posterior chamber intraocular lenses in eyes with poor capsular support. J Cataract Refract Surg 2005;31(5):903–9.
[65] Lyle WA, Jin JC. Secondary intraocular lens implantation: anterior chamber vs posterior chamber lenses. Ophthalmic Surg 1993;24:375–81.

Advances in Ophthalmology and Optometry 4 (2019) 193–210

ADVANCES IN OPHTHALMOLOGY AND OPTOMETRY

Perioperative Management of Macular Edema in the Cataract Surgery Patient

Carl S. Wilkins, MD[a,*], Ethan K. Sobol, MD[a], Robin N. Ginsburg, MD[a,b]

[a]Department of Ophthalmology, Icahn School of Medicine at Mount Sinai, One Gustave L Levy Place, New York, NY 10028, USA; [b]Department of Ophthalmology, New York Eye and Ear Infirmary of Mount Sinai, 310 East 14th Street, New York, NY 10003, USA

Keywords

• Macular edema • Cataract • Cataract surgery • Cataract extraction
• Diabetic macular edema • Uveitic macular edema • Retinal vein occlusion
• Pseudophakic macular edema

Key points

- Both macular edema and cataract are common in the overall population and often coexist.
- Topical, intravitreal, and periocular treatments for these conditions are increasingly common and effective.
- Informed consent and management of expectations is essential to the surgical course of these patients.

DIABETIC MACULAR EDEMA

Introduction

Worldwide, an estimated 285 million people have diabetes mellitus, one-third of whom have diabetic retinopathy (DR), and one-ninth of whom have vision-threatening DR [1]. The national prevalence of diabetes in America continues to rise, with Centers for Disease Control and Prevention 2015 estimates at 8.7% [2]. Diabetic eye disease is the most common cause of vision loss in American adults, with prevalence estimates even higher in black and Hispanic populations [3]. Diabetic macular edema (DME) is a common cause of vision loss

The authors have nothing to disclose.

*Corresponding author. *E-mail address:* carl.wilkins@mountsinai.org

https://doi.org/10.1016/j.yaoo.2019.04.016

among patients with DR. Among patients with diabetes over 39 years, an estimated 3.8% have DME at any time.

Despite being such a common cause of vision loss, the pathophysiology of DME is not completely understood. Broadly, damage from DR is an inflammatory process. With poorly controlled blood glucose levels, capillary walls undergo glycosylation and loss of pericytes [4]. This loss of pericytes results in the breakdown of the blood-retina barrier and egress of fluid. In addition, increased levels of vascular endothelial growth factor (VEGF), among many other cytokines, result in a general increase in porosity of microvasculature [4]. The revolution of steroid and anti-VEGF intravitreal medications targets this chronic, inflammatory pathway to improve and preserve vision.

Another common cause of vision loss among patients with diabetes is cataract progression, particularly in older patients [5]. Data from the Wisconsin Epidemiologic Study of Diabetic Retinopathy demonstrated that patients with diabetes are 2 to 5 times more likely to develop visually significant cataracts, and 15 to 20 times more likely if diagnosed before the age of 40 years [6]. Furthermore, DME has long been known to be exacerbated by cataract extraction (CE) [7,8], although overall rates of progression of severity seem to be equivalent [8]. Given the increasing incidence and prevalence of DR and DME, as well as the aging American population in need of CE, the management of DME before and after cataract surgery presents a common challenge for cataract surgeons and retinal specialists.

Diagnosis

The diagnosis of DME may be attained accurately with routine slit lamp biomicroscopy; however, imaging modalities may detect subclinical macular edema (ME). In patients who had no history of DME, it may be useful to obtain fluorescein angiography (FA) or macular optical coherence tomography (OCT) images to detect edema not apparent on clinical examination.

FA involves an intravenous injection of 2 to 3 mL of sodium fluroescein dye and allows dynamic monitoring of chorioretinal perfusion and vascular leakage. DME appears as a nonspecific retinal interstitial leakage in mid-to-late phases on angiography, and may be anatomically associated with microaneurysms (MA), which are more easily visualized on FA than fundoscopy. Early studies by the Diabetic Retinopathy Clinical Research Network (DRCR.net) defined clinically significant macular edema (CSME) as 500 μm of retinal thickening involving the fovea, exudates within 500 μm of the fovea with adjacent retinal thickening, or 1 disc diameter (DD) of retinal thickening that is within 1 DD of the fovea [9]). This aimed to identify areas that would require treatment with focal laser photocoagulation. Although this identification has fallen somewhat out of favor, FA may identify areas of extrafoveal MA that may be amenable to laser treatment before surgery. In addition, FA has high sensitivity for identifying neovascularization of the retina or disc, which may be missed, particularly in patients with more advanced cataracts or peripheral corneal lesions. Finally, FA can identify areas of retinal nonperfusion, whether from ischemic capillary dropout secondary to diabetes, retinal vein occlusion (RVO), or other pathologic origins. FA allows identification and quantification of macular ischemia, which may ultimately limit final visual acuity (VA) despite successful cataract surgery, and should be discussed with the patient.

Identification of subclinical ME with OCT is now generally the favored imaging modality given its noninvasive mechanism and rapid acquisition. OCT allows quantification of retinal thickness, mapping of location(s) of retinal edema, localization of fluid within the retina (intraretinal vs subretinal), and identification of exacerbating factors such as vitreomacular traction or epiretinal membrane [10]. Newer classification of DME favors "center-involved" DME (CIDME) to the former CSME definition [10]. ME resulting in central subfield thickness (CSF) of 275 μm or greater, or in the central 1 mm of the fovea, is considered center-involved and has high sensitivity with OCT. In the modern anti-VEGF injection era, the older definition of CSME may not adequately characterize the clinical picture or guide treatment. In addition, disorganization of the inner retinal layers (DRIL) may be identified and quantified, which may aid in the estimation of postoperative visual potential. DRIL is defined as loss of visualization of normal inner retinal laminations (ganglion cell-inner plexiform boundary, inner nuclear layer, and outer plexiform layer) on OCT, and is quantified by width in micrometers on OCT [11]. Progression and regression of DRIL is associated with final visual outcomes and severity of DR. Previous studies have demonstrated that a 50% or greater DRIL in the central 1-mm foveal zone is associated with poorer visual outcomes, even with otherwise successful anatomic results [11,12]. OCT preoperatively and postoperatively allows for serial monitoring of this quantitative metric and management of expectations in the cataract surgery patient.

Management

Primary medical management should be a priority, and both the primary care physician and ophthalmologist should work in concert to evaluate and educate the patient. The Diabetes Control and Complications Trial (DCCT) and UK Prospective Diabetes Study (UKPDS) were large prospective studies of type 1 and type 2 diabetes mellitus, respectively, and demonstrated that intensive blood glucose control resulted in long-term decreased risk of DR [13]. In the DCCT, incidence of DR was decreased by 76% and progression by 54% [13]. In the UKPDS, incidence of all microvascular events was decreased by 25%, onset of DR was decreased, as has the need for panretinal photocoagulation, vitreous hemorrhage rates, and legal blindness. A large cross-sectional study demonstrated increased risk of ME with uncontrolled blood glucose levels (odd ratio [OR] = 3.19), which increased further with poorer blood pressure control and higher cholesterol [14]. Patients must be counseled regarding continued primary medical care, irrespective of ongoing ophthalmic treatments.

Ideally, successful management of DME before cataract surgery will help attenuate postoperative inflammation and ME. Several previous DRCR.net studies aimed to identify risk factors for postoperative DME. Protocol P and Q investigated risk of postoperative CIDME in patients with and without preoperative CIDME, respectively.

Protocol P prospectively recruited patients with current CIDME who were undergoing cataract surgery. Mean CSF for study patients was 338 μm, mean VA of 55 ETDRS (Early Treatment of Diabetic Retinopathy Study) letters (~20/80), and 76% of patients had prior history of DME treatment (injection or focal laser) [15]. Although sample size was low due to difficult recruitment, overall patients did well, with an average of +12 ETDRS letters gained after CE. Only 10% of eyes experienced worsened vision, and 15% worsened ME at 16 weeks follow-up [15].

Protocol Q looked at all patients with and without preoperative eccentric DME to determine risk of subsequent postoperative CIDME. A total of 293 patients were enrolled and followed 16 weeks after CE. At final follow-up 22% of patients were found to have developed postoperative CIDME [16]. Additional analysis demonstrated increased risk of postoperative conversion to CIDME in patients who had previous history of CIDME treatment [16].

Considering this demonstrated risk, imaging and treatment before surgery is preferred, although no standard of care exists. Most studies have centered around intraoperative and postoperative management of ME in the patient with cataract. Moshfeghi and colleagues [17] recently reported outcomes of cataract surgery among patients enrolled in RISE and RIDE trials. These patients received intravitreal ranibizumab 0.3 mg, 0.5 mg, and sham monthly injections for 24 months, with the sham arm then crossing over to 0.5 mg dosing for months 25 to 36. Per protocol, all patients were injected no earlier than 7 days before cataract surgery and no more than 1 month thereafter. Patients in the treatment arms experienced a mean improvement in VA of +11.3 ETDRS letters, while sham-treated eyes demonstrated stable VA of −0.5 letters. This finding suggests that, in patients with untreated DME before cataract surgery, visual benefit from cataract surgery may be equalized by persistent or worsened ME. One limit to this study is the lack of consistent OCT measurements after cataract surgery, because the primary study protocol did not adjust for that variable.

Several studies have investigated the usefulness of intraoperative intervention for DME. One large meta-analysis found that postoperative topical nonsteroidal anti-inflammatory drug (NSAID) therapy decreased odds of ME (OR = 0.11) in patients who were nondiabetic, and combination topical NSAID and steroid therapy decreased odds of CIDME in patients with diabetes (OR = 0.17) [18]. Prospective studies in patients with diabetic ME suggest that intraoperative ranibizumab at the time of cataract surgery may help prevent postoperative CIDME in patients with and without preoperative DME [19,20]. Simultaneous intravitreal bevacizumab injection at the time of cataract surgery also has been shown in randomized controlled trials to blunt increase in ME postoperatively, as well as to result in mildly improved VA at 3 months [21]. Aflibercept (Eylea; Regeneron Pharmaceuticals) is a recombinant fusion protein to VEGF 1 and 2, and has been shown in large randomized trials (VIVID and VISTA) to be efficacious in treatment of DME [22]. Studies of intraoperative aflibercept injection at time of cataract surgery are currently ongoing, although early results are promising [23].

Intravitreal corticosteroids are encouraging for the perioperative management of DME. A randomized trial of intraoperative triamcinolone versus bevacizumab for patients with preexisting DME demonstrated efficacy of both agents, with reduction in postoperative ME [24]. However, at 6-month follow-up, only 16.7% of patients administered triamcinolone required additional intravitreal injection compared with 70.6% treated with intraoperative bevacizumab [24].

Intravitreal steroid implants have been shown to be very effective as primary treatments or as adjuncts to anti-VEGF medications, and have been studied in the perioperative period for cataract surgery. Several groups have investigated simultaneous CE and intravitreal 0.7 mg dexamethasone (Dex) implant (Ozurdex; Allergan Pharmaceuticals) for patients with DME. Panozzo and colleagues [25] prospectively followed a cohort of such patients up to 8 months after combined CE and steroid implantation, with mean improvement in VA of +18 ETDRS letters at 1 month and mean decrease in CSF 193 μm at 1 month. ME was observed to recur in 73.8% of patients between 4 and 5 months, compatible with maximum efficacy findings of other studies typically around 3 to 4 months postinjection [26–28]. A retrospective case series by Pacella and colleagues [27] demonstrated durable improvement in VA for 6 months, and in CSF for 4 months, after combined CE-Dex injection, with mean CSF returning to baseline level at 6 months.

Intravitreal 0.19 mg fluocinolone acetonide implant (ILUVIEN; Alimera Sciences) shows immense promise for long-term control of DME. Injection of this medication is similar to the Dex implant, safely done in-office, and has been shown through the multicenter FAME trial. This trial showed stable improvement in VA and CSF, which met statistical significance at the 3-year endpoint [29]. Further analysis of the FAME trial data demonstrated safety and efficacy in both phakic and pseudophakic patients, with stable improvement in VA in both groups [30].

Side-effect profiles for intravitreal steroid injection specifically include cataract formation and glaucoma. Certainly in patients undergoing CE, no concern should exist for worsened cataract; however, the risk of elevated intraocular pressure (IOP) and glaucoma should be discussed with the patient. Data from the MEAD and FAME trials show rates of incisional glaucoma surgery of 0.6% and 3.7% for Dex and fluocinolone implants, respectively [26,29]. Most steroid-responsive patients were managed with topical ocular hypotensives alone.

UVEITIC MACULAR EDEMA

Introduction

Uveitis is a significant cause of visual impairment, and is estimated to be the fifth leading cause of vision loss in developed countries [31]. In addition, uveitis is fairly common, with incidence and prevalence estimates up to 52 and 734 patients per 100,000 people, respectively [32]. Uveitis is generally divided into infectious and noninfectious causes, and categorized by anatomic location: anterior, intermediate, posterior, or panuveitis. The sequelae of uveitic disease are heterogenous, with patients at increased risk for glaucoma, corneal failure, retinal detachment, and neovascularization, among others; however, uveitic macular edema (UME) is the most common cause of vision loss and affects up to one-third of all patients with uveitis [31]. Consequently, management of UME is critical to preserving vision in these patients. It is no surprise that, given the heterogeneity of causes and presentations of UME, treatments may vary immensely.

Cataract formation is very common in patients with uveitis, with an estimated prevalence of greater than 50% [33–35]. Given a history of previous inflammatory episodes, surgery can be complicated owing to peripheral anterior synechiae with shallowing of the anterior chamber, posterior synechiae and poor dilation, pupillary membrane, and dense cataract requiring excessive phacoemulsification, among other issues. ME is common preoperatively and postoperatively, and has been known to complicate postoperative course particularly in patients with pars planitis and those with preoperative recalcitrant UME [33].

Diagnosis

Initial diagnosis and work-up of uveitis involves standard ophthalmic testing, particularly examination for anterior chamber cell and proteinaceous flare, as well as posterior segment vitreous cell and haze. Given the incidence of UME in these patients, standard work-up includes an FA and/or OCT macula. FA also may help identify unique staining patterns or peripheral neovascularization to better arrive at a diagnosis. OCT is sensitive for cystoid macular edema (CME) and quantifies CSF–particularly helpful in conditions resulting in retinal atrophy such as birdshot chorioretinopathy or masquerades such as acute macular neuroretinopathy.

The most common identified causes for UME include HLA B27-associated anterior uveitis, pars planitis, sarcoidosis, multiple sclerosis-associated intermediate uveitis, birdshot chorioretinitis, and Behcet's disease, although many cases will remain undiagnosed and categorized as "undifferentiated" [35]. In posterior uveitides in particular, UME is a common cause of patient presentation due to decreased VA, with estimates at 28% prevalence in posterior uveitis [31]. Full laboratory and imaging work-up are essential, as some causes of uveitis necessitate initial treatment with antibiotic or antiviral medication, high-dose steroids, or even immediate immunomodulatory therapy.

Management

Initial management invariably starts with topical steroids, although NSAIDs may be considered in the presence of UME given the role of prostaglandins in inflammation. Bromfenac 0.09% topical therapy has attracted interest as the medication has shown good penetration to the posterior segment, with 1 study suggesting synergistic effect if given in conjunction with intravitreal triamcinolone (IVT), but not as monotherapy [36]. Topical 0.5% indomethacin drops have shown modest visual and anatomic benefit for UME [37].

Topical corticosteroids are requisite in the initial management of any patient with uveitis with anterior segment inflammation. Steroids work broadly to decrease inflammation, targeting cytokine production and neutrophil chemotaxis, among other pathways [32]. When inflammation is intermediate and/or posterior involving, periocular or intravitreal steroids should be considered in noninfectious cases.

Periocular injection of triamcinolone has been investigated in noninfectious uveitis complicated by UME. Leder and colleagues [38] showed clinical resolution of UME in 53% and 57% of patients at 1 and 3 months after periocular injection, with only 15% of patients failing to demonstrate clinical response. A large, multicenter retrospective cohort demonstrated resolution of UME in 72.7% of patients within 6 months of periocular injection, although 15% of patients experienced IOP elevation to 30 mm Hg or greater, and 2.4% required incisional glaucoma surgery [39]. Necessity of glaucoma surgery may be somewhat confounded by the overall incidence of glaucoma in this population.

Multiple studies have demonstrated efficacy of a variety of intravitreal steroid injections. IVT has long been used in noninfectious uveitis with and without UME. One retrospective review of patients with persistent UME, despite adequate inflammatory control, showed improvement in mean VA and CME in 55% and 50% of patients, respectively [40]. One patient (5%) required incisional glaucoma surgery after IVT [40]. The PEACHTREE trial used a suprachoroidal delivery technique of triamcinolone, and demonstrated significant mean reduction in CSF, improvement in VA, and relatively lower rate of IOP elevation compared with intravitreal injection [41]. The final data on this phase 3 trial is pending.

The Multicenter Uveitis Steroid Treatment (MUST) trial is a landmark study comparing systemic immunosuppression with local control of inflammation with surgical 0.59 mg fluocinolone acetonide implant (Bausch & Lomb). The primary study randomized patients to systemic therapy-oral prednisone 1 mg/kg/d up to 60 mg with subsequent taper, or to surgical fluocinolone implantation, and followed for 2 years. Both implant and systemic therapy groups showed gain in VA, and control of inflammation was more efficacious in the implant group, with only 12% of patients experiencing continued intraocular inflammation compared with 29% of systemic therapy patients at 2 years (MUST 2 year) [42]. ME was better controlled in implant versus systemic group at 6 months (20% vs 34%), although this gap narrowed at 2 years to nonsignificance [42].

Previous studies, such as the HURON trial, demonstrated excellent efficacy of Dex implant in noninfectious uveitis, with significant improvement in final VA [43]. The POINT trial is a head-to-head randomized trial comparing periocular triamcinolone, IVT, and intravitreal Dex implant [44]. Significant reductions in CSF and improvement in VA occurred in all groups; however, gains in vision and reduction in ME were greater in intravitreal therapy compared with periocular treatment [44]. Larochelle and colleagues [45] showed that Dex implant in patients with uveitis within 4 months of CE may help attenuate postoperative exacerbation. Indeed, in patients who received the implant within 1 month of surgery, mean CSF decreased by −47.0 μm, whereas patients who received the implant between 1 and 4 months before surgery had a mean increase in CSF of 51.1 μm. Change in mean CSF from preoperative to postoperative period was +5 μm [45]. Although this study was retrospective and nonrandomized, it does suggest that Dex in the immediate preoperative period (<4 weeks) may be of benefit.

A prospective cohort study by Bélair and colleagues [46] compared incidence of CME in patients with and without uveitis undergoing CE. Patients with a history of uveitis had a 3-fold increased risk (12% vs 4%) of postoperative CME at 1-month follow-up [46]. Patients with a history of uveitis treated with oral corticosteroid taper (1 mg/kg/d of prednisone 2 days before or within 2 days postoperative) or with intraoperative IV methylprednisolone had a 7-fold decreased risk (relative risk [RR] = 0.14) in postoperative CME. In eyes with a history of uveitis, a history of active inflammation within 3 months of surgery portended an increased risk of CME (RR = 6.19). Although no large randomized prospective trial exist, these data provide strong support for tight control of inflammation within 3 months, as well as for perioperative oral steroid taper for those patients who can tolerate it.

Systemic immunomodulatory therapy may on occasion be an appropriate monotherapy for UME. In the STOP-Uveitis study, Sepah and colleagues [47] demonstrated efficacy with 2 separate doses of tocilizumab, an interleukin-6 inhibitor. At 6-month follow-up, mean VA showed significant improvement, as have intraocular inflammatory markers, and mean CSF decreased (−83.9 μm). Anti-tumor necrosis factor alpha agents such as adalimumab and infliximab have both shown suggested benefit in UME [32]. Mycophenolate mofetil has demonstrated efficacy for prevention of recurrent inflammation and improvement in ME [32]. Lastly, several European studies have demonstrated rapid improvement in recalcitrant UME with interferon alpha infusion; however, this medication is poorly tolerated due to an extensive side-effect profile. Ultimately, as these agents are typically aimed for long-term immunosuppression, they are less useful in a perioperative setting for the sole purpose of attenuating ME. In addition, immunosuppressive agents have higher risk of systemic adverse events and lack the rapid onset of local or systemic corticosteroid therapies, making them higher-risk and less-convenient modalities.

RETINAL VEIN OCCLUSION

Introduction and diagnosis

RVOs are the second most common cause of retinal vascular disease, surpassed only by diabetes mellitus. Pooled results estimate a prevalence of 4.42 and 0.80 per 1000 persons for branch retinal vein occlusion (BRVO) and central retinal vein occlusion (CRVO), respectively, suggesting that as many as 16 million people worldwide may be affected [48].

Anatomically, RVO are separated into BRVO and CRVO. Further classification into ischemic or nonischemic is based on the degree of decreased retinal perfusion--5 DD on FA for BRVO and 10 DD for CRVO [49,50]. Advanced age and hypertension are most commonly associated with RVO, although risk factors such as hyperlipidemia, diabetes mellitus, glaucoma, and other uncommon prothrombotic disorders have been implicated [49,50]. Examination findings classically seen on fundoscopy include intraretinal hemorrhages and dilated tortuous retinal vasculature, with or without cotton wool spots. Spectral domain OCT is used to assess for ME. The extent of ischemia can be evaluated with FA or OCT angiography. The prognosis for visual recovery may be estimated by the degree of foveal pathology and the presence or extent of ME and ischemia.

Management: preoperative

For ME secondary to RVO (whether BRVO or CRVO), pharmacologic management has become the mainstay of therapy. Previous studies have demonstrated the efficacy of intravitreal anti-VEGF injections compared with laser therapy [51]. After the initial injection, common practice is to repeat the injection monthly for up to 6 months, after which an extended time interval or as-needed treatment can maintain the effect. In the VIBRANT study, monthly injections of aflibercept resulted in 52.7% of eyes with ME from BRVO improving by 15 or more letters from baseline acuity [51]. The COPERNICUS and GALILEO studies, which took place in North America and Europe, respectively, demonstrated efficacy of intravitreal aflibercept for ME from CRVO with mean decrease in CSF at 24 months of −453.1 μm [52] (Integrated study). Similar results were shown for ranibizumab and BRVO, with 56.0% and 60.3% of eyes (0.3 or 0.5 mg dosing, respectively) achieving an improvement of 15 or more letters from baseline best corrected visual acuity (BCVA) [53]. Once eyes in the sham treatment arm were switched to as-needed ranibizumab at 6 months, a rapid reduction in central retinal thickness was achieved; however, the visual results did not improve to the same extent as those eyes that had initially received ranibizumab, which underscores the importance of prompt treatment on diagnosis [53]. For CRVO, similar results were demonstrated in the study by Campochiaro and colleagues [54], with visual and anatomic benefits maintained through the 12-month study period. The SCORE2 trial demonstrated that visual outcomes of bevacizumab were noninferior to aflibercept for CRVO through a 6-month follow-up period [55]. At present these studies have shown that any of the 3 current anti-VEGF agents are a reasonable and well-tolerated first-line treatment, with demonstrated benefit to early treatment on diagnosis.

In addition to anti-VEGF injections, the usefulness of triamcinolone and Dex injections have been demonstrated [56]. Use of sustained delivery Dex implantation (Ozurdex; Allergan, Inc, Irvine, CA) has been shown to improve VA in

ME from BRVO or CRVO. In the Ozurdex GENEVA study, Dex implant was both safe and well tolerated, with similar outcomes when a second treatment was required over a 12-month follow-up period [57]. Peak VA improvement was at 60 days postinjection, with an average of 10 letters of improvement. At least a 15-letter improvement from baseline was seen in 30% to 32% of patients in those who received 2 treatments. Of particular interest for the surgeon planning CE are the known side effects of increased IOP and cataract formation. In the GENEVA study, cataract progression occurred in nearly 30% of phakic patients who received 2 implants, although cataract surgery was only performed in 1.3% [57]. In the COMRADE-C study, ranibizumab was compared with Dex implantation. Although similar efficacy was observed between the 2 treatments, the effect of Dex declined after 3 months, suggesting that, when used, Dex may require retreatment intervals shorter than 6 months, consistent with previous studies [58].

Management: postoperative

Pseudophakic ME is a common vision-impairing complication after cataract surgery. Few studies have directly examined the effects of phacoemulsification and intraocular lens implantation on the severity and treatment of RVO-related ME. Although limited in scope, the studies highlighted below may provide valuable insight to surgical planning.

Cho and colleagues [59] evaluated the incidence of pseudophakic ME in 113 eyes with a history of RVO before cataract surgery. The results from this study showed that 27.4% of these eyes developed ME within 3 months of surgery, leading to significantly worse vision. Eyes that had a history of treatment of ME before cataract surgery were found to have an 11-fold increased risk (OR = 11.022) of developing CME in the postoperative period, with an even greater risk associated with a larger number of previous intravitreal treatments for ME. At 6 months, VA was no longer significantly different between the eyes that initially developed ME and those that did not [59]. These results suggest that although a greater risk of pseudophakic cystoid macular edema (PCME) exists in patients with a history of RVO, the potential for good visual outcomes remains.

In the same study by Cho and colleagues, eyes that were previously treated for ME with intravitreal injections were treated with the same drug if ME occurred after cataract surgery. If no previous treatments had been performed, eyes were treated with topical NSAIDs, IVT, or anti-VEGF. Most eyes responded to 1 treatment, and all but 2 of the 31 eyes resolved with treatment by 6 months after cataract surgery. Despite higher incidence of pseudophakic ME in this study, visual outcomes remained consistent with previous reports.

The small case series by Sze and colleagues [60] evaluated the safety and efficacy of concurrent intravitreal Dex implantation and cataract surgery in 24 eyes with ME at the time of surgery. Half of these patients had ME secondary to RVO (10 CRVO, 2 BRVO), and the remainder were diabetic in origin. Although this study demonstrated that intravitreal Dex at the time of cataract surgery was safe and effective, subgroup analysis showed that the benefits were more profound in the DME compared with the RVO group, with significant BCVA improvement and less recurrence of ME at a median follow-up time of 13 months. Yet, 75% of RVO eyes had 2 or more lines of BCVA at both 3-month and final follow-up, and central macular thickness decreased from 667.5 to 301.3 μm ($P = .003$) at the study's conclusion. Complications, particularly steroid-induced IOP elevation, occurred rarely, but still should be discussed with all patients. Given the success of Dex implantation in the GENEVA study, treatment concurrent with CE serves a reasonable choice in the perioperative period.

Limited data exist to date examining the postoperative management of RVO-associated ME in the postcataract surgery patient, due to the inherent difficulty in distinguishing between postoperative ME due to RVO versus postsurgical inflammation. In the studies that do address this issue, patients may require more, albeit similar, treatments for RVO-associated ME. Although visual outcomes with pharmacologic treatment are excellent, potential increased costs should be considered and discussed during the informed consent process.

IRVINE-GASS

Introduction

Cataract is the leading cause of blindness in the world, and PCME is the leading complications [61]. Also known as Irvine-Gass syndrome, this postoperative form of ME has been reported in up to 20% of patients after CE; however, in the absence of diabetes the incidence is near 1% [61]. The cost burden of PCME in the United States is significant, with 1 study finding near double the claims cost ($10,410 vs $5950) among Medicare patients [62]. In patients with a history of DR, including those without any history of previous DME, the underlying cause of new ME may be difficult to delineate. PCME is thought to be caused by release of inflammatory cytokines postoperatively, which is a known chronic state for patients with DME [63]. Since ME after cataract surgery may lead to disappointing visual outcomes, differentiating between isolated PCME and ME from other causes is important for patient counseling and subsequent treatment regimen.

Diagnosis

Differentiating between PCME and other causes of CME, particularly DME, UME, and CME secondary to RVO, may be difficult. As with other causes of CME, OCT and FA may be of benefit in differentiating the underlying cause. Munk and colleagues [63] evaluated the usefulness of OCT as the only diagnostic modality in differentiating PCME from DME. OCT findings that significantly favored PCME included isolated inner nuclear layer cysts, presence of subretinal fluid, and absence of epiretinal membrane. Even among mixed DME/PCME cases, masked OCT readers could accurately delineate postoperative causality in 95% of these cases [63]. A prospective observational study compared FA and OCT for diagnoses of PCME. Among patients who did not demonstrate appreciable edema on FA, 25.8% were found to have ME on OCT diagnostic of PCME [64]. This suggests that OCT may be the most efficient primary imaging modality for differentiating PCME from DME, with FA a useful additional modality in some cases.

Management

Primary management of PCME involves topical NSAID and corticosteroid therapy, intravitreal anti-VEGF and corticosteroid therapy, and periocular corticosteroid injection [65]. Although large, placebo-controlled randomized trials (RCT) are sparse, many data support the use of topical NSAID and corticosteroid medications. A large retrospective cohort study within the Kaiser Permanente system identified a 0.73% rate of PCME [66]. Among this cohort, patients received perioperative prednisolone acetate (PA) alone, PA with NSAID, or intraoperative subconjunctival triamcinolone acetonide (TA) injection alone. The PA + NSAID group had lower odds of developing PCME (OR = 0.45) compared with PA alone, and the subconjunctival TA alone group had increased odds of PCME compared with PA alone (OR = 1.21) [66]. Wielders and colleagues [18] published a systematic review of prevention of PCME among diabetic and nondiabetic populations. Topical monotherapy favored NSAID to PA treatment (OR = 0.11 and 0.05, nondiabetic and mixed populations), and combination topical NSAID + PA treatment decreased risk of PCME also (OR = 0.21 and 0.17). Preoperative intravitreal corticosteroid or anti-VEGF injection did not show additional benefit in this analysis [18]. A small RCT compared PA, NSAID, and combination PA + NSAID therapy for treatment of PCME and found significant benefit of combination treatment [67]. In addition, improvement in edema was more rapid in combination therapy [67]. Mean improvement in VA was 3.8 lines in combination therapy versus 1.6 and 1.1 lines in NSAID and PA therapy, respectively [67].

Intravitreal corticosteroids are a sensible treatment modality given the proposed proinflammatory origin of PCME. Gloth and colleagues [68] evaluated 86 eyes with postoperative CME (82 eyes with PCME) treated with a single intravitreal TA injection, and found durable benefit through a 6-month follow-up period. At 3-month follow-up, 63% of eyes had either resolution of or improvement in ME (29% and 34%), as well as improvement of 2 lines or more in VA acuity in 42.2% of patients. Intravitreal Dex implant also has been shown to be well tolerated among patients with recalcitrant PCME [69]. Subgroup analysis of patients in the Dex drug delivery system study group with persistent PCME or CME secondary to uveitis found significant improvement in VA and decrease in angiographic edema on FA [69]. A prospective case series of 27 patients with PCME refractory to topical therapy and periocular steroid injection found significant improvement in mean VA (from 20/70 to 20/25), as well as mean CSF from 454 μm at baseline to 214 μm at month 12 [70]. Only 1 patient needed reinjection, suggesting the remarkable durability of Dex implant within this patient population [71].

Furthermore, safety and side-effect profiles within this population are favorable for intravitreal implant, particularly as cataract progression is no longer a concern in these patients.

Alternative therapy includes intravitreal anti-VEGF injection in patients with or without previous history of DR. Arevalo and colleagues [71] reported significant improvement in mean VA and in CSF among patients with refractory PCME treated with bevacizumab (Avastin; Genentech) monotherapy. At 12 months, mean CSF decreased from 499.9 to 286.1 μm, with a mean of only 2.7 injections during that period. Another retrospective case series of 16 patients with PCME reported improved mean anatomic but not visual outcomes after bevacizumab injection [72]. Treatment of PCME with anti-VEGF monotherapy seems to be an option in patients with PCME refractory to topical therapy, particularly in those with previous DME or DR, although anti-VEGF monotherapy in true patients with PCME may not yet be validated.

Lastly, pars plana vitrectomy (PPV) for recalcitrant PCME has been investigated. Harbor et al. reported a retrospective case series of 24 patients with chronic PCME and evidence of vitreous adhesion (23 eyes) or iris capture (1 eye). Mean post-operative visual acuity improved by 4.7 lines with a range of one to eight lines, and time to vitrectomy was not found to portend a worse outcome [73]. Pendergast et al. examined patients with chronic PCME and without evidence of vitreous-corneal wound incarceration who underwent PPV. In this series, vitreous adhesion to posterior iris or intraocular lens, or vitreous in the anterior chamber, was present in 82.6% of patients [74]. All patients had resolution of PCME within an average of 3.3 months, and mean improvement in visual acuity was 3.3 lines [74]. For patients with vitreous incarceration, vitreous traction to iris or lens, or with altered vitreous anatomy without visible traction, PPV may be of benefit in recalcitrant PCME.

SUMMARY

Management of ME in the cataract patient is complicated, with a heterogeneous group of underlying diagnoses and specific considerations that must be made. Whether from underlying DR and DME, UME, or pseudophakic ME, the pathophysiology likely shares a common proinflammatory pathway. Even so, treatment must be tailored to the individual patient. Imaging of any patient at risk should be undertaken preoperatively, with OCT standard of care, and addition of FA in select cases. Similarly, postoperative OCT in any patient with history of ME or with unexplained decreased VA or hyperopic shift will aid in identification of PCME and differentiation from other causes of ME.

Although a paucity of high-quality supportive data exist, it is prudent to consider preoperative treatment in those patients at high risk for PCME. As discussed previously, patients with uveitis in particular seem to warrant a 3-month quiescent interval as well as preoperative topical and/or systemic corticosteroids. Studies from the DRCR.net suggest an increased risk for patients with and without central-involved DME, and thus preoperative anti-VEGF or corticosteroid injection likely is beneficial. In patients with preexisting RVO with or without ME, an increased risk of postoperative ME occurs. As a result, more frequent treatments may be required in the postoperative setting, although compelling evidence exists that visual prognosis is good with prompt diagnosis and early pharmacologic management.

Treatment of postoperative CME often is accomplished with topical therapy alone. Current studies suggest good efficacy of NSAID monotherapy, with possible additional effect of topical corticosteroids. However, in recalcitrant cases, alternate therapy should be considered on a case-by-case basis. In patients with DR, anti-VEGF treatment may be favored, whereas patients with isolated PCME without history of glaucoma may be candidates for intraocular corticosteroids. Given the underlying inflammatory state, patients with uveitis may benefit most from local control with intravitreal corticosteroids, including long-acting steroid depot. For ME in the setting of RVO, both intravitreal steroids and anti-VEGF have proven efficacious, and are likely preferable after cataract surgery as they are in patients not undergoing surgery.

References

[1] Lee R, Wong TY, Sabanayagam C. Epidemiology of diabetic retinopathy, diabetic macular edema and related vision loss. Eye Vis (Lond) 2015;2:17.

[2] National Diabetes Statistics Report, 2017. Centers for Disease Control and Prevention. Available at: https://www.cdc.gov/diabetes/pdfs/data/statistics/national-diabetes-statistics-report.pdf. Accessed February 9, 2019.

[3] Varma R, Bressler NM, Doan QV, et al. Prevalence of and risk factors for diabetic macular edema in the United States. JAMA Ophthalmol 2014;132:1334–40.

[4] Das A, McGuire PG, Rangasamy S. Diabetic macular edema: pathophysiology and novel therapeutic targets ophthalmology. Ophthalmology 2015;122:1375–94.

[5] Javadi MA, Zarei-ghanavati S. Cataracts in diabetic patients: a review article. J Ophthalmic Vis Res 2008;3:52–65.

[6] Klein BE, Klein R, Moss SE. Incidence of cataract surgery in the Wisconsin Epidemiologic Study of Diabetic Retinopathy. Am J Ophthalmol 1995;119:295–300.

[7] Menchini U, Bandello F, Brancato R, et al. Cystoid macular oedema after extracapsular cataract extraction and intraocular lens implantation in diabetic patients without retinopathy. Br J Ophthalmol 1993;77:208–11.

[8] Mittra RA, Borrillo JL, Dev S, et al. Retinopathy progression and visual outcomes after phacoemulsification in patients with diabetes mellitus. Arch Ophthalmol 2000;118:912–7.

[9] Photocoagulation for diabetic macular edema. Early Treatment Diabetic Retinopathy Study report number 1. Early Treatment Diabetic Retinopathy Study research group. Arch Ophthalmol 1985;103:1796–806.

[10] Waheed NK, Duker JS. OCT in the management of diabetic macular edema. Curr Ophthalmol Rep 2013;1:128–33.

[11] Sun JK, Lin MM, Lammer J, et al. Disorganization of the retinal inner layers as a predictor of visual acuity in eyes with center-involved diabetic macular edema. JAMA Ophthalmol 2014;132:1309–16.

[12] Soliman AZ, Radwan SH, Prager SG, et al. Spectral domain optical coherence tomography parameters associated with visual acuity in patients with resolved center-involved diabetic macular edema. Invest Ophthalmol Vis Sci 2012;53:1338.

[13] Unnikrishnan AG. Intensive glucose control: the UKPDS and DCCT revisited. Kerala J Ophthalmol 2010;22:359–61.

[14] Fenwick EK, Xie J, Man REK, et al. Combined poor diabetes control indicators are associated with higher risks of diabetic retinopathy and macular edema than poor glycemic control alone. PLoS One 2017;12:e018025.
[15] Diabetic Retinopathy Clinical Research Network. Pilot study of individuals with diabetic macular edema undergoing cataract surgery (Protocol P). JAMA Ophthalmol 2014;132: 224–6.
[16] Diabetic Retinopathy Clinical Research Network, Writing Committee, Baker CW, Almukhtar T, Bressler NM, et al. Edema after cataract surgery in eyes without pre-operative central-involved diabetic macular edema (Protocol Q). JAMA Ophthalmol 2013;131: 870–9.
[17] Moshfeghi AA, Shapiro H, Lemmon LA, et al. Impact of cataract surgery during treatment with ranibizumab in patients with diabetic macular edema. Ophthalmol Retina 2018;2: 86–90.
[18] Wielders LH, Lambermont VA, Schouten JS, et al. Prevention of cystoid macular edema after cataract surgery in nondiabetic and diabetic patients: a systematic review and meta-analysis. Am J Ophthalmol 2015;160:968–81.
[19] Yumuşak E, Örnek K. Comparison of perioperative ranibizumab injections for diabetic macular edema in patients undergoing cataract surgery. J Ophthalmol 2016;2016:7945619.
[20] Chae JB, Joe SG, Yang SJ, et al. Effect of combined cataract surgery and ranibizumab injection in postoperative macular edema in nonproliferative diabetic retinopathy. Retina 2014;34:149–56.
[21] Takamura Y, Kubo E, Akagi Y. Analysis of the effect of intravitreal bevacizumab injection on diabetic macular edema after cataract surgery. Ophthalmology 2009;116:1151–7.
[22] Heier JS, Korobelnik JF, Brown DM, et al. Intravitreal aflibercept for diabetic macular edema: 148-week results from the VISTA and VIVID studies. Ophthalmology 2016;123: 2376–85.
[23] Singh R. Prevention of Macular Edema in Patient with Diabetic Retinopathy undergoing Cataract Surgery with Intravitreal Aflibercept Injection (PROMISE). Presented at: 35th Annual Meeting of the American Society of Retina Specialists. Boston, Massachusetts, August 11–15, 2017. 2017.
[24] Lim LL, Morrison JL, Constantinou M, et al. Diabetic macular edema at the time of cataract surgery trial: a prospective, randomized clinical trial of intravitreous bevacizumab versus triamcinolone in patients with diabetic macular oedema at the time of cataract surgery preliminary 6 month results. Clin Exp Ophthalmol 2016;44:233–42.
[25] Panozzo GA, Gusson E, Panozzo G, et al. Dexamethasone intravitreal implant at the time of cataract surgery in eyes with diabetic macular edema. Eur J Ophthalmol 2017;27:433–7.
[26] Boyer DS, Yoon YH, Belfort R, et al. Three-year, randomized, sham-controlled trial of dexamethasone intravitreal implant in patients with diabetic macular edema. Ophthalmology 2014;121:1904–14.
[27] Pacella F, Ferraresi AF, Turchetti P, et al. Intravitreal injection of ozurdex implant in patients with persistent diabetic macular edema, with six-month follow-up. Ophthalmol Eye Dis 2016;8:11–6.
[28] Pareja-ríos A, Ruiz-de la fuente-rodríguez P, Bonaque-gonzález S, et al. Intravitreal dexamethasone implants for diabetic macular edema. Int J Ophthalmol 2018;11:77–82.
[29] Campochiaro PA, Brown DM, Pearson A, et al. Sustained delivery fluocinolone acetonide vitreous inserts provide benefit for at least 3 years in patients with diabetic macular edema. Ophthalmology 2012;119:2125–32.
[30] Yang Y, Bailey C, Holz FG, et al. Long-term outcomes of phakic patients with diabetic macular oedema treated with intravitreal fluocinolone acetonide (FAc) implants. Eye (Lond) 2015;29:1173–80.
[31] Fardeau C, Champion E, Massamba N, et al. Uveitic macular edema. Eye (Lond) 2016;30: 1277–92.

[32] Goldhardt R, Rosen BS. Uveitic macular edema: treatment update. Curr Ophthalmol Rep 2016;4:30–7.

[33] Elgohary MA, Mccluskey PJ, Towler HM, et al. Outcome of phacoemulsification in patients with uveitis. Br J Ophthalmol 2007;91:916–21.

[34] Agrawal R, Murthy S, Ganesh SK, et al. Cataract surgery in uveitis. Int J Inflam 2012;2012: 548453.

[35] Rothova A, Suttorp-van Schulten MS, Frits Treffers W, et al. Causes and frequency of blindness in patients with intraocular inflammatory disease. Br J Ophthalmol 1996;80:332–6.

[36] Radwan AE, Arcinue CA, Yang P, et al. Bromfenac alone or with single intravitreal injection of bevacizumab or triamcinolone acetonide for treatment of uveitic macular edema. Graefes Arch Clin Exp Ophthalmol 2013;251:1801–6.

[37] Allegri P, Murialdo U, Peri S, et al. Randomized, double-blind, placebo-controlled clinical trial on the efficacy of 0.5% indomethacin eye drops in uveitic macular edema. Invest Ophthalmol Vis Sci 2014;55:1463–70.

[38] Leder HA, Jabs DA, Galor A, et al. Periocular triamcinolone acetonide injections for cystoid macular edema complicating noninfectious uveitis. Am J Ophthalmol 2011;152:441–8.

[39] Sen HN, Vitale S, Gangaputra SS, et al. Periocular corticosteroid injections in uveitis: effects and complications. Ophthalmology 2014;121:2275–86.

[40] Androudi S, Letko E, Meniconi M, et al. Safety and efficacy of intravitreal triamcinolone acetonide for uveitic macular edema. Ocul Immunol Inflamm 2005;13:205–12.

[41] Yeh S, Kurup SK, Wang RC, et al. Suprachoroidal injection of triamcinolone acetonide, CLS-TA, for macular edema due to noninfectious uveitis: a Randomized, Phase 2 Study (DOGWOOD). Retina 2018. [Epub ahead of print].

[42] Kempen JH, Altaweel MM, Holbrook JT, et al. Randomized comparison of systemic anti-inflammatory therapy versus fluocinolone acetonide implant for intermediate, posterior, and panuveitis: the multicenter uveitis steroid treatment trial. Ophthalmology 2011;118: 1916–26.

[43] Lowder C, Belfort R Jr, Lightman S, et al. Dexamethasone intravitreal implant for noninfectious intermediate or posterior uveitis. Arch Ophthalmol 2011;129:545–53.

[44] Thorne JE, Sugar EA, Holbrook JT, et al. Periocular Triamcinolone vs. Intravitreal Triamcinolone vs. Intravitreal Dexamethasone Implant for the Treatment of Uveitic Macular Edema: The PeriOcular vs. INTravitreal corticosteroids for uveitic macular edema (POINT) Trial. Ophthalmology 2019;126(2):283–95.

[45] Larochelle MB, Smith J, Dacey MS. Dexamethasone intravitreal implant in the treatment of uveitic macular edema in the perioperative cataract setting: a case series. Am J Ophthalmol 2016;166:149–53.

[46] Bélair ML, Kim SJ, Thorne JE, et al. Incidence of cystoid macular edema after cataract surgery in patients with and without uveitis using optical coherence tomography. Am J Ophthalmol 2009;148:128–35.

[47] Sepah YJ, Sadiq MA, Chu DS, et al. Primary (Month-6) outcomes of the STOP-Uveitis Study: evaluating the safety, tolerability, and efficacy of tocilizumab in patients with noninfectious Uveitis. Am J Ophthalmol 2017;183:71–80.

[48] Rogers S, McIntosh RL, Cheung N, et al. The prevalence of retinal vein occlusion: pooled data from population studies from the United States, Europe, Asia, and Australia. Ophthalmology 2010 Feb;117(2):313–9.

[49] The Branch Vein Occlusion Study Group. Argon laser photocoagulation for macular edema in branch vein occlusion. Am J Ophthalmol 1984;98:271–82.

[50] Evaluation of grid pattern photocoagulation for macular edema in central vein occlusion. The Central Vein Occlusion Study Group M report. Ophthalmology 1995;102:1425–33.

[51] Clark WL, Boyer DS, Heier JS. Intravitreal aflibercept for macular edema following branch retinal vein occlusion: 52-week results of the VIBRANT study. Ophthalmology 2016;123: 330–6.

[52] Pielen A, Clark WL, Boyer DS, et al. Integrated results from the COPERNICUS and GALILEO studies. Clin Ophthalmol 2017;11:1533–40.
[53] Brown DM, Campochiaro PA, Bhisitkul RB. Sustained benefits from ranibizumab for macular edema following branch retinal vein occlusion: 12-month outcomes of a phase III study. Ophthalmology 2011;118:1594–602.
[54] Campochiaro PA, Brown DM, Awh CC, et al. Sustained benefits from ranibizumab for macular edema following central retinal vein occlusion: twelve-month outcomes of a phase III study. Ophthalmology 2011;118:2041–9.
[55] Scott IU, VanVeldhuisen PC, Ip MS. Effect of Bevacizumab vs Aflibercept on visual acuity among patients with macular edema due to central retinal vein occlusion: The SCORE2 Randomized Clinical Trial. JAMA 2017;317:2072–87.
[56] Scott IU, Ip MS, VanVeldhuisen PC, et al. A randomized trial comparing the efficacy and safety of intravitreal triamcinolone with standard care to treat vision loss associated with macular edema secondary to branch retinal vein occlusion: the Standard Care vs Corticosteroid for Retinal Vein Occlusion (SCORE) Study report 6. Arch Ophthalmol 2009;127:1115–28.
[57] Haller JA, Bandello F, Belfort R Jr, et al. Dexamethasone intravitreal implant in patients with macular edema related to branch or central retinal vein occlusion twelve-month study results. Ophthalmology 2011;118:2453–60.
[58] Hoerauf H, Feltgen N, Weiss C, et al. Clinical efficacy and safety of ranibizumab versus dexamethasone for central retinal vein occlusion (COMRADE C): A European Label Study. Am J Ophthalmol 2016;169:258–67.
[59] Cho HJ, Hwang HJ, Kim HS, et al. Macular edema after cataract surgery in eyes with preoperative retinal vein occlusion. Retina 2018;38:1180–6.
[60] Sze AM, Luk FO, Yip TP, et al. Use of intravitreal dexamethasone implant in patients with cataract and macular edema undergoing phacoemulsification. Eur J Ophthalmol 2015;25:168–72.
[61] Chu CJ, Johnston RL, Buscombe C, et al. Risk factors and incidence of macular edema after cataract surgery: a database study of 81984 eyes. Ophthalmology 2016;123:316–23.
[62] Schmier JK, Covert DW, Hulme-lowe CK, et al. Treatment costs of cystoid macular edema among patients following cataract surgery. Clin Ophthalmol 2016;10:477–83.
[63] Munk MR, Jampol LM, Simader C, et al. Differentiation of diabetic macular edema from pseudophakic cystoid macular edema by spectral-domain optical coherence tomography. Invest Ophthalmol Vis Sci 2015;56:6724–33.
[64] Moreira TC, Silva FCL, Vilela LR, et al. Irvine-gass syndrome - fluorescein angiography vs. optical coherence tomography. Invest Ophthalmol Vis Sci 2009;50:351.
[65] Shelsta HN, Jampol LM. Pharmacologic therapy of pseudophakic cystoid macular edema: 2010 update. Retina 2011;31:4–12.
[66] Shorstein NH, Liu L, Waxman MD, et al. Comparative effectiveness of three prophylactic strategies to prevent clinical macular edema after phacoemulsification surgery. Ophthalmology 2015;122:2450–6.
[67] Heier JS, Topping TM, Baumann W, et al. Ketorolac versus prednisolone versus combination therapy in the treatment of acute pseudophakic cystoid macular edema. Ophthalmology 2000;107:2034–8.
[68] Gloth JM, Roth DB, Yarian DL, et al. Treatment of refractory post–operative cystoid macular edema (CME) with intravitreal triamcinolone. Invest Ophthalmol Vis Sci 2005;46:1455.
[69] Williams GA, Haller JA, Kuppermann BD, et al. Dexamethasone posterior-segment drug delivery system in the treatment of macular edema resulting from uveitis or Irvine-Gass syndrome. Am J Ophthalmol 2009;147:1048–54.
[70] Sudhalkar A, Chhablani J, Vasavada A, et al. Intravitreal dexamethasone implant for recurrent cystoid macular edema due to Irvine-Gass syndrome: a prospective case series. Eye (Lond) 2016;30:1549–57.

[71] Arevalo JF, Maia M, Garcia-Amaris RA, et al. Intravitreal bevacizumab for refractory pseudophakic cystoid macular edema: the Pan-American Collaborative Retina Study Group results. Ophthalmology 2009;116:1481–7.
[72] Spitzer MS, Ziemssen F, Yoeruek E, et al. Efficacy of intravitreal bevacizumab in treating postoperative pseudophakic cystoid macular edema. J Cataract Refract Surg 2008;34(1):70–5.
[73] Harbour JW, Smiddy WE, Rubsamen PE, et al. Pars plana vitrectomy for chronic pseudophakic cystoid macular edema. Am J Ophthalmol 1995;120:302–7.
[74] Pendergast SD, Margherio RR, Williams GA, et al. Vitrectomy for chronic pseudophakic cystoid macular edema. Am J Ophthalmol 1999;128:317–23.

Section VI: Glaucoma

Advances in Ophthalmology and Optometry 4 (2019) 211–222

ADVANCES IN OPHTHALMOLOGY AND OPTOMETRY

Glaucoma at the Center of the Earth

Jean-Claude Mwanza, MD, MPH, PhD,
Donald L. Budenz, MD, MPH*

Department of Ophthalmology, University of North Carolina at Chapel Hill, 130 Mason Farm Road, 5151 Bioinformatics Building, CB #7040, Chapel Hill, NC 27599-7040, USA

Keywords

• Glaucoma • Prevalence • Incidence • Center of the Earth • Ghana

Key points

- Glaucoma is a problem of public health concern in sub-Saharan Africa based on modeling-based estimates.
- Reliable population-based studies remain scarce, but available data show a higher burden of glaucoma in West Africa than in the rest of sub-Saharan Africa.
- Prevalence and incidence data from the Tema Eye Survey conducted near the "center of the earth" indicate that West Africans may have the greatest burden globally.

INTRODUCTION

Open-angle glaucoma (OAG), simply referred to hereafter as glaucoma, is a chronic and progressive degenerative optic neuropathy that leads to characteristic changes to the optic disc with corresponding visual field deficits. Visual field deficits eventually progress to blindness if the disease is not treated or is treated inadequately. Recent estimates based on a meta-analysis indicate that glaucoma is responsible for 8.5% of blindness globally and rank glaucoma as the third main cause of blindness worldwide in persons aged 50 years and older, behind cataract (35.2%) and uncorrected refractive errors (20.3%). Glaucoma accounts for 11.7% to 14.1% in sub-Saharan Africa (SSA), where 47.6% to 56.7% of blindness is caused by preventable or curable eye diseases [1]. Despite being more prevalent than in other parts of the world, glaucoma in

Disclosure Statement: The authors have nothing to disclose.

*Corresponding author. *E-mail address:* donald_budenz@med.unc.edu

https://doi.org/10.1016/j.yaoo.2019.04.017
2452-1760/19/

SSA remains largely neglected and is not given priority with regard to community-based awareness, detection, management, and capacity building. This is likely due to the irreversible nature of the disease, lack of surveillance, and poor access to treatment. Effort has been focused on eye diseases with cost-effective treatment and for which there exist preventive and/or curative remedies, such as cataract, onchocerciasis, refractive errors, and trachoma. In Africa, as in other developing parts of the world, comprehensive eye care programs that include both detection in the community and management of glaucoma remain scarce. Although private isolated initiatives (ie, STOP Glaucoma in SSA) occur [2], a concerted effort came after the World Glaucoma Association (WGA), after many years of work, succeeded in assembling a group of eye care professionals interested in tackling glaucoma on the continent. This effort ultimately led to the First African Glaucoma Summit, held in Accra, Ghana, as a 2-day meeting where the WGA decided to recognize glaucoma as a priority eye disease and center its efforts on Africa. This article provides a review of prevalence and incidence of glaucoma in SSA, with special emphasis on data from Ghana, West Africa.

PREVALENCE OF GLAUCOMA

Modeling data

Epidemiologic characteristics of a disease, such as incidence and prevalence, are critical for a better understanding of the burden of a given disease and for studying cost-effectiveness analyses of interventions. Such studies provide essential information for policy making, planning, resource and budget prioritization and allocation, and development of detection and management programs. When empirical observation to obtain epidemiologic information is incomplete or not possible, modeling techniques become an alternative to generate epidemiologic features. The prevalence of glaucoma in most SSA countries remains unknown because of the lack of both population-based and hospital-based studies. In a few countries only partial data are available, making it difficult to obtain reliable countrywide and continent-wide prevalence data. Box 1 provides a summary of our current knowledge on modeling-based prevalence of glaucoma in SSA.

Box 1: Notes on modeling-based prevalence of glaucoma in sub-Saharan Africa

- Predictive modeling estimates indicate a trend toward increase in the number of people with glaucoma worldwide in the next 20 years, as a result of improved life expectancy and global population growth [3]
- The increase will mostly affect Africa and Asia
- Both the crude and age-specific prevalence of glaucoma will remain higher in people of African descent than others throughout this period [3,4]
- Modeling-based estimates of glaucoma prevalence in SSA between 4.2% and 4.5% (Table 1) [3–5]

Table 1
Modeling-based prevalence (%) of open-angle glaucoma in Africa and world regions

	Quigley and Broman [5], 2006	Tham et al [3], 2014	Kapetanakis et al [4], 2016	Kapetanakis et al [4], 2016
Year	2010	2013	2015	2020
Age (years)	>40	40–80	≥40	≥40
Africa	4.16	4.2	4.5	4.5
Europe	1.97	2.51	2.0	2.1
Asia	—	2.31	1.8	1.9
North America	—	3.29	1.9	2.0
Latin America	—	3.65	3.4	3.5
World	1.96	3.05	2.2	2.3

Hospital-based prevalence of glaucoma in Africa

Prevalence data are important as they may be the first line of information about hospital utilization and basic epidemiologic measures needed for efficient strategy planning, resource prioritization and allocation, and development of prevention, diagnosis, and management programs. As hospitals have been growing in importance to respond to the medical needs of communities, they also have become more valuable resources for studying disease epidemiology. Thus, in resource-limited settings such as SSA, where population-based studies (PBS) are still difficult to perform, hospital-based studies (HBS) may be the alternative for providing interim data. A review of HBS shows prevalence estimates varying across African countries (Table 2) [6–13].

Population-based prevalence

Box 2 is a summary of what was known PBS before 2006.

The tema eye survey

The impetus for the Tema Eye Survey (TES) [29,30] was the realization that at the time only few comprehensive eye disease surveys in SSA existed. Before the TES, surveys on blindness and visual impairment on the continent

Table 2
Hospital-based prevalence of glaucoma in African countries

Country	Year	Prevalence (%)
Nigeria [6]	1998–2006	4.8
Nigeria [7]	2005	6.7
Ivory Coast [8]	1998	2.1
Congo (Brazzaville) [9]	2015	1.3
Congo (Brazzaville) [10]	2014	2.4
Ghana [11]	2003	6.6
Ghana [12]	2013	7.9
Cameroon [13]	2006	3.5

Box 2: Notes on population-based studies in sub-Saharan Africa

- There is a limited number of PBS for prevalence of glaucoma in SSA despite evidence of epidemiologic [14,15] and clinical [16–21] differences between people of African descent and those of other heritages
- Reasons: Attention focused on infectious diseases, high cost to run PBS, lack of specialized equipment, and limited number of trained glaucoma specialists
- Only 7 PBS had provided population-based prevalence data on glaucoma in SSA before 2006: four with reliable data [22–25] and three with less reliable findings [26–28]
- As a result of increasing life expectancy in SSA following economic growth, and improvement in living conditions and health indicators, the number of older people is rising and the prevalence of glaucoma is expected to increase

were performed mostly in rural areas and focused on trachoma and onchocerciasis. As these 2 diseases had been greatly reduced in magnitude at the time, a need existed for a modern eye survey in Africa. The practical intent of the TES was to help the local health authorities with reliable data for future planning of eye care resources. The characteristics of the study area are summarized in Box 3.

The TES was designed to determine the prevalence of blindness, visual impairment, and glaucoma and other eye diseases in an urban, West African, adult population. A target population of 5600 was selected using a multistage random cluster sampling method. An attempt was made to examine all residents 40 years or older of the selected 40 clusters from 5 municipalities. The study steps included mapping the communities, performing a census of the randomly selected clusters, performing field examination, and complete clinical examination by glaucoma specialists for those who failed field examinations. Optic disc photos were read at Moorfields Eye Hospital Reading Center

Box 3: Study area characteristics

- Tema is an urban area, fourth most populous Ghanaian city
- May be viewed geographically as the "Center of the Earth" for its location on the Greenwich Meridian (0° longitude) and close to the Equator (0° latitude) (see Fig. 1)
- Rapid economic development made Tema the "melting pot" of the country: approximately 57% of its population were immigrants from other parts of the country, which was an opportunity to make the TES findings more generalizable to the whole country
- Changing demographic: (1) life expectancy at birth increased (58 years in 2000 to 63 years currently, with projections to reach 75 years in 2050); (2) transition from a primarily agrarian population in the 1960s to an urban population (23% in 1960% to 50% in 2010)

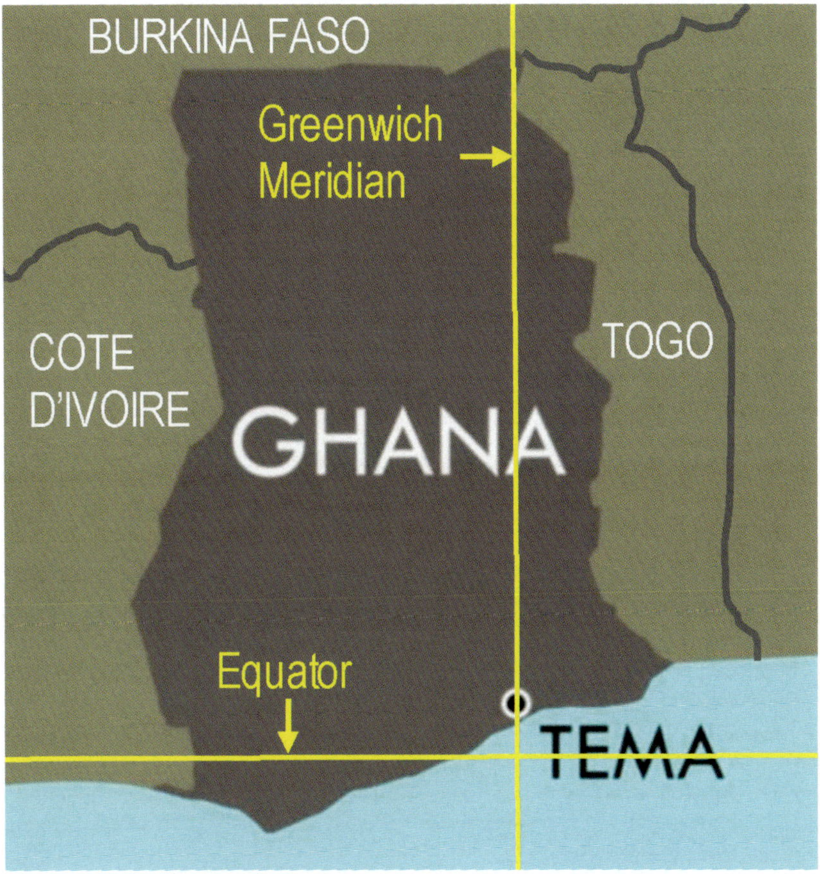

Fig. 1. Map of Ghana showing the location of Tema near the intersection between the Greenwich Meridian and the Equator.

(London, UK) and visual fields were interpreted by a United States–based glaucoma specialist. A summary of the strengths and the findings of the TES prevalence studies is given in Box 4.

Aggregating available HBS and PBS data, it is apparent that the prevalence of glaucoma in SSA is variable, likely because of differences in the definition of glaucoma. It is higher in West Africa than in East Africa and southern Africa. Wide genetic heterogeneity exists among populations, among countries, and often within the same country, which suggests a genetic explanation for the difference in prevalence rates.

INCIDENCE OF GLAUCOMA

Estimation of the incidence and determination of its predictors are important for the planning of services. Several glaucoma treatment options are available

Box 4: Key findings of Tema Eye Survey prevalence studies

Strengths

- Response rate: 82.2%, similar to other PBS as shown in Fig. 2
- Sample larger than in past PBS in SSA and in blacks outside SSA; these studies' sample sizes were 14.5% to 84% smaller than that of the TES [14,15,22–25,27,35–38]
- Sampling produced a fairly representative population of the whole country: 70% of the study population was equally distributed from other parts of the country

Visual impairment and blindness

- Based on the presenting visual acuity in the better eye, 18.3% and 1.9% of the subjects were visually impaired and blind, respectively. These rates decreased to 7.4% and 0.9% after refraction
- Glaucoma caused 14% and 20.9% of visual impairment and blindness, respectively, and was second to cataract [29]

Glaucoma

- Age and gender-adjusted prevalence of open-angle glaucoma (OAG) was 8.0%, higher than in other parts of SSA, but similar to estimates from the Caribbean and higher than in blacks outside SSA as shown in Table 3. High rates of 8.2% were reported in a rural setting of Cameroon [31], and 9.6% and 6.9% in a rural and an urban area of North Central Nigeria [32], but they are derived from studies with flawed methodologies
- The prevalence increased with age and was higher in men than women across all age groups
- Only 3% of those identified as having OAG in the study were aware they had glaucoma, similar to other areas in SSA [22–24,26,28,33], but much less than about 50% in developed countries [34]
- Among those diagnosed with glaucoma, 63.0% had a presenting intraocular pressure (IOP) less than 21 mm Hg, confirming that IOP is not a good indicator of the presence of glaucoma

in developed countries, but options such as implants and laser are either not available or infrequently available in SSA. Identification of individuals at high risk for glaucoma, therefore, is important for tailoring targeted approaches for prevention and/or treatment. In addition, incidence data are needed to plan rehabilitation services for individuals developing visual loss. The incidence of glaucoma has been investigated in a few studies worldwide, with no data from the African continent. Large variations exist in the prevalence, phenotypes, and incidence of glaucoma in different populations outside Africa, making it difficult to apply findings from other regions of the world to SSA. Alleles known to be associated with genetic glaucoma susceptibility in persons of European descent have been shown to play no role in glaucoma in people of African heritage [39].

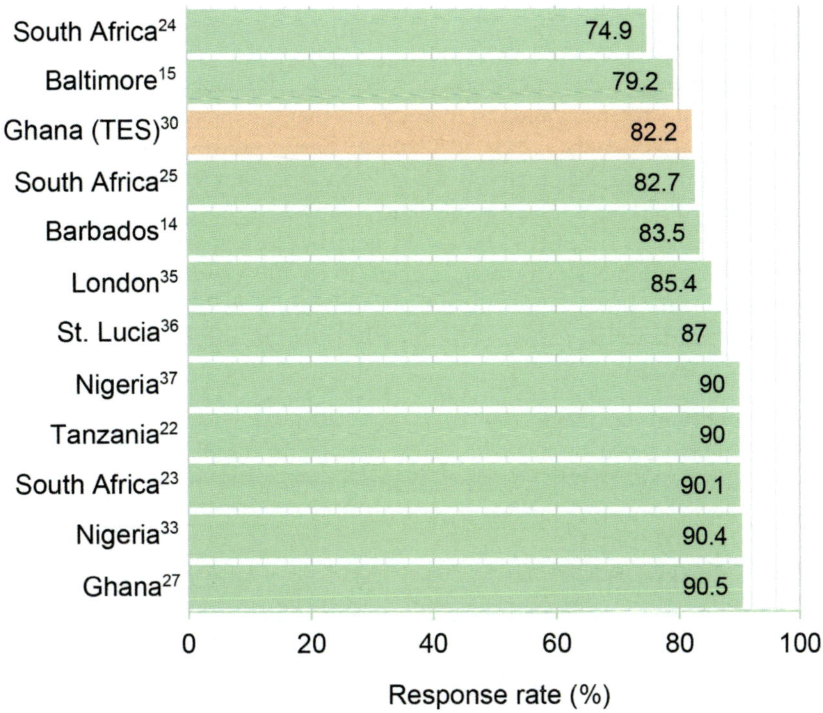

Fig. 2. Response rate in the Tema Eye Survey (TES) and other population-based studies in blacks in and outside sub-Saharan Africa.

Table 3
Population-based prevalence of glaucoma in blacks in and outside sub-Saharan Africa

Country	Prevalence (%)
Blacks in sub-Saharan Africa	
Nigeria [6]	1.5
South Africa [25]	1.5
Nigeria [33]	1.6
South Africa [23]	2.7
South Africa [24]	2.9
Tanzania [22]	3.6
Kenya [38]	4.3
Nigeria [37]	6.2
Ghana (TES) [30]	8.0
Blacks outside Africa	
London [35]	3.9
Baltimore [15]	4.4
Barbados [14]	7.4
St. Lucia [36]	9.6

Modeling-based incidence

The only attempt to estimate the incidence of glaucoma in SSA has come from Cook [17]. He used the incidence of visual loss attributable to glaucoma (0.04%) from a PBS in Uganda to hypothesize that the incidence of glaucoma would be approximately 0.04% in Central, East, and southern Africa. Of note, they cautioned that this was a very conservative estimation, and that West Africa would have a higher incidence. Outside SSA, Quigley and Vitale [40] proposed a model to estimate the incidence using prevalence data of OAG in the United States in people aged 30 to 100 years. They estimated an incidence rate of 4.2% among whites and 10.3% in blacks for the year 2000. The incidence increased more rapidly with age among blacks in comparison with whites.

Population-based incidence

Box 5 provides a take-home message on population-based incidence of glaucoma in SSA, while Fig. 3 is a representation of incidence rates of glaucoma in the TES and in blacks outside SSA [41–54].

FUTURE PERSPECTIVE

Most estimates have projected a future substantial increase in the number of people with glaucoma in SSA. However, accurate epidemiologic data on glaucoma in SSA will require country-specific PBS because of the wide heterogeneity of populations. These studies will help address not only the prevalence and incidence of glaucoma across countries but will also provide important information with regard to the natural history and risk factors of the disease in SSA. Another equally important issue to be addressed is the assessment of the efficacy of laser (ie, selective and micropulse laser trabeculoplasty) as a first-line treatment option for glaucoma [55–57]. Progression of glaucoma also will need to be studied in this setting.

Box 5: Notes on population-based studies on incidence of glaucoma in sub-Saharan Africa

- To date, the Tema Eye Survey (TES) is the only study that has provided population-based prevalence [30] and incidence [40] of glaucoma from the same cohort in SSA
- The TES incidence study was performed after an 8-year follow-up. The clinical assessment was identical at baseline and follow-up visit
- A random subset of 1500 previously normal subjects were contacted and invited, of whom 80.3% responded and were re-examined
- The age-adjusted annual incidence of glaucoma was 0.58%, higher than in nonblack populations and blacks in the Caribbean. Male sex and baseline older age, thinner central cornea, and larger vertical cup-to-disc ratio were associated with incident glaucoma
- The incidences reported in different black and nonblack populations outside SSA are shown in Fig. 3

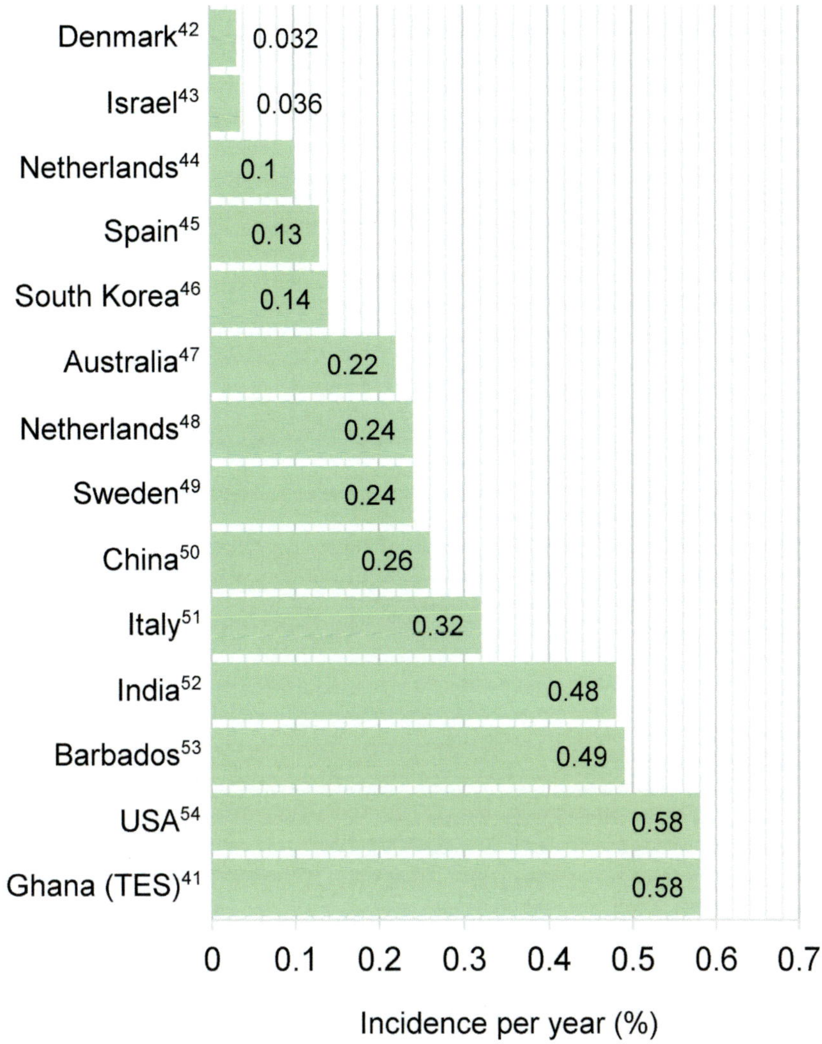

Fig. 3. Incidence of glaucoma in population-based studies around the world.

SUMMARY

OAG is more prevalent in people of African descent, particularly in those who trace their ancestry back to West Africa. Improved disease surveillance, better access to treatment, and better training in subspecialty surgery are all needed to combat the burden of blindness that will be caused by glaucoma in SSA over the next 50 years.

References

[1] Flaxman SR, Bourne RRA, Resnikoff S, et al. Global causes of blindness and distance vision impairment 1990-2020: a systematic review and meta-analysis. Lancet Glob Health 2017;5(12):e1221–34.

[2] Damji KF, Nazarali S, Giorgis A, et al. STOP Glaucoma in Sub Saharan Africa: enhancing awareness, detection, management, and capacity for glaucoma care. Expert Rev Ophthalmol 2017;12(3):197–206.
[3] Tham YC, Li X, Wong TY, et al. Global prevalence of glaucoma and projections of glaucoma burden through 2040: a systematic review and meta-analysis. Ophthalmology 2014;121(11):2081–90.
[4] Kapetanakis VV, Chan MP, Foster PJ, et al. Global variations and time trends in the prevalence of primary open angle glaucoma (POAG): a systematic review and meta-analysis. Br J Ophthalmol 2016;100(1):86–93.
[5] Quigley HA, Broman AT. The number of people with glaucoma worldwide in 2010 and 2020. Br J Ophthalmol 2006;90(3):262–7.
[6] Abba G. Prevalence of glaucoma in Nigeria. Internet J Epidemiol 2009;9(1):1–5.
[7] Omoti AE. Glaucoma in Benin-City, Nigeria. Niger Postgrad Med J 2005;12:189–92.
[8] Ahnoux-Zabsonre A, Keita C, Safede K, et al. Prevalence of primary chronic open-angle glaucoma in Ivory Coast. J Fr Ophtalmol 1998;21(9):643–7.
[9] Atipo-Tsiba PW. Profile of glaucoma patients at the University Hospital of Brazzaville. Rwanda Med J 2015;72(1):8–10.
[10] Makita C. Open-angle glaucoma and ocular hypertension in Brazzaville: 135 cases. Ann Sci Sante 2016;16(2):19–23.
[11] Ntim-Amponsah CT. Epidemiology of glaucoma: a population study in the Akwapim South district of Ghana [master's thesis]. Accra (Ghana): University of Ghana; 2003.
[12] Otabil KB, Tenkorang SB, Mac AL, et al. Prevalence of glaucoma in an eye clinic in Ghana. Russ Open Med J 2013;2(3):310.
[13] Ellong A, Mvogo CE, Bella-Hiag AL, et al. Prevalence of glaucomas in a Black Cameroonian population. Sante 2006;16(2):83–8.
[14] Leske MC, Connell AM, Schachat AP, et al. The Barbados Eye Study. Prevalence of open angle glaucoma. Arch Ophthalmol 1994;112(6):821–9.
[15] Tielsch JM, Sommer A, Katz J, et al. Racial variations in the prevalence of primary open-angle glaucoma. The Baltimore Eye Survey. JAMA 1991;266:369–74.
[16] AGIS. The Advanced Glaucoma Intervention Study (AGIS): 3. Baseline characteristics of black and white patients. Ophthalmology 1998;105(7):1137–45.
[17] Cook C. Glaucoma in Africa: size of the problem and possible solutions. J Glaucoma 2009;18(2):124–8.
[18] Girkin CA. Primary open-angle glaucoma in African Americans. Int Ophthalmol Clin 2004;44(2):43–60.
[19] Murakami Y, Lee BW, Duncan M, et al. Racial and ethnic disparities in adherence to glaucoma follow-up visits in a county hospital population. Arch Ophthalmol 2011;129(7): 872–8.
[20] Sommer A, Tielsch JM, Katz J, et al. Racial differences in the cause-specific prevalence of blindness in east Baltimore. N Engl J Med 1991;325(20):1412–7.
[21] Wang F, Javitt JC, Tielsch JM. Racial variations in treatment for glaucoma and cataract among Medicare recipients. Ophthalmic Epidemiol 1997;4(2):89–100.
[22] Buhrmann RR, Quigley HA, Barron Y, et al. Prevalence of glaucoma in a rural East African population. Invest Ophthalmol Vis Sci 2000;41(1):40–8.
[23] Rotchford AP, Johnson GJ. Glaucoma in Zulus: a population-based cross-sectional survey in a rural district in South Africa. Arch Ophthalmol 2002;120(4):471–8.
[24] Rotchford AP, Kirwan JF, Muller MA, et al. Temba glaucoma study: a population-based cross-sectional survey in urban South Africa. Ophthalmology 2003;110(2):376–82.
[25] Salmon JF, Mermoud A, Ivey A, et al. The prevalence of primary angle closure glaucoma and open angle glaucoma in Mamre, western Cape, South Africa. Arch Ophthalmol 1993;111(9):1263–9.
[26] Ekwerekwu CM, Umeh RE. The prevalence of glaucoma in an onchoendemic community in South-Eastern Nigeria. West Afr J Med 2002;21(3):200–3.

[27] Guzek JP, Anyomi FK, Fiadoyor S, et al. Prevalence of blindness in people over 40 years in the Volta region of Ghana. Ghana Med J 2005;39(2):55–62.
[28] Ntim-Amponsah CT, Amoaku WM, Ofosu-Amaah S, et al. Prevalence of glaucoma in an African population. Eye (Lond) 2004;18(5):491–7.
[29] Budenz DL, Bandi JR, Barton K, et al. Blindness and visual impairment in an urban West African population: the Tema Eye Survey. Ophthalmology 2012;119(9):1744–53.
[30] Budenz DL, Barton K, Whiteside-de Vos J, et al. Prevalence of glaucoma in an urban West African population: the Tema Eye Survey. JAMA Ophthalmol 2013;131(5):651–8.
[31] Preussner PR, Grossmann A, Ngounou F, et al. Glaucoma screening in Western Cameroon. Graefes Arch Clin Exp Ophthalmol 2009;247(12):1671–5.
[32] Durowade KA, Salaudeen AG, Akande TM, et al. Prevalence and risk factors of glaucoma among adults in rural and urban communities of Ilorin West local government area, North-Central Nigeria. Int J Clin Med 2016;3(1):6–12.
[33] Kyari F, Entekume G, Rabiu M, et al. A population-based survey of the prevalence and types of glaucoma in Nigeria: results from the Nigeria National Blindness and Visual Impairment Survey. BMC Ophthalmol 2015;15:176.
[34] Friedman DS, Wolfs RC, O'Colmain BJ, et al. Prevalence of open-angle glaucoma among adults in the United States. Arch Ophthalmol 2004;122(4):532–8.
[35] Wormald RP, Basauri E, Wright LA, et al. The African Caribbean Eye Survey: risk factors for glaucoma in a sample of African Caribbean people living in London. Eye (Lond) 1994;8(Pt 3):315–20.
[36] Mason RP, Kosoko O, Wilson MR, et al. National survey of the prevalence and risk factors of glaucoma in St. Lucia, West Indies. Part I. Prevalence findings. Ophthalmology 1989;96(9):1363–8.
[37] Ashaye A, Ashaolu O, Komolafe O, et al. Prevalence and types of glaucoma among an indigenous African population in southwestern Nigeria. Invest Ophthalmol Vis Sci 2013;54(12):7410–6.
[38] Bastawrous A, Mathenge W, Buchan J, et al. Glaucoma features in an East African population: a 6-year cohort study of older adults in Nakuru, Kenya. J Glaucoma 2018;27(5):455–63.
[39] Liu Y, Hauser MA, Akafo SK, et al. Investigation of known genetic risk factors for primary open angle glaucoma in two populations of African ancestry. Invest Ophthalmol Vis Sci 2013;54(9):6248–54.
[40] Quigley HA, Vitale S. Models of open-angle glaucoma prevalence and incidence in the United States. Invest Ophthalmol Vis Sci 1997;38(1):83–91.
[41] Mwanza JC, Tulenko SE, Barton K, et al. Eight-year incidence of open-angle glaucoma in the Tema Eye Survey. Ophthalmology 2019;126(3):372–80.
[42] Kolko M, Horwitz A, Thygesen J, et al. The prevalence and incidence of glaucoma in Denmark in a fifteen year period: a nationwide study. PLoS One 2015;10(7):e0132048.
[43] Levkovitch-Verbin H, Goldshtein I, Chodick G, et al. The Maccabi Glaucoma Study: prevalence and incidence of glaucoma in a large Israeli health maintenance organization. Am J Ophthalmol 2014;158(2):402–408 e401.
[44] de Voogd S, Ikram MK, Wolfs RC, et al. Incidence of open-angle glaucoma in a general elderly population: the Rotterdam Study. Ophthalmology 2005;112(9):1487–93.
[45] Perez-de-Arcelus M, Toledo E, Martinez-Gonzalez MA, et al. Smoking and incidence of glaucoma: The SUN Cohort. Medicine (Baltimore) 2017;96(1):e5761.
[46] Kim YK, Choi HJ, Jeoung JW, et al. Five-year incidence of primary open-angle glaucoma and rate of progression in health center-based Korean population: the Gangnam Eye Study. PLoS One 2014;9(12):e114058.
[47] Mukesh BN, McCarty CA, Rait JL, et al. Five-year incidence of open-angle glaucoma: the visual impairment project. Ophthalmology 2002;109(6):1047–51.
[48] Springelkamp H, Wolfs RC, Ramdas WD, et al. Incidence of glaucomatous visual field loss after two decades of follow-up: the Rotterdam Study. Eur J Epidemiol 2017;32(8):691–9.

[49] Bengtsson BO. Incidence of manifest glaucoma. Br J Ophthalmol 1989;73(7):483–7.
[50] Pan CW, Yang WY, Hu DN, et al. Longitudinal cohort study on the incidence of primary open-angle glaucoma in Bai Chinese. Am J Ophthalmol 2017;176(4):127–33.
[51] Cedrone C, Mancino R, Ricci F, et al. The 12-year incidence of glaucoma and glaucoma-related visual field loss in Italy: the Ponza eye study. J Glaucoma 2012;21(1):1–6.
[52] Vijaya L, Rashima A, Panday M, et al. Predictors for incidence of primary open-angle glaucoma in a South Indian population. The Chennai Eye Disease Incidence Study. Ophthalmology 2014;121(7):1370–6.
[53] Leske MC, Wu SY, Honkanen R, et al. Nine-year incidence of open-angle glaucoma in the Barbados Eye Studies. Ophthalmology 2007;114(6):1058–64.
[54] Varma R, Wang D, Wu C, et al. Four-year incidence of open-angle glaucoma and ocular hypertension: the Los Angeles Latino Eye Study. Am J Ophthalmol 2012;154(2):315–25.
[55] Realini T, Olawoye O, Kizor-Akaraiwe N, et al. The rationale for selective laser trabeculoplasty in Africa. Asia Pac J Ophthalmol (Phila) 2018;7(6):387–93.
[56] Realini T, Shillingford-Ricketts H, Burt D, et al. West Indies Glaucoma Laser Study (WIGLS): 1. 12-month efficacy of selective laser trabeculoplasty in Afro-Caribbeans with glaucoma. Am J Ophthalmol 2017;184(12):28–33.
[57] Goosen E, Coleman K, Visser L, et al. Racial differences in selective laser trabeculoplasty efficacy. J Curr Glaucoma Pract 2017;11(1):22–7.

Advances in Ophthalmology and Optometry 4 (2019) 223–243

ADVANCES IN OPHTHALMOLOGY AND OPTOMETRY

Microinvasive Glaucoma Surgeries and When to Use Them

Cara E. Capitena Young, MD*, Leonard K. Seibold, MD, Jeffrey R. SooHoo, MD, Malik Y. Kahook, MD

Sue Anschutz-Rodgers Eye Center, Department of Ophthalmology, University of Colorado Hospital, 1675 Aurora Court, F731, Aurora, CO 80045, USA

Keywords

• Microinvasive glaucoma surgery • MIGS • Ab-interno glaucoma surgery • Goniotomy/trabeculotomy • Trabecular bypass • Endocyclophotocoagulation • Suprachoroidal device

Key points

- Microinvasive glaucoma surgery (MIGS) provides new options for surgical glaucoma treatment that has excellent safety profiles and at least modest efficacy.
- MIGS procedures can be combined with cataract surgery, combined with other MIGS procedures, or performed as stand-alone procedures.
- The use of MIGS procedures may be appropriate in several clinical scenarios, including patients needing improved intraocular pressure control and/or reduction in medication burden.
- A paucity of information exists to support using one procedure over another in individual patients; however, our knowledge of ideal patient selection for each procedure is evolving.
- Additional studies are needed to further determine which MIGS approach is the most efficacious for an individual patient and if any clinical or demographic factors exist that could predict success and help us individualize treatment options.

Video content accompanies this article at http://www.advancesinophthalmology.com.

Disclosure Statement: C.E. Capitena Young and J.R. SooHoo have nothing to disclose. L.K. Seibold is a consultant to New World Medical (NWM) and Allergan. M.Y. Kahook is a consultant to Alcon, Allergan, and NWM and receives patent royalties from NWM, Alcon, and Johnson and Johnson Vision (JJV).

*Corresponding author. *E-mail address:* cara.capitenayoung@ucdenver.edu

https://doi.org/10.1016/j.yaoo.2019.04.018

INTRODUCTION

Over the last 50 years, options for the medical and surgical treatment of glaucoma have expanded. New classes of topical medications and laser procedures were added to the physician's armamentarium. Over the last decade, no sector has evolved and expanded more than surgical procedures for lowering of intraocular pressure (IOP). Traditionally, surgical intervention required creation of a new aqueous drainage pathway, one that circumvents natural outflow tracts. These filtering procedures, such as trabeculectomy and glaucoma drainage device implantation, can be highly effective. Despite advancements and modifications made over the years, however, these procedures continue to be plagued by potentially vision-threatening complications such as hypotony, choroidal hemorrhage, wound leaks, infection, implant exposure, and vision loss [1,2]. Concern over the high rate of complications associated with these options has driven surgeons and researchers alike to pursue alternative options. Subsequently, minimally invasive surgical procedures were innovated and implemented in the treatment of various forms of glaucoma and at different stages of the disease [3,4]. Later, the category of minimally invasive surgery was broadly termed "microinvasive glaucoma surgery" (MIGS).

The MIGS classification is broad and encompasses multiple innovative surgical techniques and procedures. In general, a MIGS procedure should [1] be performed via an ab interno approach, [2] cause minimal trauma, [3] be at least modestly effective at lowering IOP, [4] have an excellent safety profile and [5] allow fast visual recovery, similar to phacoemulsification. These procedures can be performed either in combination with phacoemulsification or as stand-alone procedures.

MIGS procedures and devices can be divided into different subtypes based on their target area; most of these currently focus on improving the function of the natural drainage channels by bypassing or removing tissue obstructing aqueous outflow. Many of these procedures target conventional outflow through the trabecular meshwork (TM) and Schlemm canal (SC), whereas others function by shunting aqueous into the suprachoroidal space. Still others, such as endocyclophotocoagulation (ECP), work to decrease aqueous production, thus lowering IOP by decreasing inflow. Lastly, another group of procedures bypass the natural drainage system and target the subconjunctival space. These, therefore, are similar to traditional filtering surgery in that they create a subconjunctival filtering bleb.

With the advent of numerous novel surgical techniques, surgeons are faced with the difficulty of deciding where each fits in the treatment paradigm. Given the high safety profile of MIGS, surgical intervention is being considered much earlier in the treatment pathway. Not only are they being used to improve IOP, but they also can offer medication independence for those patients intolerant to topical medications. They most often are used in combination with phacoemulsification but are increasingly being used as stand-alone procedures as well. This article outlines the current options available to surgeons as well as several emerging technologies. It reviews indications, contraindications, and various patient factors that should be considered when choosing surgical options.

TARGETING THE INFLOW SYSTEM—CYCLODESTRUCTIVE PROCEDURES

Background, safety, and efficacy

Cyclodestructive procedures are known to produce IOP lowering through ablation of the ciliary epithelium, leading to decreased aqueous production [6]. Traditional cyclophotocoagulation (CPC) performed transscleral is associated with severe, vision-threatening complications and, therefore, traditionally has been reserved for use in refractory glaucoma [6]. In contrast, ECP was designed to allow improved intraoperative control, leading to less collateral tissue damage and fewer complications [7]. Pantcheva and colleagues [6] demonstrated this histologically in human autopsy eyes. Eyes treated with ECP showed local destruction of the nonpigmented ciliary epithelium but had little to no effects noted in adjacent tissues in contrast to the CPC-treated tissue. The 810-nm diode laser procedure is performed endoscopically through a clear corneal or pars plana incision (in vitrectomized patients), which allows the surgeon to visualize the ciliary processes during treatment (Fig. 1).

Whether used alone or in combination with cataract removal, the efficacy and safety of ECP has been demonstrated by multiple studies [8–10]. As described by Kahook and colleagues [11], a second incision can be made nasally allowing access to the temporal processes to achieve a 360-degree treatment resulting in additional IOP lowering. In a recent study of 106 eyes that underwent phacoemulsification in combination with ECP, the investigators found a significant decrease in IOP at 3 years. However, the IOP-lowering effect was diminished by 3 years, with approximately 60% of eyes meeting failure criteria [10].

Complications associated with ECP are similar to those associated with phacoemulsification, including postoperative inflammation, infection, hyphema, and cystoid macular edema. A recent study showed that certain ethnic

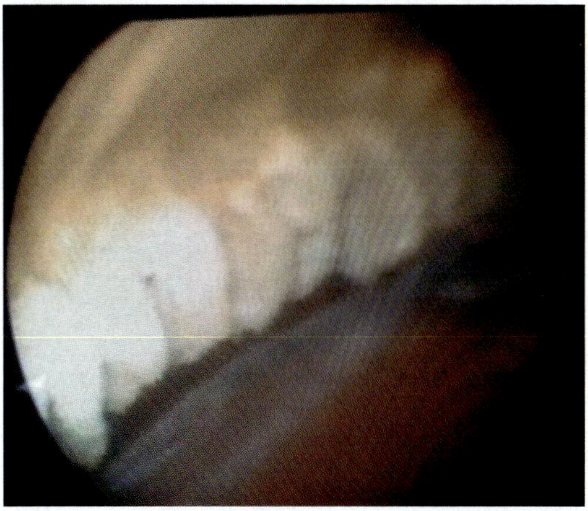

Fig. 1. Intraoperative view of ciliary processes during endoscopic cyclophotocoagulation.

groups, such as African Americans, are prone to more severe and/or prolonged postoperative inflammation [12]. More severe complications such as hypotony, choroidal detachment, retinal detachment, and malignant glaucoma, although rare, have been reported [13].

Indications, contraindications, and special considerations

Given its favorable safety and efficacy profile, the indications for ECP are broad. ECP can be performed in combination with cataract extraction or as a stand-alone procedure. When used as a solo procedure, ECP should be performed in pseudophakic or aphakic patients to avoid damaging the phakic lens. Candidates for a combined procedure are those with a visually significant cataract and either uncontrolled glaucoma or a desire to decrease medication dependence [14]. As the only MIGS procedure that targets aqueous inflow, it is indicated for use in various open-angle and angle-closure glaucoma. For this reason, it often is used in combination with other MIGS procedures, such as those that target outflow systems.

ECP also can be used in glaucoma of varying severity. Two studies have shown comparable IOP lowering and success rates between ECP and trabeculectomy as well as ECP and the Ahmed valve, respectively. It also has shown success in pediatric patients and those with refractory glaucoma, especially in patients with a history of failed filtration surgery [9,15–17]. Murakami and colleagues [18] compared ECP with a second glaucoma-drainage device in patients who had previously failed prior tube shunt surgery. They found no significant difference in postoperative IOP or glaucoma medication use between the 2 groups.

ECP is also particularly useful in patients who may be poor candidates for filtering surgery, such as those with ocular surface disease, conjunctival scarring, or a history of surgical complications [14,17]. The endoscopic nature of the procedure allows its use in patients with corneal opacities in whom angle-based surgery may not be possible due to lack of visualization.

In patients with short axial lengths, shallow anterior chambers, and/or plateau iris syndrome, filtering surgery carries a higher risk, making ECP an attractive alternative option. In these scenarios, lens extraction with ECP can be a very effective means of opening the angle and controlling IOP. Lens extraction alone can alleviate any pupillary block and angle crowding, whereas concomitant ECP can decrease aqueous production and further deepen the angle through shrinkage and posterior rotation of the ciliary processes. When used in this manner, the procedure often is referred to as endocycloplasty [17].

Because the laser targets melanin in the ciliary body, ECP may have less success in patients with pseudoexfoliation, as the white fibrillar material overlying the zonules and ciliary processes minimizes laser uptake [17]. Caution should be used in patients with a history of uveitis as well as patients with darkly pigmented eyes, given the higher risk of persistent and severe postoperative inflammation [12,14].

TARGETING THE OUTFLOW SYSTEM—TRABECULAR MESHWORK- AND SCHLEMM CANAL-BASED PROCEDURES

The TM, in particular the juxtacanalicular meshwork, has been postulated to be the site of greatest aqueous outflow resistance [19,20]. Therefore, bypassing or removing the TM should increase outflow and decrease IOP. As such, most MIGS devices and procedures currently available target traditional outflow through the TM. Traditionally, this approach has been used successfully to lower IOP in congenital glaucoma through goniotomy and trabeculotomy [21]. Because of residual TM leaflets and limited long-term success, these procedures were previously not widely used in adult glaucoma. However, novel and improved angle procedures have been developed to remove, incise, or bypass the trabecular tissue in a more efficient and complete manner. These procedures include the iStent trabecular bypass stent (Glaukos, San Clemente, CA, USA), Kahook Dual Blade (KDB) goniotomy (New World Medical, Rancho Cucamonga, CA, USA), Trabectome and Goniotome (Neomedix Corporation, Tustin, CA, USA), and gonioscopy-assisted transluminal trabeculotomy (GATT).

Trabecular tissue is not the only factor in outflow; SC and distal collector channels also play a role. Patients with primary open-angle glaucoma (POAG) have been shown to have smaller canal diameters, and canal diameter is inversely related to IOP [22]. Procedures like ab-interno canaloplasty (ABiC) attempt to lower IOP by cannulation and viscodilation of the SC. Others, such as the Hydrus Microstent (HMS) implant (Ivantis Inc, Irvine, CA, USA), attempt to address both factors by bypassing the trabecular tissue and providing a scaffold within the SC.

Good candidates for angle-based procedures should have a clear cornea and an open angle with readily identifiable structures. They should not be performed in patients with angle dysgenesis or those with active neovascularization of the angle. Angle-based procedures require patient cooperation and a clear gonioscopic view to perform safely. Patients should be able to rotate their neck approximately 30 to 45 degrees, be capable of following instructions, and be able to cease eye movements during the procedure. Lastly, although all of these procedures address either the TM or SC, they still rely on a patent downstream outflow system for optimal effect. They should not be expected to lower pressure beyond episcleral venous pressure (EVP) of 8 to 10 mm Hg [23] and, therefore, are not an appropriate choice in patients with single-digit IOP goals. Similarly, they are not indicated in patients with glaucoma due to elevated episcleral venous pressure, such as patients with Sturge-Weber syndrome [24].

Trabecular bypass

The iStent trabecular bypass was the first MIGS implant approved by the Food and Drug Administration (FDA) in the United States. This small (1.0 × 0.3 mm) titanium device (Fig. 2) is implanted within the trabecular tissue, providing a channel for aqueous outflow directly across the TM into SC. In the pivotal approval study, patients who received the iStent in conjunction

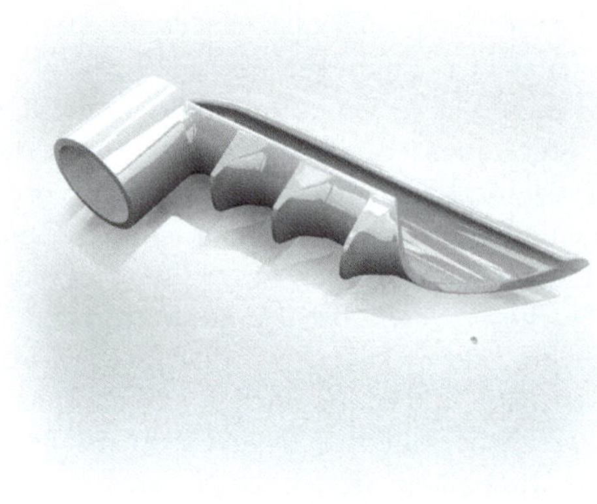

Fig. 2. First-generation iStent (Glaukos, San Clemente, CA, USA). (*Courtesy of* and used with permission from Glaukos.)

with cataract surgery were more likely to achieve greater than or equal to 20% IOP lowering without medication than those without the stent at 1-year follow-up [25]. Two-year follow-up data on these patients had similar results, although the proportion of patients who achieved this mark was less than at 1 year [26].

The iStent inject (Glaukos, San Clemente, CA, USA) is the second-generation trabecular bypass stent (Fig. 3). It is smaller in size and inserted perpendicularly to the TM, making the surgical approach simpler. Each insertion device is preloaded with 2 stents, which can both be placed into 2 TM locations through a single corneal incision. Multiple stents have been shown to be more effective at IOP reduction compared with a single stent [2,27,28]. In a prospective study of 53 patients who received 2 second-generation bypass stents in addition to continuing topical travoprost therapy (Alcon, Ft. Worth,

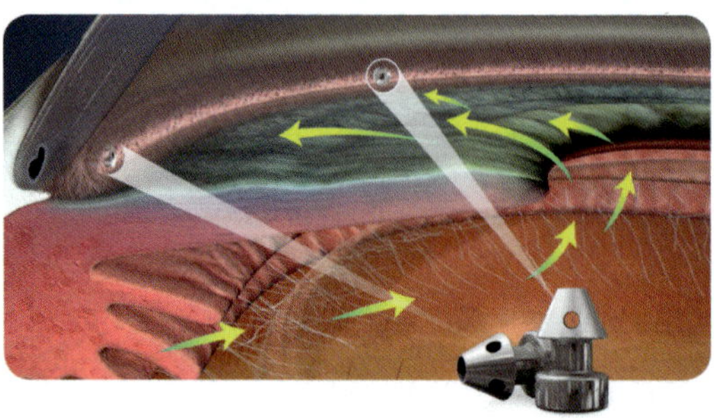

Fig. 3. iStent inject (Glaukos, San Clemente, CA, USA) and representative photo of correct placement of 2 implants. (*Courtesy of* and used with permission from Glaukos.)

TX, USA), average IOP at 1 year was less than or equal to 13 mm Hg and average IOP reduction was greater than or equal to 34% [27]. Another randomized study of 192 patients demonstrated that implantation of 2 iStent inject stents produced comparable IOP lowering to topical therapy with 2 agents (prostaglandin analogue and beta blocker) [29].

Both generation stents have excellent safety profiles. The most common adverse events are stent occlusion (4.3%) and malposition (2.6%) at 2 years. No reports of serious vision-threatening events occurred, and the rates of inflammation, macular edema, posterior capsular opacification, and corneal edema are similar to phacoemulsification [25,26]. A recent report in a small cohort of patients described fibrotic changes overlying the stent, which represents long-term biocompatibility issues, but it has not been further characterized to date [30].

Trabecular bypass stents are indicated for patients with mild to moderate open-angle glaucoma who are undergoing concomitant cataract extraction. Because access to the trabecular tissue is required to perform this procedure, it should not be used in patients with diffuse peripheral anterior synechiae (PAS) or patients with angle closure. In addition, it should not be used in patients with neovascular glaucoma or neovascularization of the angle due to the risk of bleeding. Given the modest IOP lowering and excellent safety profile, these are best used for patients with mild glaucoma on one or more medications. However, recent results from iStent inject studies suggest the new-generation device also may be appropriate for more moderate cases and patients with an IOP goal in the midteens [27,29]. The effect is limited in patients with normal-tension glaucoma or patients with severe glaucoma and a very low IOP goal [31].

Goniotomy

Goniotomy, or incision of the TM, was first described by Barkan as a way to increase aqueous outflow in children [32]. Since then, several procedures to more accurately incise TM or to fully excise a strip of TM tissue have emerged.

The Trabectome, a surgical device that incises and ablates a segment of the TM and inner wall of SC (ab-interno trabeculotomy) has been used since 2004 in the treatment of open-angle glaucoma. The device consists of a disposable handpiece with a footplate connected to an electrocautery generator. The footplate of the device is inserted into SC and cautery is applied to the TM as the handpiece is advanced across the angle. A meta-analysis of Trabectome studies demonstrated a good success rate when performed both with and without concomitant cataract extraction [33]. Neomedix recently has introduced a device that cuts TM tissue, the Goniotome, although clinical data are not available at this time.

GATT was first described by Grover and colleagues [34] in 2014. In this procedure, a 360-degree trabeculotomy is created by advancing either a suture or a microcatheter into SC circumferentially and then pulling centrally to tear through the TM. At 24 months, GATT lowered IOP 37.3% in patients with POAG and 49.8% in patients with secondary OAG. Although GATT has a better safety-profile compared with filtering surgery, a high risk of transient postoperative hyphema does exist. At 1 week postoperatively, 30% of patients still had a hyphema [34]. Another concern with the GATT procedure, as with a standard goniotomy, is the risk of reapproximation and fibrosis of the remaining TM leaflets over time, leading to closure of the cleft. Although a 360-degree incision makes closure of the cleft somewhat less likely, it often is viewed as a reason traditional goniotomies have failed in adults.

The KDB is a novel goniotomy blade designed to excise a strip of TM with minimal damage to surrounding tissue over 3 to 4 clock hours or more of the angle (Fig. 4; Video 1). A preclinical study on human corneoscleral rims demonstrated more complete TM removal histologically when compared with microvitreoretinal blade goniotomy and Trabectome [35]. Multiple studies agree that the average IOP decrease associated with KDB goniotomy is approximately 26% when performed with or without phacoemulsification, although published follow-up is currently limited to 1 year. The most common complication associated with KDB goniotomy is transient hyphema, resulting from refluxed blood at the time of treatment reported in approximately 17% of patients [36].

KDB goniotomy, Trabectome, Goniotome, and GATT all have the benefit of bypassing TM without the use of an implant. Therefore, the risk of biocompatibility issues or other implant-related complications, such as dislocation, is a nonfactor. These procedures also have broader indications and can be used as stand-alone procedures or in combination with cataract surgery in patients with ocular hypertension or those with any stage of glaucoma. They are indicated in patients with open-angle glaucoma, given the need for access to trabecular

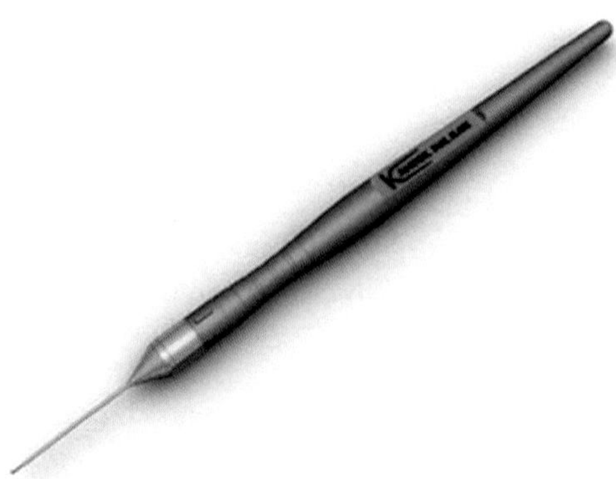

Fig. 4. Kahook Dual Blade (New World Medical, Rancho Cucamonga, CA, USA). (*Courtesy of* and used with permission from New World Medical.)

tissue and SC. Goniotomy with KDB can be performed in some patients with scattered or recently formed PAS by using the side of the blade to perform gentle goniosynechialysis before goniotomy. Trabecular removal has had particular success in patients with secondary forms of OAG, such as those with pseudoexfoliation or pigmentary glaucoma [34,36,37]. KDB goniotomy and GATT specifically have had some success in congenital glaucoma as well [38,39].

These procedures can be used in both phakic and pseudophakic patients. However, when used in a phakic patient, extreme care should be taken to avoid inadvertent damage to the lens capsule. They have been shown to produce more substantial IOP lowering than trabecular bypass devices, although prospective data are lacking [25,26,39–41]. Therefore, they should be considered in patients with ocular hypertension, mild and moderate glaucoma, and occasionally severe glaucoma. They can be considered in patients on multiple topical medications and those with previous failed glaucoma surgeries [42].

Because they all still rely on a patent downstream system, trabecular removal procedures should not be expected to lower pressure beyond EVP (8–10 mm Hg) and restraint should be used in patients with low IOP goals, especially in the single digits [23]. Although not a definitive contraindication, caution should be exercised in patients on anticoagulation therapy or those with clotting disorders, given the risk of bleeding and hyphema [34,36].

Schlemm canal–based procedures

In contrast to procedures that incise or remove TM tissue to access SC, other techniques attempt to expand or stent open the canal, which can be collapsed in POAG. Canaloplasty procedures were designed with this technique in mind. Traditional canaloplasty required scleral dissection and external access to SC, but a more modern technique has provided a different approach. ABiC uses an illuminated microcatheter to cannulate the canal 360 degrees from an ab-interno approach through 2 corneal incisions. As the catheter is withdrawn, a viscoelastic agent is injected to dilate the SC and proximal collector channels. A retrospective review of ABiC performed with and without cataract extraction showed a mean decrease in IOP of 36.1% at 36 months and a significant decrease in glaucoma medications with an excellent safety profile [43].

The HMS was based in part on this same paradigm of canal dilation but has an additional mechanism of TM bypass as well. Thus, it augments the conventional outflow system in 2 ways. The nitinol implant is threaded into SC at the time of cataract surgery and serves as a scaffold in the canal for approximately 3 clock hours of the angle across from the corneal incision. The proximal end extends across the TM to provide direct aqueous access to SC. In the HORIZON study, patients who received the HMS in addition to phacoemulsification had significantly greater IOP lowering than those who underwent phacoemulsification alone at 24 months with no difference in any safety parameters between the 2 groups. More than 77% of patients in the HMS group experienced greater than or equal to 20% IOP lowering at 2 years [44].

Similar to the previously discussed TM-based procedures, ABiC is indicated in patients with primary or secondary open-angle glaucoma. It can be used in patients of all glaucoma severities, at the time of cataract surgery or as a standalone procedure, but should not be expected to lower IOP beyond EVP. In contrast, the HMS is indicated only at the time of cataract surgery in patients with mild or moderate open-angle glaucoma.

TARGETING THE OUTFLOW SYSTEM—SUPRACHOROIDAL SPACE

Background, safety, and efficacy

Aqueous outflow occurs primarily through the conventional or trabecular pathway. However, the uveoscleral outflow pathway, which consists of the ciliary body, suprachoroidal space, and sclera, also accounts for a substantial amount of aqueous outflow and, therefore, is another potential target for glaucoma treatments [45]. Surgically, use of this space has been limited due to the risk of adverse events such as hypotony from overfiltration and drastic IOP spikes with spontaneous cleft closure [46,47]. Previous devices have attempted to access the suprachoroidal space via an ab-externo approach. Use of these devices, however, requires manipulation and dissection of both the sclera and conjunctiva and have been limited by varying success rates [48,49].

In contrast, the CyPass microstent (Alcon, Fort Worth, TX, USA) and the iStent Supra (Glaukos, San Clemente, CA, USA) target the suprachoroidal space via an ab-interno approach. The CyPass is a polyimide fenestrated tube 6.35 mm long and 0.43 mm diameter. The iStent Supra is 4 mm long and made of polyethersulfone (Fig. 5). Both implants are advanced into the suprachoroidal space intraoperatively under direct gonioscopic view. The COMPASS trial, a multicenter randomized controlled trial, evaluated the efficacy of the CyPass microstent in combination with phacoemulsification. The CyPass group had significantly greater IOP lowering compared with phacoemulsification alone at 2 years (7.4 mm Hg vs 5.4 mm Hg, $P<.001$) and approximately 85% of CyPass patients required no medication postoperatively [50]. The CyCLE study demonstrated that the CyPass microstent was effective at lowering IOP and number of glaucoma medications both when performed in combination with phacoemulsification and when used alone [51,52]. A

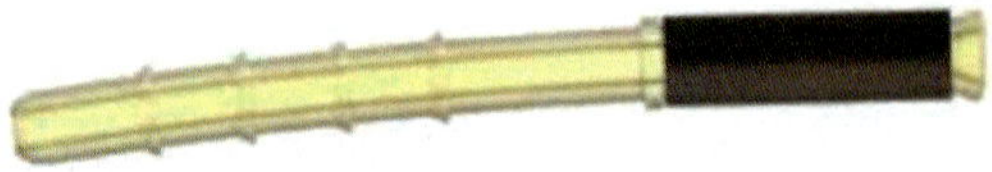

Fig. 5. iStent Supra (Glaukos, San Clemente, CA, USA). (*Courtesy of* and used with permission from Glaukos.)

multicenter randomized controlled trial is currently ongoing to investigate the safety and efficacy of the iStent Supra. However, several smaller studies have shown similar results to the CyPass in regard to the IOP-lowering ability of the iStent Supra [53,54].

Early studies on these devices demonstrated an acceptable safety profile. The COMPASS study 2-year data reported no vision-threatening microstent-related adverse events. In other studies, the most common adverse events for both implants was postoperative inflammation, need for further glaucoma procedures, obstruction of the device, and IOP elevation. Postprocedure hypotony and choroidal effusions, although usually transient, also have been reported [50–53]. However, Alcon voluntarily withdrew the CyPass device from the market in September 2018 after 5-year data from the COMPASS-XT trial showed a statistically significant decrease in endothelial cell counts in the group with the microstent compared with phacoemulsification alone [55]. Data from the ongoing iStent Supra studies, with particular attention to corneal endothelial health, will be essential in determining the safety of these devices and their future in the MIGS discussion.

Indications and contraindications

Before its removal from market, the CyPass microstent was indicated for patients with mild to moderate primary open-angle glaucoma [50]. The iStent SUPRA currently is under investigation for use in the same patient group. Because the suprachoroidal and supraciliary space bypasses the episcleral venous system, it is not limited by the EVP. Therefore, accessing this space has the potential to lower IOP more than trabecular- or SC-based devices. However, in the absence of an EVP barrier there is a greater risk of hypotony. In the COMPASS trial, 2.9% of patients experienced transient hypotony [50]. In contrast, scarring may also occur within the suprachoroidal space, which we currently have no way to modulate. Rates of PAS around the device have been reported between 3% and 10% in 2 major studies [50–52]. Scarring around devices in this space can limit their efficacy and cause extreme IOP spikes. Therefore, although these may provide additional IOP lowering compared with TM or SC procedures, surgeons must be aware of these unique risks.

Like trabecular- and SC-based procedures, angle visualization and identification of structures are essential intraoperatively in order to place and advance these devices into the correct space. All candidates for this procedure should have a clear cornea, identifiable angle structures, be able to rotate their neck by approximately 30 to 45 degrees, and be able to cease eye movements for several minutes. Further, they should not be used in patients with diffuse PAS, such as patients with either primary or secondary form of angle-closure glaucoma, as identification of angle structures is limited. These devices have not been adequately investigated in patients with uveitic, steroid-responsive, traumatic, or congenital glaucoma and, therefore, should be used with caution and monitored closely [56].

TARGETING THE OUTFLOW SYSTEM—SUBCONJUNCTIVAL SPACE

Ab interno: the Xen gel stent

Approved by the FDA in November 2016, the Xen gel stent (Allergan, Dublin, Ireland) is the first commercially available ab-interno subconjunctival stent (Fig. 6). The 6-mm implant, composed of porcine gelatin, is placed across the angle and sclera into the subconjunctival space, thus bypassing the natural outflow system. It, therefore, is similar to traditional filtering surgery in that a subconjunctival filtering bleb is created, but it is typically performed via a conjunctival sparing ab-interno approach. Whether the Xen gel stent qualifies as an MIGS procedure is debatable, as it leads to the formation of a bleb and its attendant complications such as hypotony, scarring, and bleb leaks. The device, however, was designed to be flow limiting with a 45-micron lumen and 6 mm length to prevent hypotony, as shown in preclinical studies [57]. In order to limit fibrosis, adjunctive antimetabolites such as mitomycin C and 5-fluorouracil should be used. Despite these factors, many would agree that the Xen gel stent is less invasive, technically less difficult to perform, and surgically safer with more rapid recovery when compared with traditional filtering surgery.

In a study of 65 patients with uncontrolled IOP who had previously failed filtering or cilioablative procedures, Grover and colleagues [58] showed the Xen gel stent produced greater than or equal to 20% IOP lowering in 75% of patients at 12 months. The mean decrease in IOP in their study population was 9.1 mm Hg with a decrease in the number of medications from 3.5 to 1.7. In this study the conjunctiva was opened and mitomycin C sponges were placed. In practice, however, the stent is placed without conjunctival dissection, and mitomycin C is injected into the surrounding conjunctiva. Schlenker and colleagues [59] performed a retrospective study of the Xen gel stent versus trabeculectomy in 354 eyes with uncontrolled glaucoma and no prior incisional surgery, which showed no statistically significant difference in effectiveness between the 2 procedures. Multiple small studies have confirmed these findings; however, larger comparative studies are still needed [60–62]. Data from the

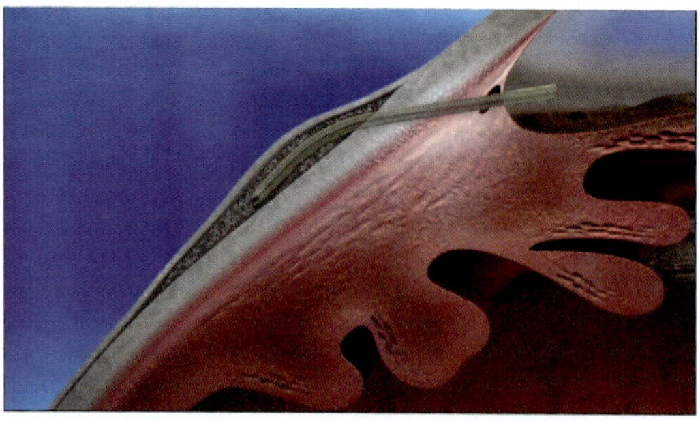

Fig. 6. Xen gel stent (Allergan, Dublin, Ireland). (*Courtesy of* and used with permission from Allergan.)

phase 4 APEX randomized controlled trial should provide additional valuable information on both the safety and efficacy of this device.

Of the complications reported, most were transient and resolved without intervention. These included postoperative visual decline, hyphema, and transient hypotony [58]. Like glaucoma drainage devices, this procedure does leave an implant in the subconjunctival space, and therefore, these implants are at risk for exposure and bleb leaks over time. Although still rare, this has been reported [63]. A common postoperative intervention needed after stent placement is postoperative bleb needling or revision. Needling rates vary somewhat between studies, but, in general, are quoted between 30.7% and 51.3% [58,61,62].

A major advantage of the Xen stent is that it can be used in a variety of types and stages of glaucoma and can be placed as a stand-alone procedure or in combination with cataract surgery with similar success rates [64]. On-label indications for the Xen gel stent include refractory glaucoma, allowing for use in a wide variety of patients. Because of its improved safety profile compared with traditional filtering surgery, surgeons are also using this implant earlier in the surgical algorithm.

Although the Xen gel stent can produce adequate IOP lowering into the low to midteen range, some surgeons find that it cannot reliably achieve an IOP as low as trabeculectomy can. Therefore, care should be taken in patients with advanced disease in whom a lower IOP is desired. However, because the stent is placed primarily in the superonasal quadrant, its presence does not preclude future filtering procedures such as tube shunts or trabeculectomies located temporal to the device. For this same reason, use of the Xen gel stent should be avoided in patients with conjunctival scarring, especially those with scarring in the superonasal quadrant. Patients at high risk for trabeculectomy failure, especially those at high risk for scarring such as young patients, and those with a history of uveitis or a history of previous filtering surgery or conjunctival inflammation are not good candidates. It is contraindicated in patients with angle-closure glaucoma, either primary or secondary, those with neovascularization of the iris or angle, and patients with anterior chamber intraocular lenses [65].

Ab externo: InnFocus microshunt

The InnFocus microshunt (Santen Pharmaceutical Co Ltd, Emeryville, CA, USA) is a novel glaucoma drainage device composed of poly(styrene-block-isobutylene-block-styrene). Although it is placed ab externo in a procedure more similar to traditional glaucoma drainage devices, it was designed as a minimally invasive implant due to its narrow lumen, which limits outflow. Similar to the Xen gel stent, it is a microtube that allows aqueous drainage from the anterior chamber into a subconjunctival bleb and also requires the use of antimetabolites intraoperatively. Clinical studies with this device are limited to date, but early results are promising. Battle and colleagues [66] reviewed 14 patients who underwent microshunt placement alone and 9 patients who underwent microshunt placement in combination with phacoemulsification. The rate of qualified success, defined as IOP less than or equal to 14 and IOP reduction greater than or equal to 20%, was 95% at 3-year follow-up. Transient hypotony was noted in some patients, but in this cohort no serious long-term adverse events occurred such as bleb leak, infection, or shunt erosion. Given the lack of clinical data currently available, indications and contraindications are still undefined but are expected to be similar to those of the Xen gel stent. Prospective randomized trials comparing the InnFocus with trabeculectomy are currently underway.

COMBINATION PROCEDURES

All of the aforementioned procedures may be performed in conjunction with phacoemulsification or as a stand-alone procedure. In the United States, however, some are only on-label for use in conjunction with cataract surgery. Although cataract surgery alone is known to lower IOP, each of these when used in combination with cataract removal has the ability to produce additional IOP lowering [10,25,50,53,67]. Patients with a visually significant cataract and either ocular hypertension or glaucoma are typically excellent candidates for an MIGS procedure at the time of phacoemulsification. The choice of MIGS depends on the surgeon and several individual patient factors including angle status, IOP goal, risk for complications, ability and desire to adhere to topical medications, and patient expectations.

Similar to using combination topical therapy to enhance multiple pathways (outflow/inflow or multiple outflow pathways) for improved IOP control, MIGS surgeries can be combined in an attempt to maximize effectiveness. The most common approach is using a combination of an inflow and an outflow procedure. The ICE procedure, which includes implantation of an iStent, cataract removal, and ECP, is a commonly used combination procedure. In a review of 70 patients with moderate glaucoma who underwent the ICE procedure, IOP was reduced from an average of 19.4 mm Hg to 15.8 mm Hg at 3 to 6 months. However, like most MIGS, this procedure was not effective in all patients [68,69]. The potential for multiple different combinations also exists. In reality, any outflow-based procedure can be combined with ECP in a pseudophakic or aphakic patient or a patient undergoing phacoemulsification.

Multiple outflow procedures also can be performed in conjunction with one another. Both Katz and colleagues [2] and Belovay and colleagues [28] demonstrated that multiple iStents have better IOP-lowering abilities than a single iStent. Surgeries that target both the conventional and nonconventional outflow pathways also could be used in conjunction with one another. For instance, a TM-based procedure could be performed in combination with a suprachoroidal or subconjunctival procedure. Although it is intuitive that combining multiple procedures could produce additive IOP lowering when compared with a single procedure, clinical data proving superior efficacy of these approaches generally are lacking, and a potentially greater risk of complications exists when performing multiple procedures.

PRESENT LIMITATIONS AND FUTURE AVENUES

Current limitations and information needed

The rapidly expanding options of MIGS procedures in recent years make it clear that a new era of glaucoma surgery is upon us. Although traditional filtering surgery such as trabeculectomies and tube shunt procedures still have an important place in the glaucoma treatment algorithm, MIGS are attempting to fill the longstanding void between conservative medical and laser therapies and surgical intervention. They offer benefits such as microincisions, short operative and patient recovery times, and an improved safety profile compared with traditional filtering surgery, while still providing meaningful IOP reduction. What is still unclear, however, is which approach is truly best in any individual patient.

Few studies adequately compare one MIGS against another. Reports that have attempted comparisons have been retrospective in nature and limited by small cohorts. For example, studies that compare Trabectome and iStent when performed with cataract surgery have had variable results. Kurji and colleagues found greater IOP lowering in the Trabectome group, whereas both Gonnerman and colleagues and Khan and colleagues identified slightly greater IOP reduction in the iStent groups [40]. A few studies have now compared the efficacy of combination phacoemulsification with KDB goniotomy and iStent respectively, although these reports also are retrospective. Both showed a greater decrease in IOP and medication usage in the KDB goniotomy cohorts [41,70]. Although comparing studies using different devices can allow one to draw certain conclusions, overall these comparisons are limited due to the heterogeneity of patient populations and a lack of randomized prospective trials in this arena [40].

Prospective comparative studies are vital. Ideally, devices and procedures within the same class of MIGS should be investigated, various classes should be compared with one another and each should be compared with traditional filtering surgery. Future studies should also investigate combination procedures, such as those that target both the inflow and outflow pathways. Further, of those comparative studies that have been published, most were performed in patients with open-angle, mild-to-moderate glaucoma. Clinical data evaluating the efficacy of MIGS in those with other forms of glaucoma or in patients with severe glaucoma are lacking. Studies that have performed subgroup analyses generally have been of inadequate power to draw strong conclusions. Therefore, clinical decision-making becomes difficult for surgeons attempting to perform the best procedure for an individual patient.

Because of the lack of comparative data, physicians must rely primarily on their clinical experience, published reports, and discussions with colleagues when choosing procedures. In some cases, the indications are intuitive. For instance, it is understood that the site of outflow resistance in patients with pigment dispersion glaucoma and pseudoexfoliation glaucoma is the TM. Thus, trabecular-based procedures such as iStent, GATT, or KDB goniotomy should effectively lower IOP in these individuals; this was supported modestly by reviews of KDB goniotomy and GATT [36,37,71]. Similarly, the benefits of phacoemulsification with ECP in patients with anatomically narrow angles, appositionally closed angles, or in patients with plateau iris syndrome makes sense anatomically and physiologically [17].

Analyses of patient and ocular demographics as factors related to surgical success or failure are limited but necessary. Variables such as race, age, coexisting conditions, preoperative IOP, and subtype of glaucoma among others may help predict the success of a certain procedure and will be important in future study directions. Reliable clinical assessments of native outflow pathways such as aqueous angiography and EVP measurements may help guide surgical choice in the future. Along these lines, Fellman and colleagues [72] demonstrated that patients with a poor episcleral fluid wave after trabectome surgery had a higher likelihood of requiring a second glaucoma surgery.

Because of their minimally invasive nature and the ability to combine these procedures safely with cataract surgery, MIGS are sometimes used earlier in the treatment algorithm in an effort to decrease medication dependence. Yet data on quality-of-life measures and cost-effectiveness are limited. A group from Ontario, Canada examined cost comparisons between glaucoma medications and Trabectome, ECP, and iStent procedures. Each MIGS investigated offered a modest cost savings per patient over glaucoma medications; however, surgeon fees were not included in this analysis [73]. A group in New Zealand found iStent with cataract surgery to be reasonably cost-effective in their health system when compared with topical glaucoma medications. Not surprisingly, this was more significant when compared with those using more expensive topical medications [74]. Another analysis compared 2 trabecular microbypass stents with selective laser trabeculoplasty (SLT) and topical medications. Initial costs were higher in the surgical group, but at 5 years, the projected cumulative cost for surgical intervention was lower than both the SLT and topical medication groups [75], which suggests that earlier surgical interventions have the ability to produce greater cost savings to patients and health care systems. It is essential that we further elucidate information on the cost-effectiveness of MIGS in larger study populations, evaluate multiple MIGS procedures, and include quality-of-life parameters.

Other avenues in the pipeline

Novel and sustained drug-delivery platforms are another exciting area of growth in glaucoma. Although many of these platforms are externally placed ocular inserts such as punctal plugs and fornix-based rings, some require an intracameral injection or intraoperative placement. Because these devices are implants, some would argue that they could be categorized as MIGS and not just as medical therapy. At the moment, where these options will fall into the MIGS discussion is evolving.

MIGS procedures are evolving rapidly and, increasingly, with guidance from evidence-based medicine and real-world data. As new devices and procedures come to market, it is important to remember that even those currently in use are still in their infancy. With growth, setbacks occur. A critical step before adoption of any procedure is to ensure patient safety. Although early safety results of all of these procedures are reassuring, long-term data on biocompatibility and safety are still needed.

SUMMARY

Medical and surgical therapies for glaucoma always have centered around lowering IOP. Traditional filtering surgeries such as trabeculectomy and tube shunts are highly effective but can lead to severe, vision-threatening complications. Although no MIGS procedure to date can completely replace filtering surgery, these newer procedures are bridging the gap between medical therapy and traditional incisional glaucoma surgery and show promise for the future management of glaucoma. The explosion of MIGS procedures has expanded options for physicians and patients alike. But having more options also makes the choice of which procedure to perform more difficult. A persistent area of debate and query is which procedure is best for each individual patient.

MIGS procedures have targeted multiple avenues for IOP reduction. TM- and SC-based procedures and suprachoroidal devices exploit a potential space that has the ability to lower IOP substantially without the limit of EVP. ECP is the only current MIGS procedure to target aqueous production as a means of IOP reduction, making it an excellent option to be used in combination with other outflow procedures. Lastly, novel ab-interno and ab-externo subconjunctival filtering devices offer exciting promise for a safer and more predictable filtering procedure. They provide the same potential for substantial IOP lowering with an improved safety profile compared with traditional trabeculectomy.

We now have a variety of safe yet effective MIGS treatment options, which provide a wide array of potential options and combinations. These procedures offer patients the potential to lower IOP, reduce medication dependence, and better control glaucoma with lower-risk profiles. Prospective comparative studies are essential to guiding surgeons and patients alike as we move forward in the era of MIGS. Long-term data on device biocompatibility and safety are needed, as are comparative data between devices and further investigation into the role of MIGS without phacoemulsification. Future data will help to better define treatment guidelines and help individualize treatments for our patients.

SUPPLEMENTARY DATA

Supplementary data related to this article can be found online at https://doi.org/10.1016/j.yaoo.2019.04.018.

References

[1] Gedde SJ, Schiffman JC, Feuer WJ, et al, Tube versus Trabeculectomy Study Group. Treatment outcomes in the Tube Versus Trabeculectomy (TVT) study after five years of follow-up. Am J Ophthalmol 2012;153(5):789–803.e2.
[2] Katz LJ, Erb C, Carceller GA, et al. Prospective, randomized study of one, two, or three trabecular bypass stents in open-angle glaucoma subjects on topical hypotensive medication. Clin Ophthalmol 2015;9:2313–20.
[3] Minckler DS, Baerveldt G, Alfaro MR, et al. Clinical results with the Trabectome for treatment of open-angle glaucoma. Ophthalmology 2005;112(6):962–7.
[4] Spiegel D, Wetzel W, Haffner DS, et al. Initial clinical experience with the trabecular micro-bypass stent in patients with glaucoma. Adv Ther 2007;24(1):161–70.
[5] Saheb H, Ahmed II. Micro-invasive glaucoma surgery: current perspectives and future directions. Curr Opin Ophthalmol 2012;23(2):96–104.
[6] Pantcheva MB, Kahook MY, Schuman JS, et al. Comparison of acute structural and histopathological changes in human autopsy eyes after endoscopic cyclophotocoagulation and trans-scleral cyclophotocoagulation. Br J Ophthalmol 2007;91(2):248–52.
[7] Pastor SA, Singh K, Lee DA, et al. Cyclophotocoagulation: a report by the American Academy of Ophthalmology. Ophthalmology 2001;108(11):2130–8.
[8] Roberts SJ, Mulvahill M, Soohoo JR, et al. Efficacy of combined cataract extraction and endoscopic cyclophotocoagulation for the reduction of intraocular pressure and medication burden. Int J Ophthalmol 2016;9(5):693–8.
[9] Chen J, Cohn RA, Lin SC, et al. Endoscopic photocoagulation of the ciliary body for treatment of refractory glaucomas. Am J Ophthalmol 1997;124(6):787–96.
[10] Smith M, Byles D, Lim LA. Phacoemulsification and endocyclophotocoagulation in uncontrolled glaucoma: three-year results. J Cataract Refract Surg 2018;44(9):1097–102.
[11] Kahook MY, Lathrop KL, Noecker RJ. One-site versus two-site endoscopic cyclophotocoagulation. J Glaucoma 2007;16(6):527–30.
[12] Edmiston AM, Soohoo JR, Seibold LK, et al. Postoperative inflammation after endoscopic cyclophotocoagulation: racial distribution and effect on outcomes. J Glaucoma 2018;27(3):266–8.
[13] Pantcheva MB, Schuman JS. Cyclodestruction. In: Kahook M, Schuman JS, editors. Chandler and Grant's glaucoma. 5th edition. Thorofare (NJ): SLACK Incorporated; 2013. p. 518.
[14] Seibold LK, Soohoo JR, Kahook MY. Endoscopic cyclophotocoagulation. Middle East Afr J Ophthalmol 2015;22(1):18–24.
[15] Francis BA, Kawji AS, Vo NT, et al. Endoscopic cyclophotocoagulation (ECP) in the management of uncontrolled glaucoma with prior aqueous tube shunt. J Glaucoma 2011;20(8): 523–7.
[16] Tan JC, Francis BA, Noecker R, et al. Endoscopic cyclophotocoagulation and pars plana ablation (ECP-plus) to treat refractory glaucoma. J Glaucoma 2016;25(3):e117–22.
[17] Francis BA, Kwon J, Fellman R, et al. Endoscopic ophthalmic surgery of the anterior segment. Surv Ophthalmol 2014;59(2):217–31.
[18] Murakami Y, Akil H, Chahal J, et al. Endoscopic cyclophotocoagulation versus second glaucoma drainage device after prior aqueous tube shunt surgery. Clin Exp Ophthalmol 2017;45(3):241–6.
[19] Tham YC, Li X, Wong TY, et al. Global prevalence of glaucoma and projections of glaucoma burden through 2040: a systematic review and meta-analysis. Ophthalmology 2014;121(11):2081–90.
[20] Grant WM. Clinical measurements of aqueous outflow. AMA Arch Ophthalmol 1951;46(2):113–31.
[21] Chang I, Caprioli J, Ou Y. Surgical management of pediatric glaucoma. Dev Ophthalmol 2017;59:165–78.

[22] Andrés-Guerrero V, García-Feijoo J, Konstas AG. Targeting Schlemm's canal in the medical therapy of glaucoma: current and future considerations. Adv Ther 2017;34(5):1049–69.
[23] Allingham RR, Damji KF, Freedman SF, et al. Shields textbook of glaucoma. 6th edition. Philadelphia: Lippincott Williams & Wilkins; 2011.
[24] Shiau T, Armogan N, Yan DB, et al. The role of episcleral venous pressure in glaucoma associated with Sturge-Weber syndrome. J AAPOS 2012;16(1):61–4.
[25] Samuelson TW, Katz LJ, Wells JM, et al. Randomized evaluation of the trabecular micro-bypass stent with phacoemulsification in patients with glaucoma and cataract. Ophthalmology 2011;118(3):459–67.
[26] Craven ER, Katz LJ, Wells JM, et al. iStent Study Group Cataract surgery with trabecular micro-bypass stent implantation in patients with mild-to-moderate open-angle glaucoma and cataract: two-year follow-up. J Cataract Refract Surg 2012;38(8):1339–45.
[27] Berdahl J, Voskanyan L, Myers JS, et al. Implantation of two second-generation trabecular micro-bypass stents and topical travoprost in open-angle glaucoma not controlled on two preoperative medications: 18-month follow-up. Clin Exp Ophthalmol 2017;45(8):797–802.
[28] Belovay GW, Naqi A, Chan BJ, et al. Using multiple trabecular micro-bypass stents in cataract patients to treat open-angle glaucoma. J Cataract Refract Surg 2012;38(11):1911–7.
[29] Fea AM, Belda JI, Rekas M, et al. Prospective unmasked randomized evaluation of the iStent inject ((R)) versus two ocular hypotensive agents in patients with primary open-angle glaucoma. Clin Ophthalmol 2014;8:875–82.
[30] Capitena Young CE, Ammar DA, Seibold LK, et al. Histopathologic examination of trabecular meshwork changes after trabecular bypass stent implantation. J Glaucoma 2018;27(7):606–9.
[31] Seibold LK, Gamett KM, Kennedy JB, et al. Outcomes after combined phacoemulsification and trabecular microbypass stent implantation in controlled open-angle glaucoma. J Cataract Refract Surg 2016;42(9):1332–8.
[32] Barkan O. Technique of goniotomy for congenital glaucoma. Arch Ophthalmol 1949;41(1):65–82.
[33] Kaplowitz K, Bussel II, Honkanen R, et al. Review and meta-analysis of ab-interno trabeculectomy outcomes. Br J Ophthalmol 2016;100(5):594–600.
[34] Grover DS, Godfrey DG, Smith O, et al. Gonioscopy-assisted transluminal trabeculotomy, ab interno trabeculotomy: technique report and preliminary results. Ophthalmology 2014;121(4):855–61.
[35] Seibold LK, Soohoo JR, Ammar DA, et al. Preclinical investigation of ab interno trabeculectomy using a novel dual-blade device. Am J Ophthalmol 2013;155(3):524–9.e2.
[36] Sieck ES, Epstein RS, Kennedy JB, et al. Outcomes of Kahook dual blade goniotomy. Ophthalmol Glaucoma 2018;1(1):75–81.
[37] Ting JL, Damji KF, Stiles MC, et al. Ab interno trabeculectomy: outcomes in exfoliation versus primary open-angle glaucoma. J Cataract Refract Surg 2012;38(2):315–23.
[38] Khouri AS, Wong SH. Ab Interno trabeculectomy with a dual blade: surgical technique for childhood glaucoma. J Glaucoma 2017;26(8):749–51.
[39] Grover DS, Smith O, Fellman RL, et al. Gonioscopy-assisted transluminal trabeculotomy: an Ab Interno circumferential trabeculotomy: 24 months follow-up. J Glaucoma 2018;27(5):393–401.
[40] Lavia C, Dallorto L, Maule M, et al. Minimally-invasive glaucoma surgeries (MIGS) for open angle glaucoma: a systematic review and meta-analysis. PLoS One 2017;12(8):e0183142.
[41] Dorairaj SK, Kahook MY, Williamson BK, et al. A multicenter retrospective comparison of goniotomy versus trabecular bypass device implantation in glaucoma patients undergoing cataract extraction. Clin Ophthalmol 2018;12:791–7.

[42] Grover DS, Godfrey DG, Smith O, et al. Outcomes of Gonioscopy-assisted transluminal trabeculotomy (GATT) in eyes with prior incisional glaucoma surgery. J Glaucoma 2017;26: 41–5.
[43] Lewis RA, Von wolff K, Tetz M, et al. Canaloplasty: three-year results of circumferential viscodilation and tensioning of Schlemm canal using a microcatheter to treat open-angle glaucoma. J Cataract Refract Surg 2011;37(4):682–90.
[44] Samuelson TW, Chang DF, Marquis R, et al. A Schlemm canal microstent for intraocular pressure reduction in primary open-angle glaucoma and cataract: the HORIZON study. Ophthalmology 2019;126(1):29–37.
[45] Alm A, Nilsson SF. Uveoscleral outflow – a review. Exp Eye Res 2009;4:760–8.
[46] Galin MA, Baras I. Combined cyclodialysis cataract extraction: a review. Ann Ophthalmol 1975;7(2):271–5.
[47] Shields MB, Simmons RJ. Combined cyclodialysis and cataract extraction. Ophthalmic Surg 1976;7(2):62–73.
[48] Skaat A, Sagiv O, Kinori M, et al. Gold micro-shunt implants versus Ahmed Glaucoma valve: long-term outcomes of a prospective randomized clinical trial. J Glaucoma 2016;25(2):155–61.
[49] Hueber A, Roters S, Jordan JF, et al. Retrospective analysis of the success and safety of Gold Micro Shunt Implantation in glaucoma. BMC Ophthalmol 2013;13:35.
[50] Vold S, Ahmed II, Craven ER, et al. Two-year COMPASS trial results: supraciliary microstenting with phacoemulsification in patients with open-angle glaucoma and cataracts. Ophthalmology 2016;123(10):2103–12.
[51] Garcia-Feijoo J. Safety and efficacy of CyPass Micro-Stent as a stand-alone treatment for open-angle glaucoma: Worldwide clinical experience. Presented at: European Society of Cataract and Refractive Surgeons (ESCRS). Milan, Italy, September 8–12, 2012.
[52] Hoeh H. Clinical outcomes of combined cataract surgery and implantation of the CyPass Micro-Stent for the treatment of open-angle glaucoma. Presented at: European Society of Cataract and Refractive Surgeons (ESCRS). Milan, Italy, September 8–12, 2012.
[53] Junemann A. Twelve-month outcomes following Ab Interno implantaton of suprachoroidal stent and postoperative administration of travoprost to treat open angle glaucoma. 31st Congress of the European Society of Cataract and Refractive Surgeons. (ESCRS) Amsterdam, Netherlands, October 5–9, 2013.
[54] Myers J, Katz J. Open angle glaucoma treated with a suprachoroidal stent and topical travoprost. 23rd Annual American Glaucoma Society Meeting. San Fancisco, CA, February 28 to March 3, 2013.
[55] Alcon announces voluntary global market withdrawal of CyPass micro-stent for surgical glaucoma.[Press Release] 8.29.2018. Alcon, Fort Worth TX. Available at: https://www.novartis.com/news/media-releases/alcon-announces-voluntary-global-market-withdrawal-cypass-micro-stent-surgical-glaucoma. Accessed November 20, 2018.
[56] Instructions for Use CyPass Microstent. 7.26.2016. Alcon, Fort Worth, TX. Available at: https://www.accessdata.fda.gov/cdrh_docs/pdf15/p150037d.pdf. Accessed November 25, 2018.
[57] Sheybani A, Reitsamer H, Ahmed II. Fluid dynamics of a novel micro-fistula implant for the surgical treatment of glaucoma. Invest Ophthalmol Vis Sci 2015;56(8):4789–95.
[58] Grover DS, Flynn WJ, Bashford KP, et al. Performance and safety of a new ab interno gelatin stent in refractory glaucoma at 12 months. Am J Ophthalmol 2017;183:25–36.
[59] Schlenker MB, Gulamhusein H, Conrad-Hengerer I, et al. Efficacy, safety, and risk factors for failure of standalone ab interno gelatin microstent implantation versus standalone trabeculectomy. Ophthalmology 2017;124(11):1579–88.
[60] Heidinger A, Schwab C, Lindner E, et al. A retrospective study of 199 Xen45 stent implantations from 2014 to 2016. J Glaucoma 2018;256(3):621–5.
[61] Galal A, Bilgic A, Eltanamly R, et al. XEN glaucoma implant with mitomycin C 1-year follow-up: result and complications. J Ophthalmol 2017;2017:5457246.

[62] Tan SZ, Walkden A, Au L. One-year result of XEN45 implant for glaucoma: efficacy, safety, and postoperative management. Eye (Lond) 2018;32(2):324–32.
[63] Santamaría-Álvarez JF, Lillo-sopena J, Sanz-moreno S, et al. Management of conjunctival perforation and XEN Gel stent exposure by stent repositioning through the anterior chamber. J Glaucoma 2018; https://doi.org/10.1097/IJG.0000000000001109.
[64] Hohberger B, Welge-lüßen UC, Lämmer R. MIGS: therapeutic success of combined Xen Gel Stent implantation with cataract surgery. Graefes Arch Clin Exp Ophthalmol 2018;256(3):621–5.
[65] Directions for use for the XEN glaucoma treatment system. Allergan. Dublin, Ireland. Available at: https://allergan-web-cdn-prod.azureedge.net/actavis/actavis/media/allergan-pdf-documents/labeling/xen/dfu_xen_glaucoma_treatment_system_us_feb2017.pdf. Accessed November 25, 2018.
[66] Batlle JF, Fantes F, Riss I, et al. Three-year follow-up of a novel aqueous humor MicroShunt. J Glaucoma 2016;25(2):e58–65.
[67] Chen PP, Lin SC, Junk AK, et al. The effect of phacoemulsification on intraocular pressure in glaucoma patients: a report by the American Academy of Ophthalmology. Ophthalmology 2015;122:1294–307.
[68] Radcliffe N, Noecker R, Sarkisian S, et al. ICE surgical technique outcomes: MIGS implantation of trabecular bypass stent, cataract extraction and endoscopic cyclophotocoagulation. 2014 American Glaucoma Society Annual Meeting. Washington, DC, February 27–March 2, 2014.
[69] Ferguson TJ, Swan R, Sudhagoni R, et al. Microbypass stent implantation with cataract extraction and endocyclophotocoagulation versus microbypass stent with cataract extraction for glaucoma. J Cataract Refract Surg 2017;43(3):377–82.
[70] Mansouri K. Comparison of the intraocular pressure lowering efficacy between a novel goniotomy blade and a trabecular meshwork device. Data presented as a poster at the XXXV Congress of the European Society of Cataract and Refractive Surgeons (ESCRS). Lisbon, Portugal, October 7–11, 2017.
[71] Schweitzer C. Pseudoexfoliation syndrome and pseudoexfoliation glaucoma. J Fr Ophtalmol 2018;41(1):78–90.
[72] Fellman RL, Feuer WJ, Grover DS. Episcleral venous fluid wave correlates with trabectome outcomes: intraoperative evaluation of the trabecular outflow pathway. Ophthalmology 2015;122(12):2385–91.e1.
[73] Iordanous Y, Kent JS, Hutnik CM, et al. Projected cost comparison of Trabectome, iStent, and endoscopic cyclophotocoagulation versus glaucoma medication in the Ontario Health Insurance Plan. J Glaucoma 2014;23(2):e112–8.
[74] Ngan K, Fraser E, Buller S, et al. A cost minimisation analysis comparing iStent accompanying cataract surgery and selective laser trabeculoplasty versus topical glaucoma medications in a public healthcare setting in New Zealand. Graefes Arch Clin Exp Ophthalmol 2018;256(11):2181–9.
[75] Berdahl JP, Khatana AK, Katz LJ, et al. Cost-comparison of two trabecular micro-bypass stents versus selective laser trabeculoplasty or medications only for intraocular pressure control for patients with open-angle glaucoma. J Med Econ 2017;20(7):760–6.

Section VII: Neuro-ophthalmology

Advances in Ophthalmology and Optometry 4 (2019) 245–257

ADVANCES IN OPHTHALMOLOGY AND OPTOMETRY

Electrophysiology in Neuro-Ophthalmology

Rustum Karanjia, MD, PhD, FRCSC, DABO[a,b],
Stuart G. Coupland, PhD[b,*]

[a]Department of Ophthalmology, David Geffen School of Medicine at UCLA, Doheny Eye Institute, 10833 Le Conte Avenue, Los Angeles, CA 90095, USA; [b]Department of Ophthalmology, University of Ottawa Eye Institute, Ottawa Hospital Research Institute, The Ottawa Hospital, 501 Smyth Box 511, Ottawa, ON K1H 8L6, Canada

Keywords

• Electrophysiology • ERG • Photopic negative response • Visual evoked potentials
• Functional vision loss • Paraneoplastic optic neuropathies
• Cancer-associated optic neuropathies • Melanoma-associated optic neuropathies

Key points

- Electrophysiology is able to help neuro-ophthalmologists diagnose patients with organic and inorganic vision loss.
- Advances in technology and the development of new protocols and standards have made testing easier and more precise.
- In this article, the authors endeavor to provide a review of the basic electrophysiological techniques and their utility for understanding and evaluating patients with common neuro-ophthalmological deficits.

INTRODUCTION

Electroretinography (ERG) of the eye typically has been the domain of retina specialist, yet it provides the ability to objectively measure the electrical activity of all components of the eye. This has relevance to subspecialties of ophthalmology, in particular those dealing with the optic nerve; namely glaucoma and neuro-ophthalmology. In this article, the authors endeavor to provide a review of the basic electrophysiological techniques and their utility for understanding and evaluating patients with common neuro-ophthalmological deficits.

Disclosure Statement: R. Karanjia has nothing to disclose. S.G. Coupland Consultant for Diagnosys LLC.

*Corresponding author. *E-mail address:* scoupland@toh.ca

https://doi.org/10.1016/j.yaoo.2019.05.002
2452-1760/19/

SIGNIFICANCE

Electrophysiology and the eye

Each component of the inner and outer retina can be electrically dissected by using various stimuli and response paradigms, which have been compiled into international standards by the International Society for Electrophysiology of Vision (ISCEV). The presence of ISCEV standards for recording techniques along with the nomenclature for all standard electroretinography and visual evoked potential recordings include flash ERG [1], photopic negative response (PhNR) [2], pattern ERG (pERG) [3], and visual evoked potentials (VEPs) [4]. Following these standards ensures that data collected at different testing sights are comparable and ensures that test is an accurate reflection of the retinal or optic nerve function using established, validated testing techniques. These standards also apply to the equipment used, and it rests with the treating physician to ensure that the testing is conducted in compliance with these standards or to understand and explain any derivations from the standards. It also is important to note that not all commercial equipment abides by the ISCEV standards.

Standard electroretinography techniques

The electrical response from the eye can be captured in a basic sense by the full field or flash ERG (ffERG) recordings (Fig. 1). The ffERG typically is recorded using a Ganzfield full field stimulator, hence the name, with cornea electrodes. The characteristic waveform has 2 major deflections. The first negative deflection is termed the a-wave and corresponds to the outer retina and the photoreceptors. The intensity of the light and the use of dark or light adaptation can help isolate the components of the ERG corresponding to rods and cones, respectively. This provides a useful objective electrical marker for the outer retina. The signal is then transferred to the bipolar cells resulting in a large positive deflection, the b-wave (see Fig. 1). Each of these components has a corresponding amplitude and implicit time.

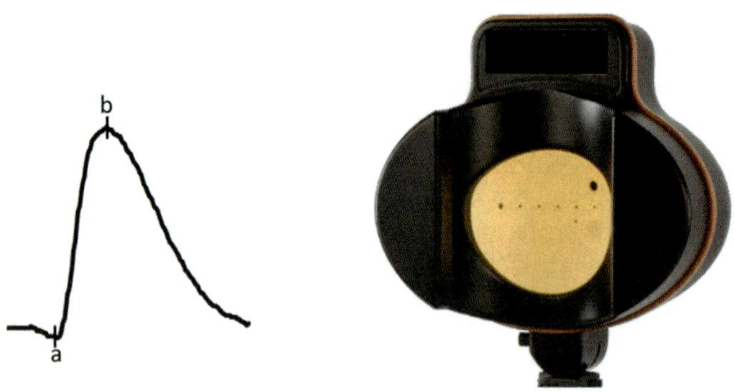

Fig. 1. ERG in response to brief flash stimulation provides an assessment of photoreceptor function reflected by the a-wave component. This is followed by the b-wave component reflecting integrity of the bipolar cell function.

Contained within the upstroke of the b-wave are oscillatory potentials (OPs), which correspond to the amacrine cells and also can be isolated by using selective electrical filtering (90–160 Hz) (Fig. 2). OPs are particularly sensitive to retinal ischemic events such as central retinal artery occlusion and diabetic retinopathy.

Inner retinal components also can be dissected by the ERGs, but the standards are less complete. To neuro-ophthalmologists, the most significant of these is the distinct electrical signal of the retinal ganglion cells (RGCs), which can be isolated using electrophysiologic techniques. The more established of these techniques is the use of pERGs. As with the ffERG, the pERG typically is recorded using corneal electrodes, but, as opposed to a Ganzfeld flash stimulus, the pERG is recorded under light-adapted conditions in response to a luminance phase-reversing grating pattern or checkerboard with an equal number of bright and dark elements. By maintaining an equal number of bright and dark elements, the mean luminance of the screen remains constant throughout the stimulus, negating any flash contribution to the pattern ERG response. The electrical response resulting from pattern stimulus takes different forms depending on the full-cycle temporal frequency of the stimulus. Low frequency (1–2 Hz; 2–4 reversals/s) elicits transient responses that have distinct components. The first positive component occurs at 50 ms after pattern reversal

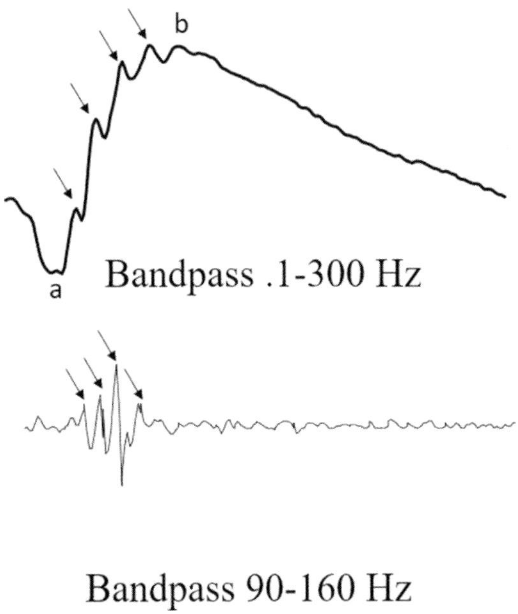

Fig. 2. The OPs are the wavelets visible on the ascending limb of the b-wave observed under broad bandpass filtering. With narrowband high-pass filtering, the high-frequency OP wavelets become more visible.

and is called P50. This is followed by a distinct negative component at 95 ms, namely the N95 (Fig. 3). Severe attenuation of the both components of the pERG occurs in animal models and human subjects who have severe glaucoma or suffered optic nerve transection [5–8]. Higher frequencies (8 Hz; 16 reversals/s) produce a steady state second harmonic response.

Although standards exist for the pERG [3], the response amplitudes are significantly smaller by a 3 orders of magnitude when compared with an ffERG (nV vs μV responses). This can result in significant signal-to-noise issues coupled with the challenges to maintain steady fixation and can limit the utility of pERG in patients with profound vision loss [9].

Another electrophysiological technique for assessing ganglion cell function was published by Viswanathan and colleagues [10]. They were able to identify a component of the flash ERG that specifically corresponded to RGC function. Called the PhNR, it followed the b-wave (Fig. 4). Experimentation with tetrodotoxin and a glaucoma model was able to show the loss of this component of the ERG, demonstrating that the PhNR is the component of the flash ERG that reflects intact RGC activity. As with pERG, an extended protocol standard also exists for the recording of the PhNR [2]. The benefit of the PhNR is that as a full field flash stimulus, it is less dependent on fixation and has a better signal-to-noise resolution when compared with the pERG. The significance of accurate objective quantification of RGC function provides a quantifiable objective metric for the evaluation of the presence and progression of diseases, and the effects of therapeutic interventions at the level of the RGC.

Retro-ocular electrical signals can be assessed using VEPs [4]. As with RGC function, the cortical activity in the primary visual cortex can be assessed to either flash or pattern stimuli. Flash VEP (fVEP) uses the same Ganzfeld stimulator as the flash ERG; however, the recording electrodes are placed in prespecified locations over the occipital lobe (Fig. 5). Detection of the characteristic waveform in an fVEP (see Fig. 5) provides evidence of at least light perception vision in an fVEP, whereas a pattern VEP (pVEP) has the

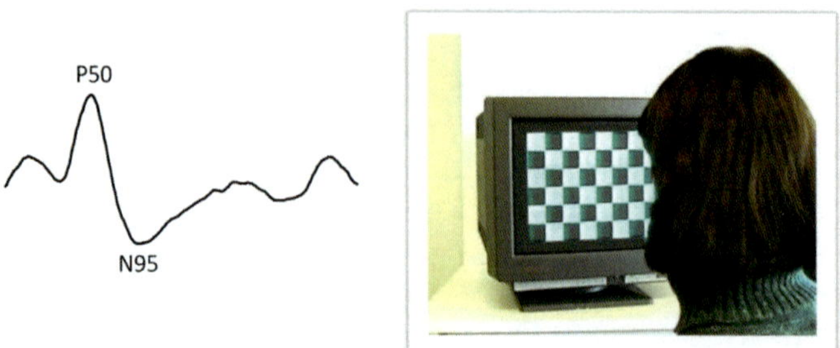

Fig. 3. The pERG is the electroretinal response resulting from pattern stimulation. The peak to trough P50-N95 amplitude reflects ganglion cell function in the inner retina.

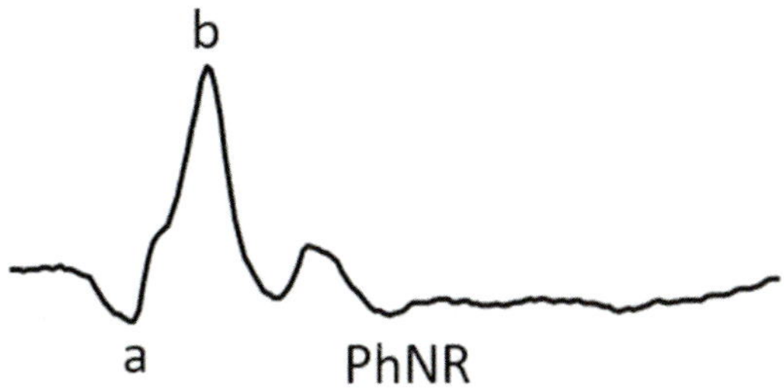

Fig. 4. The PhNR is the component following the b-wave in a ffERG. The PhNR reflects ganglion cell function and is complementary to the pERG.

added advantage of determining a minimal angle of resolution, while again suffering from the same limitations as pERG in cases of poor vision and patient fixation (Fig. 6) [11]. As with the other electrical tests discussed, ISCEV has established guidelines for the performance of both types of VEPs and provides the nomenclature with which to describe the waveforms. The fVEP has 3 major components, P1, N1, P2, of which the first negative (N1) and second positive component (P2) are the most consistent. Similarly, the P100 component of the pVEP is the most consistent across individuals, occurring at 100 ms after pattern reversal. As there is considerable difference in the thickness of the skull and contact of electrodes, the latency of VEP components typically is less variable than the amplitude. Both tests have clinical utility in neuro-ophthalmology.

PRESENT RELEVANCE, FUTURE AVENUES, AND CONCLUSIONS

In neuro-ophthalmology, electrophysiology is significant for the assessment of 3 main areas: those suspected to have inorganic vision loss, patients with autoimmune retinopathies and optic neuropathies, and diseases of the optic nerve.

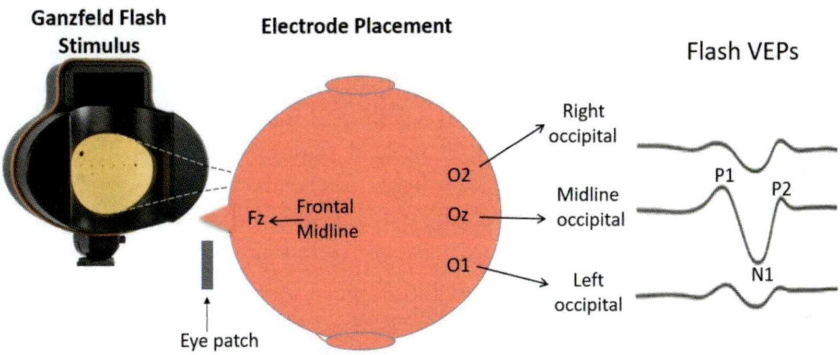

Fig. 5. The fVEP is the cortically evoked response to flash stimulation arising from the visual cortex. A normal fVEP provides objective evidence of light perception.

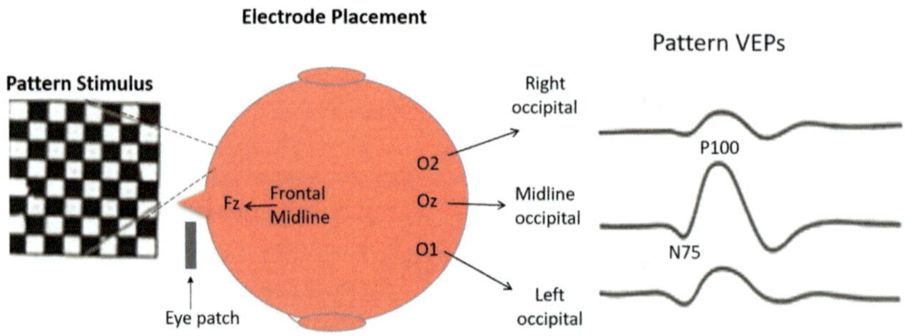

Fig. 6. The pVEP is the cortically evoked response to pattern stimulation arising from the visual cortex. A normal pVEP provides objective evidence of pattern perception and correlates with visual acuity.

Nonorganic vision loss

The presentation of nonorganic vision loss can be a diagnostic dilemma for most clinicians. Electrophysiology testing can be a useful adjunct to the clinical examination by demonstrating that the visual system is functioning normally up to the primary visual cortex. This finding, coupled with normal neuroimaging, is highly suggestive that the vision loss is nonorganic.

As the presentation of nonorganic vision loss is so varied, the type of test selected is dependent on the type of vision loss being reported. Clinically, the objective in nonorganic vision loss is to demonstrate that the vision is better than the amount reported by the patient. This is clinically more challenging the better the vision the patient has reported. For example, in a patient who claims no light perception, a flash VEP can be useful to show the system is functioning. For patients with a reported vision of 20/80 or worse, a pVEP can be useful to demonstrate better visual acuity.

As all downstream abnormalities affect the response from primary visual cortex, thus a combined evaluation of retinal as well as cortical function typically is required to assess a patient with suspected nonorganic vision loss. The presence of a normal flash or pattern ERG provides reassurance that the retinal function is intact. Traditionally this is combined with a VEP to demonstrate that the signal is getting to primary visual cortex. The VEP responses can be recorded in a variety of different ways. Full field Ganzfeld stimulation can be used to record a flash VEP [1,4]. A normal finding on a flash VEP shows that the patient can perceive at least light. Alternatively, pattern stimulation can be used to assess the minimal angle of resolution that with mathematical derivations and demonstrations can be converted into a visual acuity (see Fig. 6). One essential element in testing patients with nonorganic vision loss is to ensure the patient is correctly fixating, as all non-Ganzfeld stimuli require consistent accurate fixation. This can be monitored either directly by the test administrator or indirectly using a pupil tracker.

The work by Michael Bach and his group at the Universität Klinikum Freiburg [11] has provided a framework by which one is able to establish the minimal visual acuity for an individual using a pattern stimulated VEP (Fig. 7). One of the long-held criticisms of VEP was that it required a cooperative patient to obtain reliable results, as simply defocusing or inattention could produce an erroneous result. Building on the work by Bach's group [11] has enabled the development of a system that uses a Fourier transformation of a checkerboard pattern that substantially minimizes the effects of defocus and eye movements creating a more robust system [12,13] (see Fig. 7). This technology has been commercialized and provides a commercial method to establish that a subject can see at least the prescribed minutes of arc [12].

It is important to remember that the diagnosis of nonorganic vision loss is a diagnosis of exclusion. Hence, all appropriate tests must be performed before coming to this diagnosis, and electrophysiology can be a useful complement to this testing regimen.

Immune-mediated retinopathies and optic neuropathies

Although some consider nonorganic vision loss as a scourge on the medical system, it is important to note that other potentially life-threatening forms of vision loss can present in the same way. Key among these are the autoimmune retinopathies and optic neuropathies. As with nonorganic vision loss, the clinical presentation of these can be nondescript vision loss with the absence of objective clinical findings and typically a normal physical examination, including the absence of a relative afferent pupillary defect (RAPD). The RAPD is considered to the gold standard by which one determines if the patient has an optic neuropathy, but it is a relative test requiring a difference between the 2 eyes. This difference is not always present in autoimmune disease, as both eyes typically are affected. Electrophysiological measures thus become a key objective test to identify disruption of the electrical activity in the eyes.

Autoimmune retinopathies often present to neuro-ophthalmology, as they can develop optic nerve pallor, hyperemia, and edema [14]. The vision loss often can precede the identification of any underlying cancer. Classically, autoimmune retinopathies can be subclassified into cancer-associated (CAR),

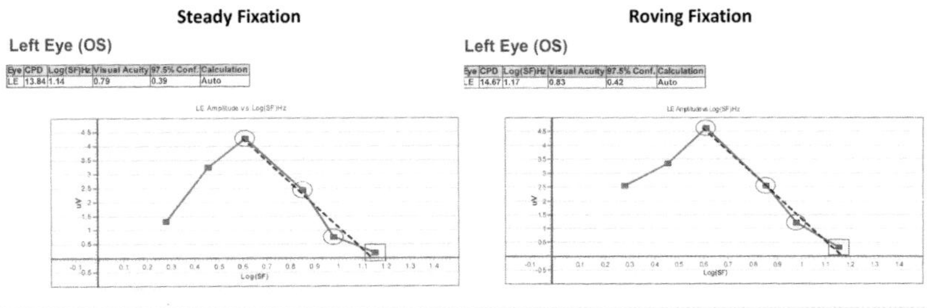

Fig. 7. Sweep VEP to low-contrast checkerboards of 6 spatial frequencies with estimated Snellen acuity under 2 fixation conditions of steady fixation and roving fixation of the 27-inch stimulus display. Estimated acuity was not compromised by fixation loss.

cancer-associated cone dysfunction (CACD), melanoma-associated (MAR), and non-paraneoplastic autoimmune (npAIR) retinopathy. Each one of these, except for npAIR, has an associated underlying neoplasm and antibodies (Table 1) [14].

The antibodies cross-react with different components of the light transduction cascade in the retina, resulting in vision loss. This can be detected in the ERG as an abnormality in the a-wave of the rod response (CAR) or cone response (CAR, CACD) or a negative ERG (loss of b-wave with preservation of a-wave), as in MAR, which has been shown to be a result of the loss of the on-bipolar response [14–16]. Functional loss of rod and cone bipolar cells can be detected by using a rapid on, slow off, saw-tooth stimulus, or a slow on, rapid off, saw-tooth stimulus, respectively (Fig. 8).

The paraneoplastic optic neuropathies (PONs) are similar diseases that primarily affect the optic nerve. They can present with normal-appearing optic nerves or signs of RGC damage, such as swelling, pallor, and atrophy of the nerve head [14]. Some of the antibodies that cause PON also cause CAR, which can further complicate the clinical picture [14,17], and patients can present with a combined autoimmune-related retinopathy and optic neuropathy syndrome [18]. The electrophysiological effects of PON are not well established, but as with any optic neuropathy, an abnormality in the ganglion cell components of the ERG (PhNR and pERG) would be expected with preservation of the outer retinal responses (a and b waves) [19]. Indeed, this has been demonstrated in human case reports and animal models of PON [17,19,20].

The clinical presentation of immune-mediated retinopathies optic neuropathies typically begin with painless progressive visual loss with photopsias, photosensitivity, and loss of color vision. These clinical findings are typically mild in the early stages and progress over time [14]. Visual prognosis is dependent on the treatment of the underlying cancer but can result in severe vision loss despite treatment, and abnormalities on ERG may persist despite recovery of normal vision [16].

Optic nerve disease

Direct assessment of ganglion cell function is becoming an area of greater interest in neuro-ophthalmology [21]. This is especially true in diseases in which the current clinical testing lacks the dynamic range or sensitivity to identify further loss or in the context of treatment, clinical improvement. For example, a patient with profound vision loss from Leber hereditary optic neuropathy is unable to complete an Early Treatment Diabetic Retinopathy Study vision, and an automated visual field; both of which are subjective tests. Similarly, the only objective measure of the optic nerve is pseudo histopathological with optical coherence tomography (OCT). Again, in that same patient, the OCT of the retinal nerve fiber layer encounters a floor effect that precludes further worsening while providing a post event marker that is unlikely to improve [22,23].

The 2 main methods of assessing the function of the RGCs, the N95 amplitude of the pERG and the amplitude of the PhNR, have both been used in

Table 1
Paraneoplastic syndromes and associated electroretinogram findings

Paraneoplastic syndrome	Common underlying neoplasms	Common circulating antibodies	ERG findings
CAR	Small-cell carcinoma of the lung, cancer of the breast, cervix, ovary, uterus and thymus, prostate, pancreas, small bowel, colon and bladder. Follicular lymphomas	Recoverin (23-kDa), retinal enolase (46-kDa), Tubby-like protein 1 (TULP1), Aryl hydrocarbon receptor protein like 1 (AIPL1), interphotoreceptor retinoid binding protein (IRBP), photoreceptor cell specific nuclear receptor (PNR), glyceraldehyde 3-phosphate dehydrogenase (GAPDH [36-kDa]), aldolase C (40-kDa), Heat shock protein 60 and 70 transducin-α	Decreased rod and cone a-wave response
CACD	Small-cell endometrial cancer, primary cervical intraepithelial neoplasia, occult small-cell lung carcinoma, and laryngeal carcinoma	Recoverin	Decreased cone response (a-wave) with preserved rod response
MAR	Melanoma	Transient receptor potential cation channel subfamily M member 1 (TRMP1), α-enolase, recoverin, heat shock protein 70, Bestrophin, myelin basic protein, rod outer segment proteins	Negative ERG (loss of b-wave with preservation of a-wave) Loss of On-Bipolar response
npAIR	None	α-enolase, recoverin, Heat shock protein 70	Loss of a-wave or negative ERG

(*continued on next page*)

Table 1
continued

Paraneoplastic syndrome	Common underlying neoplasms	Common circulating antibodies	ERG findings
PON	Adenocarcinoma, small-cell lung cancer, cancer of the prostate, stomach, colon, and thymus; melanoma	Collapsin response mediator protein 5 (CRMP-5), Aquaporin 4, recoverin, enolase, myelin oligodendrocyte glycoprotein (MOG), myelin basic protein (MBP)	Decreased PhNR with normal a-wave and b-wave (animal models) or decreased outer and inner retinal function (ARRON)

Abbreviations: CACD, cancer-associated cone dysfunction; CAR, cancer-associated retinopathy; MAR, melanoma-associated retinopathy; npAIR, non-paraneoplastic autoimmune retinopathy; PhNR, photopic negative response; PON, paraneoplastic optic neuropathy.

Data from Bogucki ZA, Kownacka M. Immunopathogenesis of ophthalmological paraneoplastic syndromes: recent findings. Adv Clin Exp Med 2018;27(10):1441–1445.

neuro-ophthalmology. The N95 component of the pERG has been demonstrated to decrease in patients with glaucoma, Leber hereditary optic neuropathy (LHON), and other optic neuropathies [8,18,19] Work by Graham Holder [24] demonstrated that the N95 component of the pERG decreased in patients with LHON, yet Porciatti's group at Bascom Palmer [25,26] were unable to demonstrate any correlation in patients with LHON whose vision improved or worsened, suggesting that limitations still exist to the signal-to-noise ratio and dynamic range of the technology.

The PhNR amplitude has been shown to be decreased in patients with LHON, and significantly showed a difference in asymptomatic carriers compared with controls [27]. More importantly, the PhNR has been shown to clinical decrease with RGC function, corresponding to the degree of optic nerve swelling in idiopathic intracranial hypertension (IIH) [20]. Further, by using a flash stimulus, the PhNR is not limited by the challenge of refractive correction and consistent fixation required for pERG, but are a challenge for patients who have a central scotoma, a common feature for most optic neuropathies [9]. Understanding the different components of the electrical response has resulted in an improvement in the ability in detecting pre-perimetric glaucomatous optic nerve damage and to better understand and track the progression of optic nerve diseases, such as LHON and IIH.

Electrophysiology has a well-established role to play in diagnosing patients with nonorganic vision loss, distinguishing this from immune-mediated retinopathies and optic neuropathies. As neuro-ophthalmology evolves from a field of diagnosticians to therapeutics, the availability of objective outcome measures becomes important. As more treatments are being developed for patients with optic neuropathies, the ability to detect preperimentric changes and to

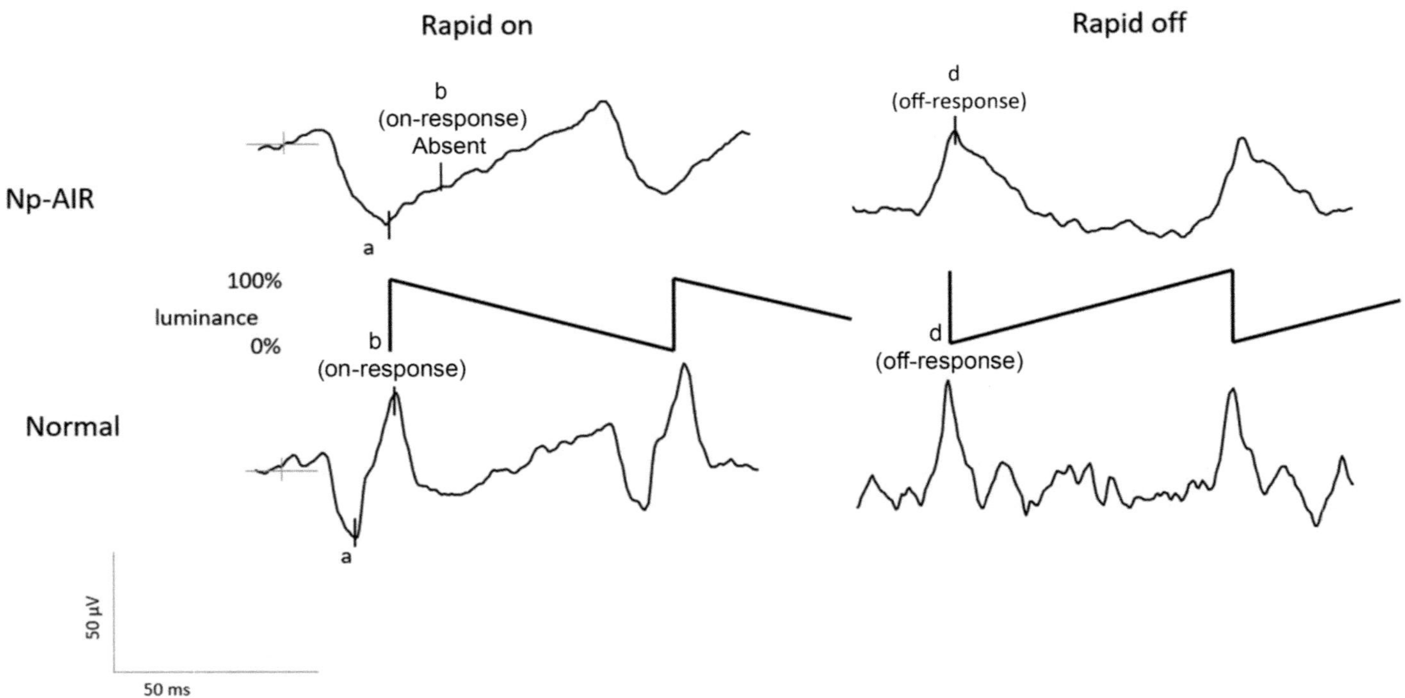

Fig. 8. On and off responses in a patient with npAIR and a normal patient. The on-response of the patient with npAIR has a diminished b-wave, suggesting dysfunction in the on-bipolar cells.

objectively follow patients with profound vision loss is becoming more important not only for expanding the therapeutic window but also allowing for objective clinical outcome measures. Electrophysiology, specifically PhNR and pERG, will likely have an important role for objectively assessing RGC function and should prove useful in future clinical studies.

References

[1] McCulloch DL, Marmor MF, Brigell MG, et al. ISCEV standard for full-field clinical electroretinography (2015 update). Doc Ophthalmol 2015;130(1):1–12.
[2] Frishman L, Sustar M, Kremers J, et al. ISCEV extended protocol for the photopic negative response (PhNR) of the full-field electroretinogram. Doc Ophthalmol 2018;136(3):207–11.
[3] Bach M, Brigell MG, Hawlina M, et al. ISCEV standard for clinical pattern electroretinography (PERG): 2012 update. Doc Ophthalmol 2013;126(1):1–7.
[4] Odom JV, Bach M, Brigell M, et al. ISCEV standard for clinical visual evoked potentials: (2016 update). Doc Ophthalmol 2016;133(1):1–9.
[5] Viswanathan S, Frishman LJ, Robson JG. The uniform field and pattern ERG in macaques with experimental glaucoma: removal of spiking activity. Invest Ophthalmol Vis Sci 2000;41(9):2797–810.
[6] Berardi N, Domenici L, Gravina A, et al. Pattern ERG in rats following section of the optic nerve. Exp Brain Res 1990;79(3):539–46.
[7] Johnson MA, Drum BA, Quigley HA, et al. Pattern-evoked potentials and optic nerve fiber loss in monocular laser-induced glaucoma. Invest Ophthalmol Vis Sci 1989;30(5): 897–907.
[8] Bach M, Hoffmann MB. Update on the pattern electroretinogram in glaucoma. Optom Vis Sci 2008;85(6):386–95.
[9] Preiser D, Lagreze WA, Bach M, et al. Photopic negative response versus pattern electroretinogram in early glaucoma. Invest Ophthalmol Vis Sci 2013;54(2):1182–91.
[10] Viswanathan S, Frishman LJ, Robson JG, et al. The photopic negative response of the macaque electroretinogram: reduction by experimental glaucoma. Invest Ophthalmol Vis Sci 1999;40(6):1124–36.
[11] Bach M, Maurer JP, Wolf ME. Visual evoked potential-based acuity assessment in normal vision, artificially degraded vision, and in patients. Br J Ophthalmol 2008;92(3):396–403.
[12] Strasser T, Nasser F, Langrova H, et al. Objective assessment of visual acuity: a refined model for analyzing the sweep VEP. Doc Ophthalmol 2019;138(2):97–116.
[13] Sacai PY, Berezovsky A, Rocha D, et al, editors. Sweep-VEP acuity as a clinical tool in the diagnosis of functional visual loss. Association for Research in Vision and Ophthalmology; Investigative Ophthalmology & Visual Science 2013;54:4379.
[14] Bogucki ZA, Kownacka M. Immunopathogenesis of ophthalmological paraneoplastic syndromes: recent findings. Adv Clin Exp Med 2018;27(10):1441–5.
[15] Sustar M, Holder GE, Kremers J, et al. ISCEV extended protocol for the photopic On-Off ERG. Doc Ophthalmol 2018;136(3):199–206.
[16] Tian JJ, Coupland S, Karanjia R, et al. Melanoma-associated retinopathy 28 years after diagnosis. JAMA Ophthalmol 2017;135(11):1276–7.
[17] Saito M, Saito W, Kanda A, et al. A case of paraneoplastic optic neuropathy and outer retinitis positive for autoantibodies against collapsin response mediator protein-5, recoverin, and alpha-enolase. BMC Ophthalmol 2014;14:5.
[18] Almarzouqi SJ, Morgan ML, Carvounis PE, et al. Autoimmune-related retinopathy and optic neuropathy accompanied by anti-GAD antibodies. Neuroophthalmology 2015;39(4): 195–200.
[19] Carboni G, Forma G, Bond AD, et al. Bilateral paraneoplastic optic neuropathy and unilateral retinal compromise in association with prostate cancer: a differential diagnostic challenge in a patient with unexplained visual loss. Doc Ophthalmol 2012;125(1):63–70.

[20] Locri F, Cammalleri M, Pini A, et al. Further evidence on efficacy of diet supplementation with fatty acids in ocular pathologies: insights from the EAE model of optic neuritis. Nutrients 2018;10(10) [pii:E1447].
[21] Porciatti V. Electrophysiological assessment of retinal ganglion cell function. Exp Eye Res 2015;141:164–70.
[22] Asanad S, Tian JJ, Frousiakis S, et al. Optical coherence tomography of the retinal ganglion cell complex in leber's hereditary optic neuropathy and dominant optic atrophy. Curr Eye Res 2019;44(6):638–44.
[23] Hwang TJ, Karanjia R, Moraes-Filho MN, et al. Natural history of conversion of Leber's hereditary optic neuropathy: a prospective case series. Ophthalmology 2017;124(6): 843–50.
[24] Holder GE. The pattern electroretinogram in anterior visual pathway dysfunction and its relationship to the pattern visual evoked potential: a personal clinical review of 743 eyes. Eye 1997;11(Pt 6):924–34.
[25] Guy J, Feuer WJ, Porciatti V, et al. Retinal ganglion cell dysfunction in asymptomatic G11778A: Leber hereditary optic neuropathy. Invest Ophthalmol Vis Sci 2014;55(2): 841–8.
[26] Lam BL, Feuer WJ, Schiffman JC, et al. Trial end points and natural history in patients with G11778A Leber hereditary optic neuropathy: preparation for gene therapy clinical trial. JAMA Ophthalmol 2014;132(4):428–36.
[27] Karanjia R, Berezovsky A, Sacai PY, et al. The photopic negative response: an objective measure of retinal ganglion cell function in patients with Leber's hereditary optic neuropathy. Invest Ophthalmol Vis Sci 2017;58(6):BIO300–6.

Advances in Ophthalmology and Optometry 4 (2019) 259–274

ADVANCES IN OPHTHALMOLOGY AND OPTOMETRY

Advances in Teleophthalmology

Is It Ready for Neuro-Ophthalmology?

Isabella Irrcher, PhD, MSc,
Martin William ten Hove, MEng, MD, FRCSC*

Department of Ophthalmology, Kingston Health Sciences Centre-HDH Site, Queen's University, 166 Brock Street, Kingston, Ontario, Canada

Keywords

• Teleophthalmology • Screening • Models of health care • Artificial intelligence (AI) • Digital imaging systems • Review • Patient engagement • Physician engagement

Key points

- Ophthalmology is well suited for widespread adoption of telemedicine because of the specialty's reliance on diagnostic imaging for screening, disease diagnoses, and treatment decisions.
- Many recent technological advances have improved the scope and accuracy of teleophthalmology as a model of eye care delivery.
- Engaging end users in the development of teleprograms by understanding the factors that predict acceptance will ensure long-term viability.

INTRODUCTION

Telemedicine is an umbrella term that refers to a modality of health care delivery that uses digital technologies to provide and support the exchange of personal health information (PHI) between a health care provider and a patient who are in separate locations. This evolving modality is now pervasive throughout medicine; with applications in patient care, education, research, and public health.

The term "tele" was first used in a medical context by the Dutch physician Einthoven in 1906 when he referred to a successful telephonic transmission of

Disclosures: The authors have no disclosures to declare.

*Corresponding author. Department of Ophthalmology, Kingston Health Sciences Centre-HDH Site, Brock2 Room 230, 166 Brock Street, Kingston, Ontario K7L 5G2, Canada. *E-mail address:* tenhove@queensu.ca

https://doi.org/10.1016/j.yaoo.2019.04.019
2452-1760/19/

an electrocardiogram as a "telecardiogram" [1]. Since then, telemedicine's scope and sophistication has evolved significantly and has been aided by advancements in technology and infrastructure, most notably the creation of the World Wide Web in 1990. Smartphone apps are an example of how telemedicine has been able to capture several types of PHI. Advancements in the portability and connectivity of medical diagnostic equipment, coupled with the development of cloud-based storage and improved data transmission, have expanded the domain of telemedicine to include screening programs, remote diagnostic and treatment programs, and home monitoring.

Many drivers exist that incentivize the widespread adoption of telemedicine. Perhaps the greatest of these is the ever-increasing financial constraints imposed on the health care system experienced by developed and developing nations. Telemedicine has the potential to significantly reduce both transportation and infrastructure costs associated with the conventional delivery of health care. Additional drivers include the increasing clinical demands of an aging population with high expectations, and the inconvenient truth that many people still do not have equal access to the highest quality of health care. These drivers have led to an urgent need to innovate our current health care system by incorporating services and programs that are easy to use, cost-effective, scalable, and improve the quality and accessibility of care. Adopting digital technologies may represent an important innovation in this context.

Within ophthalmology, telemedicine now is able to address many elements of care that are required for macular degeneration, diabetic retinopathy, and glaucoma. However, beyond these main vision-threatening diseases, progress has been much slower. Subspecialties, such as neuro-ophthalmology, have lagged behind mostly due to the underlying complexity and scope of the neuro-ophthalmic examination. The slower progress may also be due to the diagnostic assessments that are either not yet portable, digital, or suitable for untrained personnel to perform. Innovative technological advances are closing these gaps rapidly, yet some physicians still are reluctant to embrace telemedicine. This hesitation is largely due to insufficient evidence of the platform's effectiveness and efficiency–particularly in situations in which the examination and/or provision of treatment is complex. These challenges will continue to constrain telemedicine's full-scale deployment until they are addressed. This review summarizes the latest advances in teleophthalmology and discusses limitations as they apply to the neuro-ophthalmological workup in the teleophthalmology setting.

Teleophthalmology applications

The application of telemedicine as a model of care in ophthalmology was first described in the peer-reviewed literature by Rose and Grant in 1975 [2]. Today, teleophthalmology uses a broad array of ocular imaging devices that relay PHI from a remote clinic to a treating ophthalmologist. Remote teleophthalmology clinics now are ubiquitous throughout the world and have been established in at least one country on every continent [3]. Multinational efforts (where patients are seen in one country and assessed in another) have been deployed, with the greatest number established by North American and European organizations. These global initiatives provide screening, triage, consultations, treatment, and follow-up [3]. Although the ultimate goal is to provide a complete vision and ocular assessment in every clinic mode, teleophthalmology is currently focused on screening programs for specific disease entities. Diabetic retinopathy (DR) screening programs are by far the most common [3,4]. Although some programs have been clinically validated with criteria established by American Telemedicine Association (ATA) [5], even more programs remain unclassified [3].

Screening programs

Telemedicine-based DR screening programs were born of an urgent need to improve screening and surveillance rates of one of the leading causes of avoidable visual impairment worldwide [6]. This need was further supported by the established efficacy of laser photocoagulation and anti-vascular endothelial growth factor therapies in preventing visual loss from DR [7–11], and the availability of evidence-based clinical guidelines for diagnosis and management of DR [12,13]. The establishment of DR telescreening guidelines by the ATA and Ocular Telehealth Special Interest Group [5] provided a framework to better define the program's goals and the level of clinical validation (Table 1). Notwithstanding screening program goals and levels of clinical validation, at the most basic level, each program must have the ability to acquire a diagnostic image of the fundus and have the capability of storing and transmitting data to a reader where the image is subsequently graded for referral recommendations.

Diagnostic imaging. The development of high-resolution retinal photography has led to the creation of image-acquisition devices with improved performance, portability, and affordability, most of which exploit smartphone imaging technology. Some of the most commonly used devices are described in Table 2. However, before these devices can be used in screening programs, image acquisition-protocols and quality checks first require validation. To meet the clinical practice standard, an image-capture device must provide an image of sufficient resolution comparable with that achieved with standard fundus cameras, scanning multiwave laser ophthalmoscopy, and/or optical coherence tomography.

Image storage and transmission. Telemedicine-based DR screening programs almost exclusively use store and forward transmission (SFT): a 2-step process that involves the acquisition and storage of several images, typically as much as 35 to 50 MB of clinical information at point of care, and the subsequent retrieval of images at the point of evaluation. When implementing an SFT system, server size, transmission speed, bandwidth, and packet loss are all characteristics to be considered, in addition to other infrastructure and geographic determinants [6].

Image interpretation. Image reading and interpretation strategies range from human readers to the use of image-reading algorithms. At present, image-reading algorithms process high-resolution clinical images and attempt to identify disease

Table 1
American Telemedicine Association Telescreening Guidelines; programs reviewed in Tozer and colleagues [4]

Level	General Telescreening guideline	Diabetic retinopathy screening program	Program	Country/Year of deployment	Setting
1	Disease identification without disease severity stratification	Identifies patients with no or very mild NPDR	Ophdiat EyePACS Digiscope	France, 2012 USA, 2009 USA, 2002	H PCO PCO
2	Level 1 + disease severity stratification	Identifies patients ± sight-threatening DR	EyeCheck NHS	The Netherlands, 2005 UK, 2003	PCO PCO/H
3	Level 2 + sufficient accuracy for appropriate decision making	Identifies patients with NPDR, PDR, and ME, makes treatment decisions	JVN U of Alberta	USA, 2014 Canada, 2000	PCO/H PCC/H/P/OO
4	System replaces clinical exam	System equals or exceeds the ability of ETDRS photographs to identify DR lesions	N/A	N/A	N/A

Abbreviations: DR, diabetic retinopathy; ETDRS, early treatment diabetic retinopathy study; H, hospital; JVN, Joslin Vision Network; ME, macular edema; N/A, not applicable; NHS, National Health Service; NPDR, nonproliferative DR; OO, optometry office; P, pharmacy; PCC, primary care clinic; PCO, primary care office; PDR, proliferative DR; U, university.

Table 2
Examples of smartphone-based retinal imaging systems

Fundus Imaging system	Description	App/solutions	Country of origin/ reference
PaxosScope (DigiSight)	Lens attachment to smartphone (anterior/posterior images) FDA class II 510(k) exempt	Paxos Checkup Paxos Analytics	USA
Volk iNView	iPhone fundus camera	Volki Nview	USA [47]
D-EYE posterior	Apple smartphone-based digital ophthalmoscope	D-EYE app	Italy/USA [48]
Peek Retina	Smartphone attachment CE-registered class I medical device	Peek Retina	UK [49]
iExaminer	Smartphone-based imaging adaptor system (iPhone 4 + Welch Allyn PanOptic Ophthalmoscope + iExaminer app FDA approved	iExaminer	USA [50]
oDocs visoScope	3D printed lens adapting imaging system	iPhone camera, FiLMiC Pro app	NZ [51]

and flag appropriate cases for specialist referral. When validated with the appropriate levels of specificity and sensitivity, this "first pass" approach to eliminating patients with no retinal pathology is a good example of how artificial intelligence (AI) can reduce workload by 30% to 70% [14]. However, in order for AI to be used with image-reading algorithms, the image quality obtained at the point of care must be standardized. Image quality depends on many factors including the camera's ease of use, resolution, the technical proficiency of the photographer, and the clarity of the patient's ocular media. Although AI predictive image analysis is compelling, human readers still remain the gold standard for image interpretation. Readers are often not ophthalmologists but trained nonmedical professionals and/or primary care physicians [3,15].

Telescreening programs for DR are the most common teleophthalmology programs to date. Their cost-effectiveness [4,16] and diagnostic accuracy [17] are well-established. Other disease entities suitable for effective telescreening programs include age-related macular degeneration (AMD), glaucoma, amblyopia, and strabismus [18]. Some screening programs for these conditions are currently operational [3]. Although these single-disease screening programs have been a step in the right direction, screening capabilities for multiple diseases with similar workflows and resource requirements, is a logical progression for teleophthalmology. Indeed, the cost-effectiveness of a combined screening strategy with respect to DR and AMD has already been described [18–20].

As imaging capabilities improve with time, remote screening centers with validated protocols will likely be developed for other conditions including cataracts, refractive errors, and strabismus [18]. The adoption of the ATA guidelines to validate new screening programs is recommended. All screening programs should ideally be scalable and capable of expanding their scope to accommodate the anticipated increase in eye disease and the relative decline in the number of eye care providers. The magnitude of eye disease burden will not only affect screening programs but also programs that offer triage, consult, and follow-up.

Emergency/triage programs

Rural triage programs are designed to reduce unnecessary health care and travel costs by decreasing unnecessary patient transfers. This is especially relevant in rural areas where hospital closures are now common, and there is a paucity of primary care physicians and specialists [21,22]. An effective triage program must be designed to have high sensitivity to correctly identify patients who require immediate assessment (which may involve travel of either the patient or physician). Many successful triage/emergency programs located in small rural areas have been deployed worldwide [3]. These programs also function as a value-add service for emergency medicine departments and urgent care centers where reliable fundoscopic evaluation may not be available. Emergency department triage programs have proven to be equivalent or superior in providing a diagnosis and reducing unnecessary patient transfers [23]. One such example is located at the University of Pittsburgh where emergency physicians, equipped with a smartphone and an ophthalmoscope adaptor, routinely acquire images of sufficient quality that off-site ophthalmologists can make accurate and safe triage decisions [23].

Consult/follow-up programs

Teleconsult and follow-up programs, especially in rural areas, are similar to emergency/triage and screening programs in that they are meant to reduce health care and travel costs, as well as wait times. Nearly half of the teleconsultation programs described in the literature function as a general screening service conducted by an optometrist who performs the clinical examination, acquires appropriate images, and then consults with an ophthalmologist to determine the appropriate treatment and management [3]. Teleophthalmology consult programs can be helpful in managing patients with preexisiting conditions, providing peer-to-peer consultations or primary care provider-to-ophthalmologist consultations [3].

Synchronous versus asynchronous transmission

Teleophthalmology generally uses 1 of 2 methods to transmit PHI. Real-time transmission (RTT) (often referred to as synchronous transmission) and SFT (referred to as asynchronous transmission). As "real-time" implies, the patient-physician interaction occurs live. SFT does not require the physician and patient to be simultaneously available; on the contrary, clinical images and some medical data are acquired, and then subsequently stored and recalled at a later time. A hybrid model also exists in which a patient visits a remote clinic to have images taken and then later returns to a site for live consultation. The component of the eye examination determines which transmission mode is most suitable and, by extension, the required transmission speed and bandwidth. Technical barriers such as bandwidth, packet loss, and storage limitations have largely been overcome in recent years (in developed countries) [23]. As of 2017, the average data transfer rate in the Americas, Asia, and Europe ranges between 14 and 28 mbps [24]. Although these rates are sufficient for SFT, RTT may require rates as high as 24 mbps for high-resolution video [25]. As long as the transmission speed is sufficient, the diagnostic accuracy of RTT generally is comparable with face-to-face consultation; however, important dynamic information may be lost if transmission is lost or slow. Many countries are not able to consistently provide these high data transfer rates [26]. In some cases, multiple wireless data providers can be combined to overcome transmission speed bottlenecks [27]. The use of AI in teleophthalmology may add further demands for rapid data transfer depending on whether the predictive analytics takes place at the point of care or at a central server. Image analytics is an example of machine learning in which a computer is trained to recognize elements of an image. Implementation of AI technology has the potential to further reduce costs and decrease wait times [28].

Teleneuro-ophthalmology: are we ready for it?

Although retinal diseases, such as macular degeneration and DR, are ideal for telemedicine screening protocols, relatively few prevalent neuro-ophthalmologic conditions justify the development of a screening protocol. One exception may be to include a screening protocol for strabismus into a well-baby check. Beyond screening for strabismus, detecting other ocular disorders within a pediatric population would be challenging because imaging the optic nerve and fundus under sedation would be necessary. Another potential screening opportunity would be the development of a headache screening protocol to assist primary care providers and emergency physicians. The most ominous cause of a headache is raised intracranial pressure that manifests in the eye as papilledema. Most physicians are not confident with their fundoscopy skills, and papilledema often is missed by nonophthalmologists. Digital cameras already are being used in emergency rooms to determine whether papilledema is present [29]. The gold standard of detecting papilledema involves stereo viewing of the disc. However, a skilled observer using remotely acquired high-resolution images would provide the next best level of diagnostic accuracy and would likely be superior to the diagnostic certainty that many primary care providers have identifying this important finding.

Establishing a new neuro-ophthalmic diagnosis using the telemedicine platform would be difficult. Most diagnoses are complex and require a skilled clinician to conduct a detailed and thoughtful history that is technical and sometimes highly tailored to the patient under examination. The history-taking process is inherently interactive and would be difficult to accomplish using a formulated SFT approach. However, components of the history (as with all areas of ophthalmology) exist that would be amenable to intelligent assistance (IA), such as the family history, past medical history, and the review of systems. Similarly, IA could be applied to the history of the presenting problem by using preliminary questions generated from iterative paradigms that could improve time efficiency for the clinician [30].

The neuro-ophthalmic examination usually begins with an assessment of the visual pathway including visual acuity and visual field. Although there are devices and apps to assess Snellen acuity using SFT (Table 3) [31,32], subtle clues may be missed that clinicians pick up with conventional examination techniques that help to detect and localize a small central visual field defect (eg, hemianopia, hemi-field split, or a central scotoma). Amsler grid apps will allow patients to detect, record, and upload their own metamorphopsia to provide information about the central field and macula [33,34]. Similarly, apps exist to perform color vision screening [35]. Few color vision apps allow for calibration, therefore results need to confirmed with conventional color tests such as the D-15. Nevertheless, color testing apps can detect and quantify an optic neuropathy if there is an intereye performance difference or a monocular change over time.

Automated perimetry is ubiquitous in ophthalmology and is well suited to the RTT and SFT modes of telemedicine with several devices and programs that provide either screening or diagnostic data. Some studies suggest that confrontation visual field testing is not reliable; however, many clinicians use the interactive confrontation field technique to augment the information derived from automated perimetry [36]. For example, confrontation visual field assessment helps to uncover nonphysiological vision loss. The technique could be performed using a large monitor and conventional video conferencing (RTT mode), but this approach has yet to be studied to measure its viability and reliability.

The examination of the pupil involves accurate measurements of the diameter under scoptic and photoptic conditions and careful observation of the dynamics of the pupil. Measuring the pupil is subject to errors from parallax [37] and inconsistent illumination. Commercially available pupillometers provide higher precision but are expensive and technique dependent. The dynamics of pupillary constriction requires the magnification and controlled illumination of a slit lamp. A team of investigators and engineers recently have developed a drone slit lamp that is remotely controlled using keyboard signals sent via the Web to servo motors on the slit lamp to adjust all of the illumination and observation components (Fig. 1) [38]. A clinical validation of this instrument has been performed, and its ability to quantify cell and flare in anterior chamber was found to have substantial agreement with the conventional slit lamp performance (MW ten Hove, unpublished data, 2019). For the first time a remote-controlled slit lamp can provide a clinician with an RTT ability to examine the anterior segment–including the subtle dynamics of the pupillary movement (eg dilation lag and veriform movements). However, because it is controlled in real-time by a physician, the drone slit lamp is not amenable to SFT.

Table 3
Neuro-ophthalmic examination components and their suitability for teleophthalmology

Examination component	RTT	SFT	Limitation
Visual pathway			
Visual acuity	VC	iExaminer [31]	Validation
Snellen/LogMAR		Eye Handbook [32]	Missed behavioral clues
Pinhole visual acuity			
Refraction	Autorefractor	Autorefractor	Cost/training
Color (Ishihara/color saturation)	VC	PseudoChromatic Color Test app [35]	Validation Calibration
Distortion (Amsler)	VC	Amsler Grid app [33] Eyecare-Amsler [34]	Storage
Visual field testing	HFDT DICOM Specvis Confrontation fields	HFDT DICOM Specvis [52] NA	Cost
Pupils			
Size/reaction	VC[a]	Photos/pupillometer Drone slit lamp PupilX [40]	Parallax technique dependent
RAPD	VC[a]	Goggles PupilX [40]	PupilX pupillometer requires validation
Pharmacologic test	VC[a]	Photos, videos	
Anterior segment			
	Drone slit lamp	NR	Cost/ maintenance
Oculomotor functioning			
Ductions/versions	VO	9 Gaze app [53] eyeTilt app [54]	
Ocular alignment	Hirschberg Alternative cover test	In development Video	
Eyelid movement	VO	Still photos/video	
Nystagmus	VO	Video	
Saccades/pursuit/OKN/VOR	VO	Video	

Abbreviations: DICOM, digital imaging and communications in medicine; HFDT, Humphrey frequency doubling technology; NA, not available; NR, not ready; OKN, optokinetic nystagmus; RTT, real-time transmission; SFT, store and forward; VC, video conference; VO, video observation; VOR, vestibulo-ocular reflex.

[a]Trained personnel required.

Video-based acquisition of eye movements also can be performed; however, the nature of this assessment often requires the observation of the eye movement while the head is moving (eg, checking for the vestibular ocular reflex), making it difficult to obtain a video that remains in focus. Another challenge

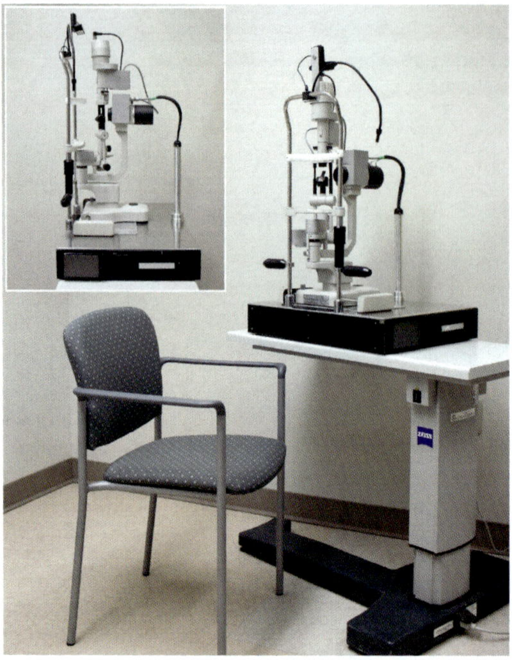

Fig. 1. Drone slit lamp set up. The remotely located specialist sees the patient via two video feeds: the first video feed is provided atop the patient's head to provide live feedback on the patient's positioning at the slit lamp. The second video feed provides a view of the patient's eye through the slit lamp camera. The patient hears the specialist through a speaker box built into the base of the slit lamp. A trained technician is always present in the room to assist with the clinical examination and to instill fluorescein drops to the patient's eye.

is measuring the degree of ocular misalignment, a skill that can be performed only by well-trained personnel (using loose prisms and/or the Risley prism). Head-worn goggles that can record eye movements using infrared technology have been developed; however, such a device is not yet commercially available.

Video-based binocular pupil recording devices that provide an expert with the ability to detect relative afferent defects in an SFT mode exist, but are expensive and require clinical validation [39,40]. One such device is the PupilX, which provides an automated measurement using a flexible eye mask that excludes all ambient light. Two video cameras enable simultaneous measurements of both pupils using proprietary algorithms. Visual stimulation, in the form of a uniformly illuminated field, can be applied independently to each eye [40].

Several limitations of teleophthalmology occur that are difficult to circumvent in the context of a neuro-ophthalmic examination. For example, elements of the complete neurologic example exist that cannot be performed remotely. Assessing the strength of the orbicularis oculi muscle is a tactile exercise that is not amenable to having an assistant perform at the point of care. Other examination skills, such as observing gait, eliciting reflexes, checking sensory perception, and conducting a mental status assessment are important elements of the neuro-ophthalmic assessment that are sometimes critical for establishing a diagnosis. These skills could conceivably be taught to an assistant who would then be required to attend every consultation assessment using teleophthalmology.

Despite these significant challenges, it is possible that in a few years teleophthalmology may be applied to perform much of the conventional neuro-ophthalmic examination and diagnose and manage several common disorders (Box 1). As with all areas of ophthalmology, the management of patients with neuro-ophthalmologic conditions frequently includes some education. For example, patients with vascular lesions need to be counseled about the reduction of vascular risk factors. Teleophthalmology could be configured to provide this service either synchronously with RTT or asynchronously by sending the patient and family educational materials electronically to be viewed at a later time. Another potential use of teleophthalmology would be to monitor the recovery of cranial neuropathies causing diplopia. The patient could simply use an eye movement app to send to their eye care provider according to a prearranged time schedule [39].

Present relevance and future directions

Telemedicine, in all of its forms including teleophthalmology, has benefited greatly from the rapid assimilation of new technology. Although most screening, triage, and consultation programs are meant to provide care to patients in remote areas, telemedicine programs also exist that span only within a few kilometers of a patient's home in urban settings. Digital connectivity and its integration with health care has the potential to improve patient-physician collaboration, increase patient satisfaction, and, importantly, reduce costs at all levels within the health care system.

Telemedicine is gaining acceptance based on its ability to deliver care that is equal or superior to a traditional clinic visit as perceived by the patient and the physician, and its ability to be cost-effective. Despite these achievements, some physicians and patients are reluctant to embrace telemedicine. Fifty-nine percent of ophthalmologists reported "low confidence" in their ability to make decisions based on fundus images without performing their own supplemental examination [41]. User satisfaction often is used as a main patient outcome; however, this falls short of providing important insights to the predictors of adoption and acceptance [42]. Furthermore, many more patients have yet to understand what telemedicine is and how it can address their health care needs.

Predictors and barriers to telemedicine adoption. Various theoretic models have been applied to understand what factors predict technology acceptance and adoption. In particular, the Technology Acceptance Model has been used to build a predictive model of telemedicine user acceptance. In their research model, Hu

Box 1: Possible telemedicine applications of the conventional neuro-ophthalmic examination

Screening for common neuro complaints

- Sudden vision loss
- Visual field defects
- Double vision
- Headache

Consult/diagnosis (eg, red eye)

- Acute monocular vision loss (VL) (optic neuropathies)
- Acute/chronic binocular VL (stroke, optic neuropathies)
- Transient VL (amaurosis, migraine)
- Acute/chronic diplopia
- Oscillopsia
- Anisocoria
- Head/ocular pain
- Ptosis/proptosis

Emergency/triage (eg, open eye; pupil involved 3rd nerve palsy [NP])

- Acute VL (giant cell arteritis [GCA])
- Acute diplopia (3rd NP)
- Potential stroke
- Trauma
- Pituitary apoplexy
- Acute/chronic headache (rule out papilledema)

Follow-up (eg, resolving central retinal vein occlusion; resolving 6th)

- Resolving nonarteritic anterior ischemic optic neuropathy
- Stable/treated GCA
- Stable/treated myasthenia
- Resolving ischemic cranial nerve
- Resolving 7th nerve paresis
- Monitoring stroke-related VL

Abbreviations: CN, cranial nerve; CRVO, central vein retinal occlusion; GCA, giant cell arteritis; NAION, nonarteritic ischemic optic neuropathy; NP, nerve palsy; R/O, rule out; VL, vision loss.

et al., hypothesized that the degree to which technology is easy to use by physicians affects both their perception of the usefulness of the technology and their attitude toward using the technology in general. The authors found that, contrary to their hypothesis, the ease of use of the platform had no significant effect on the physician's attitude toward using it. However, the perceived usefulness of the platform was found to have a significant and strong influence on physicians' intentions. This suggests that, for a telemedicine application to be accepted, its ability to fill the needs of the physician must be demonstrated [43].

Other theoretic models have been used to identify additional predictors of adoption. These include: (1) a positive link with a policy level sponsor, (2) successful structural integration, (3) cohesive cooperative groups, and (4) integration at the level of professional knowledge and practice [44]. Other factors impeding a more rapid adoption of telemedicine include physicians' views on the medical liability, reimbursement, and legal/regulatory issues [45].

Patient perspective. We have a limited understanding of patients' perceptions of telemedicine, yet their attitudes, concerns, and perceptions are critical considerations in the design of an effective and sustainable program. Only with patient input can we design tailored programs that target the appropriate patient population, who have both the need for the health care service and likelihood to use it. Valikodath and colleagues [42], consulted a patient population largely unfamiliar with telemedicine to explore attitudes, perceptions, and willingness to participate in the context of a DR screening program. Surprisingly, patient demographic factors such as older age had no association with the willingness to participate, perception of convenience, or the physician-patient relationship. Patients who valued convenience or who had more systemic health problems were more willing to participate in telemedicine. Willingness to participate in telemedicine also was strongly influenced by how much patients valued the relationship they had with their primary care physician; the better the relationship the less likely they would be to participate.

Similar to physician acceptance of technology, theoretic models also have been applied to predict technology adoption in patient populations. The Unified Theory of Acceptance and Use of Technology suggests that adoption is affected by performance expectancy (technology will enhance quality of life performance), ease of use, social influence, and the patient's belief that the organizational and technical infrastructure exists [46]. Ultimately, user acceptance is a critical success factor for telemedicine adoption. If telemedicine is meant to disrupt the ailing health care systems of the world and provide access to better health outcomes, then perhaps the biggest strides in telemedicine adoption will be made once the beliefs, attitudes, and intentions are explored. Technology will continue to provide us with innovative and cost-conscious products. However, if the consumer stands firm in their belief that telemedicine will not be useful to them, technology adoption will continue to languish.

SUMMARY/DISCUSSION

Recent technological advancements have significantly enabled the evolution of teleophthalmology. The development of apps that leverage high-resolution smartphone cameras (up to 48 megapixels), the miniaturization of diagnostic equipment, the availability of affordable cloud-based storage, and the improvement of data transmission have all played a role in the expansion of telemedicine into all branches of medicine. Teleophthalmology now is a well-established platform for screening programs for conditions such as macular degeneration, DR, and glaucoma. A teleophthalmology platform that is able to conduct a complete eye examination, including the anterior and posterior segment of the eye, has not yet been developed, but with the advent of a drone slit lamp, it may soon be possible. Neuro-ophthalmology as a subset of the complete eye examination offers some additional challenges–most notably a way to observe, measure, and document ocular motility disorders. The development of new apps and increased data transmission speeds will help to overcome these barriers. Additional efforts are needed to better understand and overcome the reasons behind the reluctance that some physicians have to embrace teleophthalmology. Similarly, patient biases need to be addressed so that teleophthalmology can find its rightful place in the health care system and ease the fiscal pressures on a system that is, struggling to meet the demands of an aging population with high expectations and unequal access.

References

[1] Einthoven W. [The telecardiogram]. [Het telecardiogram]. Ned Tijdschr Geneeskd 1906;50:1517–47.

[2] Rose H, Grant TW. The use of a travelling ophthalmic technologist in a remote, sparsely populated region. Can J Ophthalmol 1975;10:201–4. Available at: https://www.ncbi.nlm.nih.gov/pubmed/?term=Rose+and+Grant+and+Canadian+Journal+of+Ophthalmology+and+1975. Accessed May 23, 2019.

[3] Caffery L, Taylor M, Gole G, et al. Models of care in tele-ophthalmology: a scoping review. J Telemed Telecare 2019;25(2):106–22.

[4] Tozer K, Woodward MA, Newman-Casey PA. Telemedicine and diabetic retinopathy: review of published screening programs. J Endocrinol Diabetes 2015;2(4); https://doi.org/10.15226/2374-6890/2/4/00131.

[5] Li HK, Horton M, Bursell S-E, et al. Telehealth practice recommendations for diabetic retinopathy, second edition. Telemed J E Health 2011;17(10):814–37.

[6] Cuadros JA. Telemedicine-based diabetic retinopathy screening programs: an evaluation of utility and cost-effectiveness, Smart Homecare Technology and TeleHealth 2015;2:119–27.

[7] Massin P, Bandello F, Garweg JG, et al. Safety and efficacy of ranibizumab in diabetic macular edema (RESOLVE study): a 12-month, randomized, controlled, double-masked, multicenter phase II study. Diabetes Care 2010;33:2399–405.

[8] Korobelnik JF, Do DV, Schmidt-Erfurth U, et al. Intravitreal aflibercept for diabetic macular edema. Ophthalmology 2014;121:2247–54.

[9] Elman MJ, Ayala A, Bressler NM, et al. Intravitreal ranibizumab for diabetic macular edema with prompt versus deferred laser treatment: 5-year randomized trial results. Ophthalmology 2015;122:375–81.

[10] Photocoagulation for diabetic macular edema. Early treatment diabetic retinopathy study report number 1. Early Treatment Diabetic Retinopathy Study research group. Arch Ophthalmol 1985;103(12):1796–806.

[11] Treatment techniques and clinical guidelines for photocoagulation of diabetic macular edema. Early treatment diabetic retinopathy study report number 2. Early Treatment Diabetic Retinopathy Study Research Group. Ophthalmology 1987;94:761–74.

[12] Grading diabetic retinopathy from stereoscopic color fundus photographs–an extension of the modified Airlie House classification. ETDRS report number 10. Early Treatment Diabetic Retinopathy Study Research Group. Ophthalmology 1991;98:786–806.

[13] Wilkinson CP, Ferris FL, Klein RE, et al. Proposed international clinical diabetic retinopathy and diabetic macular edema disease severity scales. Ophthalmology 2003;110: 1677–82.
[14] Bernardes R, Serranho P, Lobo C. Digital ocular fundus imaging: a review. Ophthalmologica 2011;226:161–81.
[15] Kassam F, Yogesan K, Sogbesan E, et al. Teleglaucoma: improving access and efficient for glaucoma care. Middle East Afr J Ophthalmol 2013;20:142–9.
[16] Sharafeldin N, Kawaguchi A, Sundaram A, et al. Review of economic evaluations of teleophthalmology as a screening strategy for chronic eye disease in adults. Br J Ophthalmol 2018;102:1485–91.
[17] Shi L, Wu H, Dong J, et al. Telemedicine for detecting diabetic retinopathy: a systematic review and meta-analysis. Br J Ophthalmol 2015;99:823–31.
[18] Chew E, Schachat A. Should we add screening of age-related macular degeneration to current screening programs for diabetic retinopathy? Ophthalmology 2015;122:2155–6.
[19] Kawaguchi A, Sharafeldin N, Sundaram A, et al. Tele-ophthalmology for age-related macular degeneration and diabetic retinopathy screening: a systematic review and meta-analysis. Telemed J E Health 2018;24:301–8.
[20] Chan C, Gangwani R, McGhee S, et al. Cost-effectiveness of screening for intermediate age-related macular degeneration during diabetic retinopathy screening. Ophthalmology 2015;122:2278–85.
[21] Rosenblatt RA, Hart LG. Physicians and rural America, West. J Med 2000;173:348–51.
[22] Fleming P, Sinnot M-L. Rural physician supply and retention: factors in the Canadian context. Can J Rural Med 2018;23:15–20.
[23] Rathi S, Tsui E, Mehta N, et al. The current state of teleophthalmology in the United States. Ophthalmology 2017;124:1729–34.
[24] Wikipedia. List of countries by Internet connection speeds, (n.d.). Available at: https://en.wikipedia.org/wiki/List_of_countries_by_Internet_connection_speeds. Accessed May 23, 2019.
[25] Scanlon PH. The English National Screening Programme for diabetic retinopathy 2003–2016. Acta Diabetol 2017;54:515–25.
[26] Tan IJ, Dobson LP, Bartnik S, et al. Real-time teleophthalmology versus face-to-face consultation: a systematic review. J Telemed Telecare 2017;23:629–38.
[27] Qureshi A, Shih E, Fan I, et al. Improving patient care by unshackling telemedicine: adaptively aggregating wireless networks to facilitate continuous collaboration. AMIA Annu Symp Proc 2010;2010:662–6.
[28] Korot E, Wood E, Weiner A, et al. A renaissance of teleophthalmology through artificial intelligence. Eye 2019;3–5; https://doi.org/10.1038/s41433-018-0324-8.
[29] Lamirel C, Bruce B, Wright D, et al. Non-mydriatic digital ocular fundus photography on the iPhone 3G: the FOTO-ED study. Arch Ophthalmol 2012;130:939–40.
[30] M. Empower MD. Transcription. No Title. (n.d.).
[31] I. Welch Allyn. Welch Allyn iExaminer Pro, (n.d.).
[32] Cloud Nine Development LLC. Eye Handbook, (n.d.). Available at: https://itunes.apple.com/ca/app/eye-handbook/id335546959?mt=8. Accessed May 23, 2019.
[33] Konan Medical USA. Amsler Grid App. Available at: https://itunes.apple.com/ca/app/amsler-grids/id982604083?mt=8. Accessed May 23, 2019.
[34] Eyecare, eyecare-Amsler Grid Eye Test, (n.d.). Available at: https://www.amslerapp.com/. Accessed May 23, 2019.
[35] Cassiopeia Information Techonlogies. PseudoChromatic ColorTest App. Available at: https://itunes.apple.com/ca/app/pseudochromatic-colortest/id375608394?mt=8. Accessed May 23, 2019.
[36] Johnson LN, Baloh FG. The accuracy of confrontation visual field test in comparison with automated perimetry. J Natl Med Assoc 1991;83(10):895–8, Key words * confrontation testing * automated perimetry * visual field defects.

[37] Murray NP, Hunfalvay M, Bolte T. The reliability, validity, and normative data of interpupillary distance and pupil diameter using eye-tracking technology. Transl Vis Sci Technol 2017;6:2.

[38] Taneja M, Gonzalez A, Rowaan C, et al. Comparative functional evaluation of a stereoscopic robotized teleophthalmic drone slit lamp with conventional slit lamp, ARVO Annual Meet. Orlando, Florida, May 4–8, 2014. 55. [Abstract].

[39] Nowak W, Zarowska A, Szul-Pietrzak E, et al. System and measurement method for binocular pupillometry to study pupil size variability. Biomed Eng Online 2014;13:69.

[40] Cayless A, Bende T. First results of automated RAPD-SWIFT method in dynamic pupillometry. Z Med Phys 2016;26:143–9.

[41] Shaw J. Teleophthalmology: ready for prime time? EyeNet Mag 2016;41–5. Available at: https://www.aao.org/eyenet/article/teleophthalmology-ready-prime-time. Accessed May 23, 2019.

[42] Valikodath NG, Leveque TK, Wang SY, et al. Patient attitudes toward telemedicine for diabetic retinopathy. Telemed J E Health 2017;23:205–12.

[43] Hu PJ, Chau PY, Sheng ORL, et al. Examining the technology acceptance model using physician acceptance of telemedicine technology. J Manag Inf Syst 1999;16:91–112.

[44] May C, Harrison R, Finch T, et al. Understanding the normalization of telemedicine services through qualitative evaluation. J Am Med Inform Assoc 2003;10:596–604.

[45] Rogers EM. Diffusions of Innovations. 5th Edition. New York: The Free Press A division of Macmillan Publishing Co., Inc; 2003.

[46] Cook EJ, Randhawa G, Sharp C, et al. Exploring the factors that influence the decision to adopt and engage with an integrated assistive telehealth and telecare service in Cambridgeshire, UK: a nested qualitative study of patient "users" and "non-users. BMC Health Serv Res 2016;16; https://doi.org/10.1186/s12913-016-1379-5.

[47] Volk iNview, (n.d.). Available at: https://volk.com/index.php/volk-products/ophthalmic-cameras/volk-inview.html. Accessed May 23, 2019.

[48] D-EYE Posterior, (n.d.). Available at: https://www.d-eyecare.com/#vision. Accessed May 23, 2019.

[49] Peek Retina, (n.d.). Available at: https://www.peekvision.org/en_GB/peek-solutions/peek-retina/buy-peek-retina/. Accessed May 23, 2019.

[50] iExaminer, (n.d.). Available at: https://www.welchallyn.com/en/microsites/iexaminer.html. Accessed May 23, 2019.

[51] oDocs VisoScope, (n.d.). Available at: http://www.odocs-tech.com/visoscope/#. Accessed May 23, 2019.

[52] Dzwiniel P, Gola M, Wójcik-Gryciuk A, et al. Specvis: free and open-source software for visual field examination. PLOS ONE 2017;12(10):e0186224.

[53] L. See Vision, 9 Gaze, (n.d.). Available at: https://itunes.apple.com/us/app/9-gaze/id1173442389?mt=8. Accessed May 23, 2019.

[54] L. See Vision, eyeTilt, (n.d.). Available at: https://itunes.apple.com/us/app/eyetilt/id1262715223. Accessed May 23, 2019.

Section VIII: Cornea and External Diseases

Advances in Ophthalmology and Optometry 4 (2019) 275–282

ADVANCES IN OPHTHALMOLOGY AND OPTOMETRY

Neurotrophic Keratopathy

A Review of New and Emerging Therapies

Krishi Peddada, MD, Brett Campbell, MD, Briana Ply, MD, An Vo, MD*

Department of Ophthalmology, Drexel University, Drexel University College of Medicine, 219 North Broad Street, 3rd Floor, Philadelphia, PA 19107, USA

Keywords

- Neurotrophic keratopathy • Nicergoline • Corneal neurotization
- Regenerating agents (RGTAs) • Substance P • Insulinlike growth factor 1 (IGF-1)
- Nerve growth factor • Thymosin beta-4

Key points

- Neurotophic keratopathy (NK) is a degenerative disease of the corneal epithelium that occurs as a result of impairment of trigeminal innervation, leading to a decrease or loss of corneal sensitivity.
- Early diagnosis is essential and treatment largely depends on disease stage and severity.
- The management of NK continues to be a challenge, due to the lack of treatments targeting nerve regeneration.
- Experimental and clinical evidence show that several novel treatments, such as growth factors and corneal neurotization, may improve the clinical management and outcomes of this disease.

INTRODUCTION

Neurotrophic keratopathy (NK) was first described in 1824, with the observation that transection of the trigeminal nerve leads to degenerative changes in the cornea [1]. These corneal changes are secondary to altered cellular metabolism, which leads to accumulation of metabolites and subsequent tissue swelling, loss of vitality, and desquamation [2]. Reduction in corneal sensitivity or complete corneal anesthesia is the hallmark of NK and can lead to epithelial keratopathy, ulceration, and perforation [3]. Causes of NK include a wide

The authors declare that there is no conflict of interest regarding the publication of this article.

*Corresponding author. *E-mail address:* an.vo@mooreeye.com

https://doi.org/10.1016/j.yaoo.2019.05.003
2452-1760/19/

variety of ocular and systemic conditions that damage trigeminal innervation. Some etiologies include herpetic keratitis, diabetes, chemical damage, multiple sclerosis, and neurosurgical procedures [3,4]. NK can be difficult and challenging to manage due to the lack of treatments that target nerve regeneration. Recently, novel medical and surgical treatments have been developed and are currently being investigated. These primarily include topical administration of nerve growth factor (NGF) and surgical corneal neurotization. The prognosis depends on a wide range of factors, including the etiology behind corneal sensitivity impairment, the severity of trigeminal damage, and the presence of concomitant ocular surface diseases.

EPIDEMIOLOGY

Many ocular and systemic diseases can damage the fifth corneal nerve anywhere from the trigeminal nucleus to peripheral corneal nerve endings. The most common cause of NK is herpetic viral keratitis and the second most common is trigeminal nerve damage from either intracranial neoplasia or neurosurgical procedures [4]. Traumatic causes include ocular thermal burns, ocular chemical burns, and contact lens misuse. In addition, systemic conditions such as diabetes, multiple sclerosis, and leprosy can damage the corneal nerves and cause NK. Other causes include medications such as antipsychotics and antihistamines [5]. The incidence and prevalence of NK is not definitively known, but it is estimated at less than 1.6 per 10,000 patients. NK has a prevalence of 1.22 per 10,000 in herpes simplex keratitis and 0.02 per 10,000 in postsurgical trigeminal neuralgia patients [6].

PATHOPHYSIOLOGY

The pathophysiology of NK is complex. Novel animal models, which replicate the pathophysiology of NK by transection of the trigeminal nerve or by trigeminal nerve stereotactic electrolysis, provide a greater understanding of this disease [7]. In NK, the number of mitoses is diminished, leading to impaired epithelial healing that results in recurrent erosions and ulcerations [8]. Loss of corneal sensitivity can lead to intracellular swelling of epithelial cells, loss of microvilli, and abnormal production of basal lamina [8]. Delayed rate of healing, fewer desmosomes, and excessive exfoliation of epithelial cells result in epithelial defects [9].

Careful observations of patients have led to an understanding of the sequence of changes that are set into motion when innervation to the cornea is cut [10]. First, the lack of trophic neuromediators leads to the slowing of epithelial mitosis and maturation at the limbus. This leads to epithelial irregularity because older, pre-exfoliating cells in the center of the cornea cannot withstand the shear forces of every eyelid blink. Because of the epithelial irregularities, the mucin distribution over the tear film and the composition of the tear film are significantly altered. This leads to chronic epithelial instability with loss of effective tight junctions and zona occludens. In addition, there is usually a reduced ability of limbal stem cells to migrate to the central cornea.

This creates a central epithelial defect made up of rolled borders of cells unable to adhere to the basement membrane. The local cytokine activity, surface damage, and epithelial damage make the underlying stroma susceptible to activity by matrix metalloproteases. Activity of matrix metalloproteases can result in stromal melts as well as perforation if left unchecked [10].

STAGING

The most common staging system for NK is based on Mackie [11]. Stage 1 is characterized by corneal epithelial hyperplasia, stromal scarring, dellen formation, superficial punctate keratopathy, and decreased tear break-up time. Stage 2 is characterized by a persistent epithelial defect of the cornea with Descemet folds and stromal swelling. Stage 3 is characterized by corneal ulcer and corneal perforation. Treatment of NK is guided by the stage. For stage 1, treatment aims to optimize the ocular surface with usage of preservative-free artificial tears, punctual plugs, cyclosporine 0.05% solution, and autologous serum tears. For stage 2, treatment involves therapeutic contact lenses, surgical tarsorrhaphy, and amniotic membrane transplantation. For stage 3, treatment involves tarsorrhaphy, conjunctival flap, lamellar keratoplasty, or penetrating keratoplasty [6].

EXAMINATION

In addition to external examination, slit-lamp examination, and staining with vital dyes, a few other diagnostic modalities can be specifically helpful in patients with NK [10]. One is the quantification of corneal sensation, which is measured in several areas of the corneal surface with either the Cochet-Bonnet aesthesiometer or the Belmonte noncontact gas aesthesiometer. The Cochet-Bonnet aesthesiometer has a nylon filament can be extended from 5 mm to 60 mm to vary the force on the corneal surface from 200 g/mm to 11 g/mm. The longer the filament is extended, the less force that is applied, and the greater the corneal sensitivity is [12]. The Belmonte noncontact gas aesthesiometer stimulates the cornea with a calibrated gas emission kept close to the cornea. Mechanical, chemical, and thermal sensitivities of the cornea are measured by altering the flow, temperature, and composition of the gas [13].

Imaging modalities can be helpful as well. Image analysis programs of in vivo confocal microscopy can help determine nerve density, tortuosity, angulation, thickness, and reflectivity [14]. The subbasal corneal nerves can be altered significantly in corneas presenting with severe NK [15]. The sensitivity of in vivo confocal microscopy to detect changes can be profound. In diabetics, the corneal sensitivity is associated with decreased subbasal nerve and basal epithelium density [16]. In herpes simplex virus, a relationship exists between corneal sensitivity and changes in subbasal plexus and endothelial morphology [17,18]. Anterior segment optical coherence tomography provides a unique perspective on the ocular surface and morphology. This modality can measure tear meniscus and epithelial thickness for Stage 1 NK. In advanced stages of NK, anterior segment optical coherence tomography can measure the depth of stromal ulcerations and stromal thickness changes [20].

NEW THERAPIES

Several new therapies are being developed and used for NK. The active ingredients in topical therapies for NK have their basis in neuromodulators, extracellular matrix proteins, and tissue repair proteins involved in cell growth. They assist in developing and promoting the cellular signaling pathways that allow nerve regeneration to take place. A new oral therapy uses nicergoline, an agent that increases blood flow to the brain in cognitive disorders. Surgical techniques include transposition of the supraorbital, supratrochlear, infratrochlear, and sural nerves to the cornea to provide new innervation (Box 1).

Topical therapies

Extracellular matrix proteins are the basis of one of the topical therapies. Regenerating agents (RGTAs) are chemically engineered polymers that are designed to replace heparan sulfate and currently are in a phase III clinical trial [5]. RGTAs work by inducing cell migration and adhesion via a microenvironment that ultimately promotes healing of the epithelium. One recent study showed promising results with RGTA topical treatment, yielding complete corneal ulcer healing in 73% of 11 patients with NK [21]. A more recent prospective case series of 6 patients, however, resulted in failure of corneal healing in 67% of patients [22].

Another approach to corneal epithelial healing utilizes neuromodulators. The combination of substance P (SP), a neuropeptide that stimulates angiogenesis and fibroblast proliferation, and insulinlike growth factor 1 (IGF-1), an anabolic hormone, is being studied. A study in the 1990s involving corneal

Box 1: New treatments for neurotophic keratopathy

- Topical therapy with RGTAs, chemically engineered polymers that are designed to replace herapan sulfate, helps induce cell migration and adhesion by rebuilding cellular connections to the extracellular matrix
- Topical neuromodulators, including SP and IGF-1, promote epithelial migration to the cornea
- Topical therapy with thymosin beta-4, an intracellular protein that helps regulate actin polymerization, assists in suppression of apoptosis and inflammation, synaptogenesis, and axon growth
- Topical therapy with NGF, a neurotrophin that promotes the growth and survival of neurons in addition to the restoration of injured neurons
- Oral therapy with nicergoline, a drug that increases blood flow to the brain, has been efficacious in NK through increasing concentration of NGF.
- Surgical techniques, known as corneal neurotization, that involve direct transposition of the supraorbital and supratrochlear nerves, indirect transposition of sural nerve grafts, or use of the infraorbital nerve

epithelial growth of the rabbit cornea found the combination of the 2 agents induced epithelial migration of the cornea [23]. Several newer studies have tested the effect of this combination as a topical therapy. The clinical efficacy of an substance P-derived peptide and phenylalanine -glycine-leucine-methionine (FGLM)-amide, with IGF-1 as treatment was examined in 11 patients with persistent epithelial defects with NK for 28 days [24]; 89% of patients who received full therapy (8 of 9) had complete epithelial resurfacing, and no adverse effects were observed [24]. Another similar study yielded similar results; 73% of patients had complete epithelial resurfacing without any adverse side effects [25].

A third therapy being studied for NK is thymosin beta-4, an intracellular protein, which plays a role in regulation of actin polymerization. Thymosin beta-4 is involved with multiple wound healing processes, including suppression of apoptosis and inflammation, synaptogenesis, and axon growth [26]. An open study involving 9 patients with NK demonstrated some efficacy of thymosin beta-4 as 6 (66.67%) patients had a reported complete healing of corneal ulcers [5,26]. There currently is an ongoing randomized control trial for the topical treatment of thymosin beta-4 in NK patients.

One of the most promising topical therapies to date for NK is NGF, a neurotrophin that promotes the growth, survival, and restoration of neurons [27]. It initially was studied as a potential treatment of peripheral neuropathy. NGF's role in ocular surface disease has become a more recent focus as it has been tested in both animal models and patients affected by neurotrophic ulcers [28–31]. The first open-label studies tested murine-derived NGF in patients with moderate (stage 2) and severe (stage 3) NK. All patients experienced corneal healing, improved corneal sensitivity, improved tear production, and improved visual acuity without any marked adverse effects [5,30,31]. A subsequent recombinant human NGF eye drop displayed a good safety profile in phase I trials [28]. More recently, two independent, double-masked, randomized, multicentered clinical control trials displayed the efficacy of the recombinant human NGF treatment known as cenegermin [32,33]. In the European study, 72.0% of patients in the treatment arm had complete healing of the cornea versus 33% of those in the control arm. The United States study saw similar results, with 65% of the treatment arm versus 16.7% of the control arm achieving complete healing. Cenegermin was approved by the European Union for moderate to severe NK in July of 2017, and was recently approved by the Food and Drug Administration in the United States on August 22, 2018.

Oral therapy

Currently, oral therapy using nicergoline is being pursued for NK. Nicergoline increases blood flow to the brain and it is currently used in the treatment of cognitive, affective, and behavioral disorders [34]. Animal studies have shown that nicergoline promotes corneal healing by increasing NGF in the cornea. One prospective, noncomparative interventional study has showed promising results in patients with NK unresponsive to conventional therapy. The study included 24 patients who took oral nicergoline for 2 weeks and found that 23 of 24 corneal epithelial defects healed completely between 7 days and 30 days of treatment [35]. In addition, significant improvement also occurred in mean corneal sensitivity, best corrected visual acuity, and tear nerve growth [35], signifying the potential use of this medication as an alternative treatment of NK.

Surgical techniques

New surgical procedures, known collectively as corneal neurotization, involve rerouting healthy nerves to innervate the cornea [5]. Direct corneal neurotization involves transposition of a nearby supraorbital or supratrochlear nerve [5,17,18], whereas indirect corneal neurotization involves anastomosis of a nerve graft to one of the nearby nerves [19]. Animal studies have demonstrated the efficacy of corneal neurotization by showing that there is increased sensitivity and wound healing of the cornea after the procedure [36].

The direct technique has been accomplished in human patients by using the contralateral supraorbital and the supratrochlear nerves, which are obtained using a large corneal incision and then inserted on the limbus of the affected cornea via a tunnel across the nose bridge. One study demonstrated that a total of six patients with unilateral facial nerve palsy and corneal anesthesia were noted to have improved corneal sensation, improved vision, and no future ulcers after this procedure was done [37]. Another individual case in which a patient with combined cranial nerves V and VII palsies underwent the same procedure had notable improvement in corneal health and visual acuity [38].

Similar positive results have been seen with use of the indirect neurotization, in which the sural nerve graft is anastomosed to the supratrochlear nerve and tunneled through the upper eyelid to the cornea. In indirect corneal neurotization, much smaller incisions of the cornea are required [5]. A 2014 study involving 4 eyes that had undergone treatment using this technique saw marked corneal sensation improvement in 3 of the eyes at 6 months [39]. A more recent study of patients who underwent indirect sural nerve graft neurotization for severe NK demonstrated that 83% of patients had improved VA and 50% had no need for further surgical intervention [40]. With low reported complication rates, as well as notable benefits, these surgical procedures may be the future mainstays of treatment.

SUMMARY

NK is a degenerative disease of the corneal epithelium that occurs as a result of impairment of trigeminal innervation, leading to a decrease or loss of corneal sensitivity. Early diagnosis is essential and treatment largely depends on disease stage and severity. The management of NK continues to be a challenge, due to the lack of treatments targeting nerve regeneration. Experimental and clinical evidence shows that several novel treatments, such as growth factors and corneal neurotization, may improve the clinical management and outcomes of this disease.

References

[1] Magendie J. De la influence de la cinquime paire nerfts sur la nutrition et les functions de 1664 l'oeil. J Physiol 1824;4:176–82.
[2] Klein M. Contact lens in cases of neuroparalytic keratitis. Br J Ophthalmol 1943;27:221–2.
[3] Wells JR, Michelson MA. Diagnosing and treating neutrophic keratopathy. EyeNet 1910 Magazine 2008 American Academy of Ophthalmology.
[4] Sacchetti M, Lambiase A. Neurotrophic factors and corneal nerve regeneration. Neural Regen Res 2017;12(8):1220–4.
[5] Versura P, Giannaccare G, Pellegrini M, et al. Neutrophic keratopathy: current challenges and future prospects. Eye Brain 2018;10:37–45.
[6] Sacchetti M, Lambiase A. Diagnosis and management of neutrophic keratopathy. Clin Ophthalmol 2014;8:571–9.
[7] Ferrari G, Chauhan SK, Ueno H, et al. A novel mouse model for neutrophic keratopathy: trigeminal nerve stereotactic electrolysis through the brain. Invest Ophthalmol Vis Sci 2011;52(5):2532–9.
[8] Bonini S, Rama P, Olzi D, et al. Neurotrophic keratitis. Eye (Lond) 2003;17(8):989–95.
[9] Araki K, Ohashi Y, Kinoshita S, et al. Epithelial wound healing in the denervated cornea. Curr Eye Res 1994;13:203–11.
[10] Dua HS, Said DG, Messmer EM, et al. Neuroparalytic keratitis. Prog Retin Eye Res 2018;66:107–31.
[11] Mackie IA. Neuroparalytic keratitis. In: Fraunfelder F, Roy FH, Meyer SM, editors. Current ocular therapy. Philadelphia: WB Saunders; 1995. p. 452–4.
[12] Chao C, Stapleton F, Badarudin E, et al. Ocular surface sensitivity repeatability with Cochet-Bonnet esthesiometer. Optom Vis Sci 2015;92(2):183–9.
[13] Tesón M, Calonge M, Fernández I, et al. Characterization by Belmonte's gas esthesiometer of mechanical, chemical, and thermal corneal sensitivity thresholds in a normal population. Invest Ophthalmol Vis Sci 2012;53(6):3154–60.
[14] Lambiase A, Sacchetti M, Mastropasqua A, et al. Corneal changes in neurosurgically induced neutrophic keratopathy. JAMA Ophthalmol 2013;131(12):1547–53.
[15] Mastropasqua L, Nubile M, Lanzini M, et al. In vivo microscopic and optical coherence tomography classification of neutrophic keratopathy. J Cell Physiol 2019;234(5):6108–15.
[16] Rosenberg ME, Tervo TM, Immonen IJ, et al. Corneal structure and sensitivity in type 1 diabetes mellitus. Invest Ophthalmol Vis Sci 2000;41(10):2915–21.
[17] Hamrah P, Cruzat A, Dastjerdi MH, et al. Corneal sensation and subbasal nerve alterations in patients with herpes simplex keratitis: an in vivo confocal microscopy study. Ophthalmology 2010;117(10):1930–6.
[18] Hillenaar T, Weenen C, Wubbels RJ, et al. Endothelial involvement in herpes simplex virus keratitis: an in vivo confocal microscopy study. Ophthalmology 2009;116(11):2077–8, e1-2.
[19] Sridhar MS, Martin R. Anterior segment optical coherence tomography for evaluation of cornea and ocular surface. Indian J Ophthalmol 2018;66(3):367–72.
[20] Sharma N, Singhal D, Maharana PK, et al. Spectral Domain Anterior Segment Optical Coherence Tomography in Fungal Keratitis. Cornea 2018;37(11):1388–94.
[21] Aifa A, Gueudry J, Portmann A, et al. Topical treatment with a new matrix therapy agent (RGTA) for the treatment of corneal neurotrophic ulcers. Invest Ophthalmol Vis Sci 2012;53(13):8181–5.
[22] Arvola RP, Robciuc A, Holopainen JM. Matrix regeneration therapy: a case series of corneal neurotrophic ulcers. Cornea 2016;35(4):451–5.
[23] Nishida T, Nakamura M, Ofuji K, et al. Synergistic effects of substance P with insulin-like growth factor-1 on epithelial migration of the cornea. J Cell Physiol 1996;169(1):159–66.
[24] Nishida T, Chikama T, Morishige N, et al. Persistent epithelial defects due to NK treated with a substance p-derived peptide and insulin-like growth factor 1. Jpn J Ophthalmol 2007;51(6):442–7.

[25] Yamada N, Matsuda R, Morishige N, et al. Open clinical study of eye-drops containing tetrapeptides derived from substance P and insulin-like growth factor-1 for treatment of persistent corneal epithelial defects associated with neutrophic keratopathy. Br J Ophthalmol 2008;92(7):896–900.
[26] Dunn SP, Heidemann DG, Chow CY, et al. Treatment of chronic nonhealing neurotrophic corneal epithelial defects with thymosin beta4. Ann N Y Acad Sci 2010;1194:199–206.
[27] Levi-Montalcini R. The nerve growth factor 35 years later. Science 1987;237(4819): 1154–62.
[28] Ferrari MP, Mantelli F, Sacchetti M, et al. Safety and pharmacokinetics of escalating doses of human recombinant nerve growth factor eye drops in a double-masked, randomized clinical trial. BioDrugs 2014;28(3):275–83.
[29] Lambiase A, Mantelli F, Sacchetti M, et al. Clinical applications of NGF in ocular diseases. Arch Ital Biol 2011;149:283–92.
[30] Bonini S, Aloe L, Bonini S, et al. Nerve growth factor (NGF): an important molecule for trophism and healing of the ocular surface. Adv Exp Med Biol 2002;506:531–7.
[31] Lambiase A, Rama P, Bonini S, et al. Topical treatment with nerve growth factor for neurotrophic corneal ulcers. N Engl J Med 1998;338:1174–80.
[32] Bonini S, Lambiase A, Rama P, et al, for the REPARO Study Group. Phase II randomized, double-masked, vehicle-controlled trial of recombinant human nerve growth factor for neutrophic keratopathy. Ophthalmology 2018;125:1332–43.
[33] Chao W, Benitez Del Castillo JM, Dana R, et al. Healing of persistent epithelial defects or corneal ulcer by recombinant human nerve growth factor eye drops in patients with Stage 2 or 3 neutrophic keratopathy. Presented at the Congress of the European Society of Ophthalmology (SOE). Barcelona, Spain, June, 10–13, 2017.
[34] Fioravanti M, Flicker L. Efficacy of nicergoline in dementia and other age associated forms of cognitive impairment. Cochrane Database Syst Rev 2001;(94):CD003159.
[35] Lee YC, Kim SY. Treatment of neutrophic keratopathy with nicergoline. Cornea 2015;34(3): 303–7.
[36] Catapano J, Antonyshyn K, Zhang JJ, et al. Corneal Neurotization improves ocular surface health in a novel rat model of neutrophic keratopathy and corneal neurotization. Invest Ophthalmol Vis Sci 2018;59(11):4345–54.
[37] Terzis JK, Dryer MM, Bodner BI. Corneal neurotization: a novel solution to neutrophic keratopathy. Plast Reconstr Surg 2009;123(1):112–20.
[38] Allevi F, Fogagnolo P, Rossetti L, et al. Eyelid reanimation, neurotisation, and transplantation of the cornea in a patient with facial palsy. BMJ Case Rep 2014;2014 [pii: bcr2014205372].
[39] Elbaz U, Bains R, Zuker RM, et al. Restoration of corneal sensation with regional nerve transfers and nerve grafts: a new approach to a difficult problem. JAMA Ophthalmol 2014;132(11):1289–95.
[40] Ezekiel W, Avi R, Ahmed RAG, et al. Sural nerve graft for neutrophic keratopathy: early results. Can J Ophthalmol 2018;53(1):24–9.

Section IX: Oculoplastics

Advances in Ophthalmology and Optometry 4 (2019) 283–304

ADVANCES IN OPHTHALMOLOGY AND OPTOMETRY

Acellular Dermal Matrix in Eyelid and Socket Reconstruction

Ran Stein, MD[a,*], Sara Núñez Márquez, MD[b,c], Evan Kalin-Hajdu, MD[d], Yasser Khan, MD[b,c]

[a]Ophthalmic Plastic Surgery, Shamir (Assaf-Harofeh) Medical Center, affiliated to Tel-Aviv University, Tel-Aviv, Israel; [b]Orbital and Ophthalmic Surgery, McMaster University, Hamilton, Ontario, Canada; [c]Carrot Eye Clinic, 284 Queen Street East, Brampton, Ontario L6V 1C2, Canada; [d]Centre Universitaire d'Ophtalmologie, Hôpital Maisonneuve-Rosemont, 5415 boul. de l'Assomption Montréal, Montréal, Québec H1T 2M4, Canada

Keywords

• Acellular dermal matrix • Eyelid reconstruction • Socket reconstruction

Key points

- Acellular dermal matrices (ADMs) comprise alternative graft materials for eyelid and socket reconstruction while providing advantages, such as abundancy, ease of use, reduced surgical time, and absence of secondary donor site complications.
- Various ADMs have been implemented in diverse oculoplastics procedures with varying levels of success.
- Outcomes are affected by contraction, compatibility of material to procedure, and surgical technique but in some instances deliver excellent results with minimal rate of complications.

INTRODUCTION

Periocular and socket reconstruction may require the use of adjunctive materials and substances to restore the integrity and the functionality of the original structure. These materials can be either autologous (hard palate graft, ear cartilage grafts, nasal septum, buccal mucosa, temporalis fascia, fascia lata, periosteum, dermis, or dermis fat) or homologous (bank sclera or amniotic membrane). Alternatively, synthetic materials, such as polytetrafluoroethylene

Disclosure Statement: The authors have nothing to disclose.

*Corresponding author. *E-mail address:* steinran@gmail.com

https://doi.org/10.1016/j.yaoo.2019.04.011

(Gore-Tex) and porous polyethylene (Medpor), can be used. In the past 20 years, the use of acellular dermal matrices (ADMs) has been studied and clinically implemented in diverse reconstructive procedures with variable levels of success.

ADM usually comprises tissue harvested from human cadavers or from animals that is then processed to exclude cells and cellular components to create an inert, antigen-free substance. Unlike autologous grafts, which usually are limited in size and shape, the use of ADMs provides unlimited amounts and easy-to-handle graft material. It also obviates a secondary surgical site and its related complications and patient discomfort. It spares surgical time by avoiding the harvesting of the autologous graft, and by the quick and easy handling of the ADM grafts.

This article reviews the application of the more common ADM products used in various oculoplastics procedures.

THE MOTIVES FOR EMERGING OF TISSUE SUBSTITUTES

The introduction of ADMs into Oculoplastics occurred due to absence of a perfect graft or implant for use either in primary or reconstructive oculoplastics procedures. This is reflected by the numerous materials that have been commonly implemented, without a consensus substance for many procedures [1].

The ideal graft is expected to be accessible and affordable and to require short preparation time. It should be easy to handle, shape to fit, and place securely within the tissue. After implantation, the implant should provoke minimal inflammation, exhibit minimal change in size and shape, and allow for native tissue ingrowth to become indistinguishable [2,3]. The graft should be malleable to fit for a desired contour and rigid enough to provide tensile strength, with a surface that is appropriate to interface with adjacent tissue.

In cases of posterior lamella augmentation, for example, the implant should resemble tarsal conjunctiva to provide both structural support and a smooth interface with the ocular surface [2]. The best solutions are a tarsoconjunctival flap and free graft; however, these are limited in both horizontal and vertical dimensions and may cause healthy tissue morbidity [4]. Complication rates have been reported as high as 10% and include wound dehiscence, upper lid retraction, and cicatricial ectropion [5]. If used in conjunction with eyelid-sharing techniques, such as a Hughes flap, the integration phase usually requires occluding the eye completely. Therefore, it is not suitable is cases of a single functioning eye or during the amblyogenic period.

Commonly used graft materials for posterior lamella include auricular cartilage and hard palate mucosal grafts [4]. Hard palate for eyelid reconstruction is often considered the gold standard for posterior lamella replacement [6]. It is a composite material, with thickness and texture similar to tarsus [7] and composed of a firm stromal tissue covered by a layer of mucous membrane, which facilitates conjunctival coverage. Palatal grafts deliver excellent eyelid appearance and function due to relative flexibility, with reliable and stable outcome owing to minimal shrinkage [2]. Disadvantages, however, include relative coarse harvesting, bleeding, donor site morbidity, fistula formation, candidiasis, pain and patient discomfort, and possible persistent keratinization of the graft surface–thus, the search for alternatives [6,8].

Ear cartilage graft is easy to obtain and provides excellent structural support; however, its rigidity is occasionally associated with inadequate fitting with the eyelid contour as well as reduced motility of the lower eyelid [9,10]. The graft may cause corneal irritation due to the absent of epithelial surface, until the conjunctival migration over the graft is complete [8].

Other autologous materials have been used either as a spacer or a scaffold. Temporalis fascia was used as a spacer with some favorable results; however, paralysis of the temporal branch of the fascial nerve is a risk during harvesting [4]. Nasal cartilage no longer is commonly used due to difficulty in graft handing to match eyelid contour and donor site complications, including septal perforation [4]. Dermis-fat grafts have been used as a spacer in a variety of procedures for eyelid and orbit reconstruction; however, they may be associated with unpredictable volume loss, central necrosis, infection, and hair growth [4]. Buccal mucosa is composed of nonkeratinized stratified squamous epithelium and of elastic fibers; it is easy to obtain, but is too soft to provide structural support [5].

In addition, in all cases in which autologous material is required, obtaining and processing the tissue prolong surgical time. Even without subsequent complications, handling a secondary surgery site is a burden on both surgeon and patient.

To address the obstacles related to autologous grafts, some homologous materials have been introduced. Banked sclera was shown to deliver good outcome as a spacer; however its structural support is less than that of hard palate graft, and shrinkage and absorption are significant [8,10]. Amniotic membrane graft is a valid alternative as a barrier or for coverage, but it dissolves quickly and is incapable of providing any structural support. Furthermore, in either case of homologous grafting, there is a risk for disease transmission [4].

Synthetic materials, such as Medpor and Gore-Tex, have been used as alternatives for human-derived grafts. They are abundant, inert, sterile, stable, and easy to handle; nevertheless, extrusion and unfavorable outcomes have limited their practice [11,12].

Into this gap between the desired graft material and the ones available in the authors' practice, ADM products have emerged as a viable alternative that is accessible and easy to handle. Most of all, they are effective and safe.

CHARACTERISTICS OF ACELLULAR DERMAL MATRIX

ADMs were first used clinically for the treatment of full-thickness burns in 1992 [3]. Since then they have been widely implemented in various oculoplastics settings. Their aforementioned benefits have been challenged throughout the years with complaints of contraction and resorption, leading to unpredictable results, and with the potential risk of inflammatory or allergic reactions and disease transmission [6]. Additionally, the price of these products, occasionally exceeding hundreds of dollars per item, comprise a substantial drawback.

ADMs differ from one another in their tissue source, processing, arrangement and content of the final product, and level of prehydration. Biophysical characteristics vary as well and may affect the suitability for specific indications. Most of the products have been designed for use in plastic surgery, such as burn injuries and full-thickness wounds. Some subsequent products aimed to comply with the specific characteristics and needs of the periocular tissue. The main types of ADM products are listed in Table 1.

ADMs are produced from either human or animal tissue that is treated to leave an acellular substance composed mainly of collagen and elastin proteins. Processing differs between products, is largely franchised and undisclosed [13], and includes enzymatic digestion, hypertonic solutions or detergents washing, cross-linking, and/or irradiation. Animal models of ADMs exhibited incorporation of the graft into the native tissue with variably minimal inflammation, followed by encapsulation, inflammatory cell infiltration, and eventually fibrovascular ingrowth, providing durable soft tissue replacement [13]. Clinically, this process is characterized by inflammation and initial resorption followed by stabilizing of size and shape. Processing methods affect the inflammatory response and graft incorporation and eventually influence its endurance, rigidity and support [13,14].

Microscopic analysis of the products reveals architecture that is variably similar to the original tissue. AlloDerm (LifeCell Corporation, Woodlands, Texas / Branchburg, NJ, USA), for example, comprises normally oriented collagen bundles with discrete elastin fibers. The basement membrane is intact but the epidermis is absent, and no internal cellular structures remain [15]. The matrix is repopulated by host cells and human keratocytes, and the basement membrane provides a natural substrate for epithelial migration; histology shows fibroblast infiltration, neovascularization, and neoepithelialization without rejection [16].

The infectious potential of ADMs should not be overlooked. The products are either aseptic or sterile; however, intact bacterial DNA was found in both and theoretically could comprise a risk for disease transmission [17]. Various ADM materials have been used, however, in hundreds of thousands of procedures across several disciplines, without any evidence of direct transmission of any infectious factors. ADM material is screened and processed carefully to eliminate this risk of bacterial or viral infection, including hepatitis and HIV. All cells and cellular components are eliminated, reducing capability of inflammatory stimulation. The theoretic risk of prion transmission still exists, due to difficulties in prion screening and decontamination. No cases of prion transmission through an acellular dermal product, however, has been reported [2].

As for the financial aspect of these materials, this is still a matter of debate; however, some investigators postulate that reduced operating time, easy

Table 1
Main types of acellular dermal matrix products used in oculoplastics

Product Name	Source	Sterility	Structure and Content	Product Properties	Hydration
AlloDerm Regenerative Tissue Matrix* LifeCell Corporation, Woodlands, TX/Branchburg, NJ, USA	Human cadavers	Aseptic	Dermis like + basement membrane	Thin (0.33–0.76 mm) or thick (0.78–2.2 mm) 1 cm × 2 cm, 1 cm × 4 cm, and 2 cm × 4 cm sheets	Rehydration in 2 saline baths, minimum 10 min each
AlloMax Bard, Warwick, RI, USA	Human cadavers	Sterile (Tutoplast process, Gamma irradiation)	Dermis like + basement membrane	AlloMax 1 mm (thickness 0.8–1.2 mm); various dimensions between 5 cm × 8 cm and 16 cm × 20 cm AlloMax Surgical Graft (thickness 0.8–1.8 mm); various dimensions between 2 cm × 4 cm and 16 cm × 20 cm	Rehydration in saline for 5 min
DermaMatrix Synthes, West Chester, PA, USA	Human cadavers	Aspetic	Dermis like + basement membrane	Ultrathin (0.2–0.4 mm), thin (0.4–0.8 mm), thick (0.8–1.7 mm), and ultrathick (>1.8 mm); various dimensions between 1 cm × 1 cm and 20 cm × 25 cm	Rehydration in saline up to 20 min
ReDerm Jayya Company, Beijing, China	Human cadavers	Sterile (Gamma irradiation)	Dermis like + basement membrane	0.8 mm thickness, 2 cm × 3 cm	Hydrated (moist) —no need for rehydration Lyophilized (dry) sheets—10 min hydration in saline

(*continued on next page*)

Table 1
(continued)

Product Name	Source	Sterility	Structure and Content	Product Properties	Hydration
BellaDerm Musculoskeletal Transplant Foundation, Edison, NJ	Live human	Aseptic	Dermis like + basement membrane	Three thicknesses: 0.4–0.8 mm, 0.8–1.7 mm, and 1.8–4 mm; various dimensions between 1 cm × 2 cm and 10 cm × 20 cm	Prehydrated
SurgiMend Integra, Plainsboro, NJ, USA	Fetal bovine	Sterile (Ethylene oxide)	Homogenous	Various dimensions between 6 cm × 16 cm and 15 cm × 15 cm	Rehydration in saline for 5 min
Enduragen Stryker CMF, Newnan, GA, USA	Porcine	Sterile (Gamma irradiation)	Homogenous	1-mm thickness in 4 cm × 1 cm, 5 cm × 2 cm, 8 cm × 3 cm sheets	Prehydrated
Permacol Covidien, Dublin, Ireland				0.5-mm thickness in 2-cm × 5-cm sheets	
TarSys IOP Inc., Costa Mesa, CA, USA	Porcine small intestine	Sterile (Ethylene oxide)	8/12 layers	Thickness 1–2 mm, in 1-cm × 4-cm sheets	Hydration in saline for 20 min
Integra Integra LifeScience, Plainsboro, NJ, USA	Bovine tendon	Sterile (Gamma irradiation)	Bilayer: Dermal-like layer Epidermal-like layer made of polisiloxane	Various dimensions between 5 cm × 5 cm and 20 cm × 25 cm	Prehydrated

*Alloderm Ready-To-Use (RTU) is a sterile, prehydrated version available since 2012 but is not mentioned in this study.

postoperative care, and lack of donor site discomfort and morbidity balance out the extra cost of the product [18].

APPLICATIONS OF ACELLULAR DERMAL MATRIX

As defined by Rubin and colleagues [3], the use of ADMs can be divided into 2 indications: (1) barrier/scaffolding–such as orbital implant patch grafts, spacer grafts, lining of exenterated socket or filling, for full-thickness skin defects, and (2) volume augmentation–such as in repair of superior sulcus or tear trough defects.

Lower eyelid retraction

Lower eyelid retraction is defined as an inferior malposition of the lower eyelid margin without eversion [19]. It can result from contraction or impaired structure and/or integrity of either of the eyelid lamella. Factors, such as lower lid laxity, eyeball protrusion, and cheek descend, and specific anatomic variations, mainly negative vector eyelid topography, predispose to this condition [1,7]. Lower lid retraction may result from thyroid-associated orbitopathy, trauma, thermal or chemical injuries, paralysis, and lower blepharoplasty. It also may be related, however, to aging or anatomic variations [9].

Lower lid retraction poses both aesthetic and functional concerns; severe symptomatic or aesthetically concerning retraction requires intervention, according to the severity. Mild cases can be treated with recession of the lower eyelid retractors and/or horizontal tightening through lateral tarsal strip [20]. Severe retraction, defined as greater than 2 mm, usually requires spacer grafts to elongate the posterior lamella, while recessing the capsulopalpebral fascia, pushing the lower eyelid margin upward and supporting the lid structurally [20]. When midface descend is involved, a preperiosteal malar fat pad elevation or midface lift may be necessary as an adjunctive procedure [19].

Traditionally, posterior lamella lengthening has been achieved using autologous grafts, mainly hard palate or auricular cartilage, although various other autologous, homologous, or synthetic materials, as discussed previously, have been used for the same purpose [6,20–22]. ADM products were introduced as an alternative to these, with a structure resembling tarsoconjunctival graft in thickness, stability, and surface characteristics. The technique used is similar to that used for autologous spacer grafts and usually includes lateral canthotomy and cantholysis, conjunctival incision at the inferior tarsal border, dissection or resection of the retractor muscles and placement of the graft between the inferior tarsal border, and the cut edge of the conjunctiva. Adjunctive procedures were performed as needed (Fig. 1). Due to anticipated graft contraction, the size of the graft used is usually 1.5-fold to 2-fold the extent of the retraction [20] or in other cases placed to overcorrect the position of the lower eyelid margin by 1 mm. When using a polar material, such as AlloDerm and DermaMatrix (Synthes, West Chester, PA, USA), the dermal side is placed facing the surgical wound, whereas the basement membrane side is aligned with the conjunctiva.

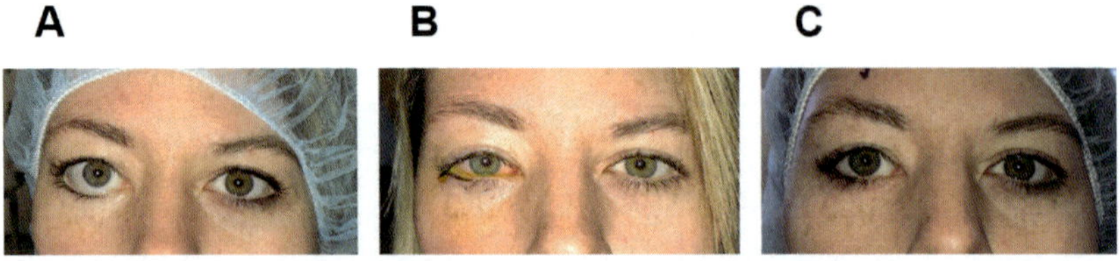

Fig. 1. Paralytic right lower lid retraction, reconstructed with AlloMax. (*A*) Day of surgery. Note severe lower lid retraction and ocular asymmetry. (*B*) One week postoperative. Excellent lower lid position with minimal chemosis. (*C*) Nine weeks postoperative. Mild residual retraction. The patient was scheduled for revision, that was canceled due to satisfactory outcome. (*Courtesy of* Dr. Kalin-Hajdu, Université de Montréal, Montreal, Quebec, Canada)

AlloDerm was one of first available ADM products and is probably the most studied in oculoplastic surgery, introduced initially for surface grafting in 1992 and then for oral and otolaryngeal procedures in 1995 [3], AlloDerm exhibited characteristics, which seemed similar to hard palate graft: its polarity provides one surface to act as a basement membrane for epithelial migration and population, whereas the other faces the inner layers of the eyelid [22]. In 1999, Rubin and colleagues [3] presented their outcomes in utilizing AlloDerm graft for various procedures: 7 cases of lower lid retraction repair exhibited good results after 6 months of follow-up. A year later, Shorr and colleagues [16] published a large retrospective review of 92 eyelids of 52 patients with lower lid retraction, mainly after blepharoplasty, reconstructed with AlloDerm spacer graft and suborbicularis oculi fat (SOOF) lift. Results were good, with only 3 cases requiring revisions and 13 patients with residual inferior scleral show despite improvement in eyelid position. Favorable outcomes also were published by Chang and colleagues [23], Bee and colleagues [24], and Kim and colleagues [20], with a total of 65 of 69 cases defined as successful. The latter presented an impressive reduction in margin reflex distance (MRD) 2, from a mean of 7.38 in 13 cases preoperatively to 5.46 mm at 6 months postoperatively [20]. No infection, inflammation, allergic reaction, or rejection was seen in any of the studies. Mild corneal punctate erosions and transient lid swelling were described [23]. The graft was noted to be fully epithelialized within 3 weeks [16] and indistinguishable from its surrounding tissue [3,24].

AlloDerm also was proved effective in a retrospective study comparing decompression accompanied by AlloDerm as spacer graft to decompression with inferior retractors recession or decompression alone [25]. In the AlloDerm group, comprising 36 eyes of 20 patients, preoperative MRD2 was the highest (mean 8.0 mm) and exhibited the greatest improvement after the surgery–mean 2.7 mm at 4 months' to 6 months' follow-up. No complications were evident in the AlloDerm group, except for transient chemosis in 1 patient.

Some comparative studies have been published as well. Chang and colleagues [22] demonstrated satisfactory, equivalent results when using either

AlloDerm (7 eyelids) or dermis fat graft (4 eyelids) as part of the en-glove technique. Two studies compared AlloDerm and hard palate graft for post-blepharoplasty lower-lid retraction repair as spacer grafts, along with canthopexy and midface lift (Madam Butterfly procedure). Sullivan and Dailey [8] demonstrated 6 of 7 successful cases when using AlloDerm, and 5 of 6 successful cases when using hard palate graft. The study looked into graft contraction and noted contraction range 30% to 73% (average 55%) for AlloDerm and 0% to 44% (average 19%) for hard palate. Resorption did not correlate to failure. When comparing AlloDerm (35 eyelids) to hard palate graft (25 eyelids) Li and colleagues [7] showed satisfactory outcomes in both groups with a trend to better results with the latter. In a consecutive retrospective study performed by similar researchers, thick AlloDerm (1-mm thickness) delivered outcomes equivalent to those of hard palate graft when used for the same indication and within the same procedure [2].

Parallel to the growing implementation of AlloDerm in oculoplastics use, other materials and products have been introduced for the same purpose, with variable outcomes.

DermaMatrix also is derived from cadaveric human dermis and incorporates a structure similar to that of AlloDerm. Lee and colleagues [26] presented 7 of 9 successful cases implanted with DermaMatrix spacer graft as part of lower lid retraction repair, without any complications. BellaDerm (Musculoskeletal Transplant Foundation, Edison, NJ, USA) is derived from live human donors, aiming to improve its biophysical characteristics. In a prospective study including 15 eyelids, Scruggs and colleagues [6] demonstrated mean MRD2 change from 7 mm preoperatively to 4.8 mm after average follow-up of more than 15 months. There was transient postoperative inflammation and 1 pyogenic granuloma. The investigators proposed that either improved integrity attributed to live donor harvesting or alternate processing techniques of this ADM tissue may have contributed to its clinical success. tarSys (IOP Inc., Costa Mesa, CA, USA) is a decellularized porcine-derived membrane, made specifically for eyelid retraction repair. Liao and Wei [10] used tarSys for Graves' ophthalmopathy related lower eyelid retraction in 37 eyelids of 32 patients. Graft height was 4:1 correlated to the extent of retraction. Mean MRD2 prior to surgery was 7.1 mm and at 6 months' follow-up 5.6 mm. Complications included transient lower lid swelling in 6 cases, and 1 conjunctival granuloma. The investigators noted graft resorption and contraction; nevertheless, the clinical results were satisfactory.

Enduragen (Stryker CMF, Newman, GA, USA) is a porcine-derived ADM, which incorporates increased durability and rigidity compared with AlloDerm [27]. Its efficacy was evaluated in 2 large retrospective studies. In the first, McCord and colleagues [28] used either an anterior or a posterior approach for placing the Enduragen spacer graft in 104 cases of lower lid retraction. More recently, Dailey and colleagues [21] used the same material for lower lid retraction repair in 160 eyelids (100 patients) not associated with previous surgery. Outcomes were satisfactory in both studies. Complication rates were

12% to 14% and included the need for revision, infections, pyogenic granuloma, graft exposure or rejection, and prolonged inflammation. Nevertheless, both studies concluded that Enduragen is a reliable graft for this purpose and integrates well and even superior to other graft materials. When the implant was rejected or had to be removed, retraction did not recur. Owing to the rigid structure of this material, McCord and colleagues [28] recommended placing the graft low, away from the cornea, and emphasized the importance of adequate, round trimming.

The efficacy of Enduragen was also compared with that of SurgiMend (bovine ADM; Integra, Plainsboro, NJ, USA) and autologous ear cartilage graft in 11, 12, and 19 cases of lower lid retraction, respectively [9]. Preoperative mean MRD2 was 7.5 mm, reduced to 5.0 mm 6 months postoperatively. Success and complications rate were not statistically significant between the 3 groups: corneal abrasion seen in 17% of eyes, revision surgery in 14%, one case of pyogenic granuloma. Postoperative swelling at week 1 was significantly higher in the ear cartilage group, followed by SurgiMend and then Enduragen. The investigators noted that Enduragen was easier to handle and is prehydrated, therefore more convenient to use.

Upper eyelid retraction

Eyelid retraction most commonly is the result of thyroid orbitopathy, usually Graves disease; however, it can occur after overcorrected ptosis repair and traumatic injuries. Although increasing the palpebral aperture, upper eyelid retraction leads to dry eye, ocular irritation, and in severe cases may cause lagophthalmos followed by corneal ulcers and perforation. Thyroid-related retraction occasionally is accompanied by temporal flare and associated with an aggressive appearance [29]. Surgical correction has been described using Müller muscle excision, levator recession or myotomy, full-thickness blepharotomy, and levator lengthening with or without a spacer graft [29]. Several spacer materials have been studied throughout the years, among them scleral graft, mersilene mesh, deep temporal fascia, and conchal cartilage.

Both AlloDerm and Enduragen have been used as spacers for upper eyelid lengthening in thyroid-related orbitopathy. The graft usually was placed between the upper tarsal border and the detached levator aponeurosis and anterior to intact conjunctiva. AlloDerm was used for this indication by Rubin and colleagues [3] and Shorr and colleagues [16], who presented total of 5 cases, with subsequent good eyelid position and improvement. McCord and colleagues [28] presented good results with Enduragen graft used in 8 cases. No complications were seen in neither of the studies.

In a recent study, Sun and colleagues [29] used bovine acellular graft (similar to SurgiMend) for thyroid-related severe upper eyelid retraction in 32 eyelids (26 patients). Average MRD1 improved from 7.7 mm preoperatively to 3.3 mm at 6 months after surgery, accompanied by resolution of lagophthalmos and improvement in symptoms in most patients.

Cicatricial entropion

Cicatricial entropion occurs after vertical contraction of the posterior lamella. The subsequent inner rotation of the lid margin and the anterior lamella leads to posterior migration of keratinized epithelium and trichiasis.

The condition is caused by thermal or chemical (mostly caustic) injuries, conjunctival infections (trachoma and herpes), inflammatory diseases (ocular pemphigoid and Stevens-Johnson syndrome), allergies, membranous or pseudomembranous conjunctivitis, and pseudopemphigoid after long-term use of certain eye drops [30].

Surgical repair of cicatricial entropion usually relies on splitting the anterior from the posterior lamella and/or rotating of the lid margin, occasionally while using grafts to minimize consecutive contraction and scarring. Procedures that lengthen the posterior lamella by grafting sometimes are favored because they target the anatomic abnormality [30]. This has been done using tarsoconjunctiva, nasal cartilage, sclera or hard palate mucosal graft, and acellular dermal products.

Gu and colleagues [30] used ReDerm (Jayya Company, Beijing, China) graft for posterior lamella lengthening in 16 eyelids (14 patients) with severe cicatricial entropion, mostly due to trachoma. Cure was achieved in 14 cases, whereas 2 cases, both related to thermal burn, required revisions due to contraction. Postoperative inflammation resolved in most cases within 3 weeks, and epithelialization was complete 2 months postoperatively.

Full-thickness eyelid defects

Reconstruction of large full-thickness eyelid defects usually comprises various techniques aimed to recruit both anterior and posterior lamella, mostly involving mobilizing adjacent tissue and/or transferring tissue from the ipsilateral or the contralateral eyelid complex or from remote areas. Upper eyelid reconstruction is more difficult because it must provide greater functionality in terms of mobility and compatibility to the ocular surface than the lower eyelid [5]. Challenge is greater when defects involve the entire vertical or horizontal extent or when the damage–usually tumor, severe trauma, burn, or necrosis–affects both upper and lower eyelids [31].

Reformation of the posterior lamella with substances with similar qualities is crucial for the integrity and function of the eyelid [31]. Acellular dermal products have been used as an alternative to tarsoconjunctiva with varying outcomes. These usually are complex cases, however, in which traditional methods for reconstruction also tend to deliver varying results.

AlloDerm was used as a posterior lamella graft for reconstruction of 3 eyelids after either basal cell carcinoma excision or traumatic injury [32]. The thick (0.78–1.78 mm) graft was shaped 30% in excess to compensate for the anticipated contraction. Anterior lamella was recruited through Cutler-Beard procedure for the upper eyelids and advancement flap in the lower eyelid. No complications were noted, except for minimal inflammation. The grafts were covered by conjunctiva within 6 weeks and were well incorporated into the native tissue. No corneal irritation was noted and a mucocutaneus junction was formed with excellent cosmesis.

Hayek and colleagues [33] presented their experience with thin (0.2-mm) AlloDerm as a posterior lamella sandwich graft along with Cutler-Beard procedure for anterior lamella in 5 cases of full-thickness eyelid defects after tumor resection. Excellent functional and cosmetic outcome was seen in 3 patients, whereas the 2 others had satisfactory outcome. No allergic reaction, rejection, or infectious transmission was noted.

In a recent, larger study, extensive eyelid defects were reconstructed using either AlloDerm (3 cases) or SureDerm (Hans Biomed Corp, Seoul, Korea) (7 cases) as posterior lamella graft [31], combined with various procedures for anterior lamella formation. The implant size measured twice the size of the deficit; in contrast to the procedure reported in the former study, the graft was not covered by conjunctiva. Excellent cosmetic and functional outcome were seen in 7 patients, and 3 required reoperation. No complications were seen, including corneal irritation; conjunctivization was completed in all patients, and 1 month to 2 months postoperatively the allografts were indistinguishable from the surrounding tissue.

ReDerm was used as tarsal substitute for reconstruction of large full-thickness marginal upper eyelid defects resulting from either burns or mechanical trauma in 2 studies. In the first [5], ReDerm was used as composite graft along with buccal mucosa posteriorly and placed within a full blepharotomy incision, while covered anteriorly by orbicularis bipedicle flap and free skin graft. In the second [34], a similar technique was applied but with amniotic membrane graft covering the graft posteriorly in cases where there was insufficient conjunctiva. Results were good in 21 of 23 patients in both studies. Full conjunctivization of the surface was seen within 2 weeks (Fig. 2).

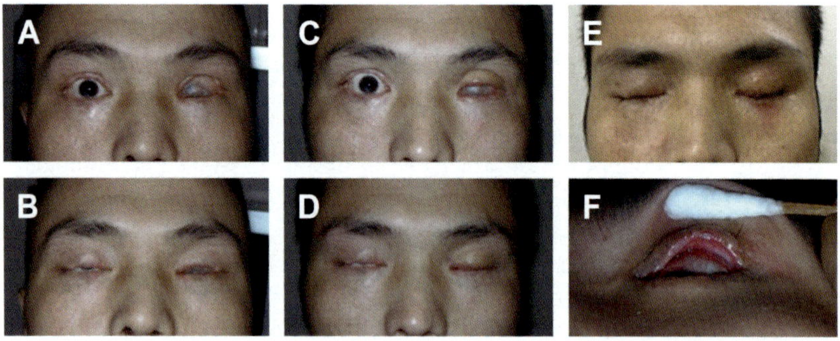

Fig. 2. Left eye full-thickness defect of the upper eyelid after thermal injury reconstructed with ReDerm. (*A, B*) Before reconstruction. Note irregular eyelid margin with wide full-thickness deficit (A) and lagophthalmos (B). (*C, D*). Six months after reconstruction, presenting smooth eyelid margin (C) and complete eye closure (D). (*E*) Two years after reconstruction, with preserved outcome. (*F*) ReDerm graft is seen incorporated into the native eyelid tissue. (*Courtesy of* Dr. Jiaqi Chen, Zhongshan Ophthalmic Center, Sun Yat-sen University, Guangzhou, China)

Periocular full-thickness skin defects

Periocular full-thickness skin defects can be managed by primary closure or secondary intention in cases of small, well located deficits [35]. In other instances, autologous skin grafts or local flaps can be used. In cases of extensive traumatic damage or burn injuries or in cases of severe comorbidities, however, these measures may be inappropriate or insufficient. Large defects with loss of deep tissue down to the bone often necessitates complex reconstruction that may be disfiguring [35,36]. The use of acellular dermal products enriches a surgeon's options for reconstruction and occasionally simplifies or eliminates the need for consecutive procedures using flaps or grafts [35].

AlloDerm was used by Levin and colleagues [38] for reconstruction of large periocular cutaneous defects in 6 patients after wide tumor or extensive trauma. Complete epithelialization occurred in all cases. Results were good in all but 1 patient, who required cicatricial ectropion repair. Nevertheless, the investigators noted the unpredictable and less aesthetic outcome compared with full-thickness skin grafts, attributed to the former's tendency for contraction and scarring.

Integra (Integra LifeScience, Plainsboro, NJ, USA) for reconstruction of periocular full-thickness skin defect was first presented in 2012 [36]. Integra Bilayer Matrix Wound Dressing was used to fill the remaining defect involving the left upper eyelid, brow, and temporal fossa, 8 cm $\times$ 5 cm. At 3 weeks' follow-up, the silicone layer was removed, exposing rich vascularized bed within the dermal layer of the graft. Meshed clavicular skin graft was then placed to cover the implant. Final outcome was excellent, aesthetically and functionally.

Chen and colleagues [35] presented their experience with Integra Dermal Regeneration Template for reconstruction in 4 patients in whom primary flap was suboptimal. In 2 patients, complete closure of the defect was seen 1 month after reconstruction. One patient experienced greater than 50% reduction in the defect dimensions, which allowed for complete closure using undermining and advancement. The fourth patient was seen with 80% reduction in defect size and eventually healed completely without further intervention.

Socket reconstruction—contracted socket

Epithelial lining of the anophthalmic socket, composed mainly of bulbar and palpebral conjunctiva and Tenon capsule, may be limited in extent due to previous trauma or surgery, thermal or chemical burn, infection or inflammation, or radiotherapy [38]. Insufficient lining may pose a challenge when attempting to fit an orbital implant after evisceration or exenteration and later on can affect the stability of the prosthesis due to shortening of the fornices.

Nevertheless, progressive socket contraction can occur even with outstanding technique and excellent surgical outcome. Management usually involves extension of the socket lining by placing grafts, such as buccal mucosa, temporalis fascia, periosteum, amniotic membrane, and dermis fat graft or hard palate graft [39]. ADM comprises an abundant, accessible alternative.

In a retrospective study, AlloDerm was used for deepening of the fornix of contracted sockets [23], delivering 8 of 10 successful cases. After release of adhesions, the graft was placed as a spacer and sutured to the conjunctiva. In a prospective study aimed at evaluating graft contraction, Sullivan and Dailey compared AlloDerm to hard palate for use as a spacer graft [8] for repair of socket contraction. AlloDerm was used in 5 cases: 2 were considered successful and 2 partially successful, and 1 was concluded a failure. One case of hard palate graft was successful. Graft contraction ranged 45% to 71% for AlloDerm, average 61%, whereas in the single case using hard palate graft in this setting, the graft maintained its original size. The investigators noted the high success rates achieved for hard palate in previous studies and concluded that these grafts are superior to AlloDerm for this indication. When AlloDerm is still used for socket repair, they recommended using oversized grafts.

In a retrospective comparative study, either Permacol (Covidien, Dublin, Ireland; 10 cases) or buccal mucosa graft (44 cases) was used for secondary reconstruction of contracted anophthalmic socket [40]. Mean preoperative fornix depth was 4.4 mm and 5.8 mm at the Permacol and buccal mucosa groups, respectively, increasing to 9.1 mm and 14.9 mm at 6 months' follow-up. The investigators concluded that Permacol failed to deliver as good outcome as the buccal mucosal graft, owing to graft contraction and inflammatory reaction, and recommended using oversized grafts with this substance.

Socket reconstruction—primary/secondary implant coverage

Protrusion of the orbital implant, exposure, and infection are more common using porous implants [39,40], likely secondary to mechanical irritation from their rough surface, and may occur in up to one-third of cases [38]. These are best managed in advance by using specific wrapping materials or different implants [41] and by maintaining meticulous technique: adequate-size implant and tension-free closure Tenon and the conjunctiva [42].

In cases of exposure of the implant, reconstruction usually requires release of both conjunctiva and Tenon capsule and complete coverage of the implant. This may be challenging in cases of insufficient lining and thus necessitates using a patch graft.

ADMs are a viable alternative to the traditional grafts used in this setting. An animal model demonstrated that AlloDerm wraps support fibrovascularization of both hydroxyapatite and porous polyethylene implants, with minimal inflammation [43]. At the same time, the graft acts as a barrier, separating the conjunctiva from the potential mechanical abrasion by the implant, thereby reducing the chance of recurrent exposure.

Rubin and colleagues [3] described their initial experience with AlloDerm grafts for anterior coverage of polyethylene orbital implants. They noted good results with primary and with secondary orbital implants, as long as the graft was covered completely by conjunctiva. However, 2 cases in which the conjunctiva was insufficient to cover the graft completely were characterized by slow advancement of the conjunctiva and melting of the graft. The investigators hypothesized that complete coverage with conjunctiva would bring about good outcome. In a different study, in which the AlloDerm graft was completely covered by conjunctiva, only 1 case of 27 patients cases of exposure was seen [38].

Rubin and colleagues' assumption may have been challenged in a retrospective review, in which AlloDerm patch graft was used during either primary evisceration (7 cases) or secondary enucleation (after implant exposure, 5 cases) when there was insufficient conjunctiva for closure over the porous implant [42]. The graft was placed over the central exposed sclera or implant while the surrounding conjunctiva overlapped its periphery and was sutured onto it. With a mean follow-up of 24 months, no exposure was seen. Two patients required reoperation for fornix reconstruction. Park and colleagues [44] demonstrated good results when implementing the same technique in 6 cases of evisceration. Conjunctivization pace correlated with age, with slower progression with increasing age.

In a small cases series [45], Permacol patch graft was used in 3 cases while not covered completely by conjunctiva, which resulted in meltdown and erosions. When Enduragen graft was used, however, covered by both Tenon capsule and conjunctiva [39], there was no sign of re-exposure. The investigators concluded that, despite previous reports, with improved surgical technique, Enduragen is safe and effective for this indication.

Exenterated socket

Exenterated sockets usually are reconstructed with split-thickness skin grafts when there is no involvement of sinonasal or intracranial cavity. When orbital bone is removed or postoperative radiotherapy is planned, regional flaps or free flaps are used but they limit the option of prospect prosthesis [4,18]. These measures prolong surgical time and are associated with infections, loss of the graft or the flap, and donor site morbidity. The eyelid-sparing exenteration technique eliminates the need for grafts or flap; however, it is associated with complications, such as dehiscence, fluid accumulation, and regional disfigurement [18]. Spontaneous granulation is a simple, viable alternative; however, this process takes months and frequent office visits for follow-up and débridement and is associated with high rate of sinonasal fistula [4,18].

Integra was introduced as an alternative to the traditional lining of the socket. The dressing is placed firmly against the bone and remaining tissue and sutured to the surrounding soft tissue. The silicone layer is removed within 3 weeks to 4 weeks, exposing a well vascularized dermal layer, which is then left for secondary epithelialization. Alternatively, a split-thickness skin graft can be placed at this point.

Rafailov and colleagues [4] described excellent results in 7 cases of exenteration reconstructed with Integra Matrix Wound Dressing. One case had used adjuvant radiotherapy, with no apparent effect on the graft or the integrity of the socket. Ozgonul and colleagues [18] presented equivalent outcomes while using Integra Dermal Regeneration Template in 5 patients for the same indication. In all cases, the sockets were completely granulated by 4 weeks and completely epithelialized in 6 weeks to 8 weeks. No infection, bone exposure, inflammation, or necrosis was seen during the follow-up. In a case report published recently, Integra Dermal Regeneration Template was used for socket lining after exenteration due to invasive basal cell carcinoma [46], followed by placement of full-thickness skin graft 3 weeks thereafter to allow for proximate radiotherapy. The investigators concluded that Integra is an ideal graft for this setting. It delivers excellent results, while allowing for urgent radiotherapy without compromising the integrity of the newly reconstructed socket (Fig. 3).

Volume augmentation

Periocular volume augmentation is used mostly for aesthetic purposes and also addresses postoperative or traumatic defects. This has been traditionally achieved by local flaps, such as orbicularis flaps, or fat transposition or grafts, such as free autologous fat or dermis fat, each with its own disadvantages. Recently, specially designed implants made of various material, such as Medpor, have become available. At the same time hyaluronic acid fillers, which have gained increased popularity for cosmetic purposes, also have proved beneficial for sculpting larger deficits. The potential risks and the temporary nature of hyaluronic acid fillers, however, limit its use for this indication [47].

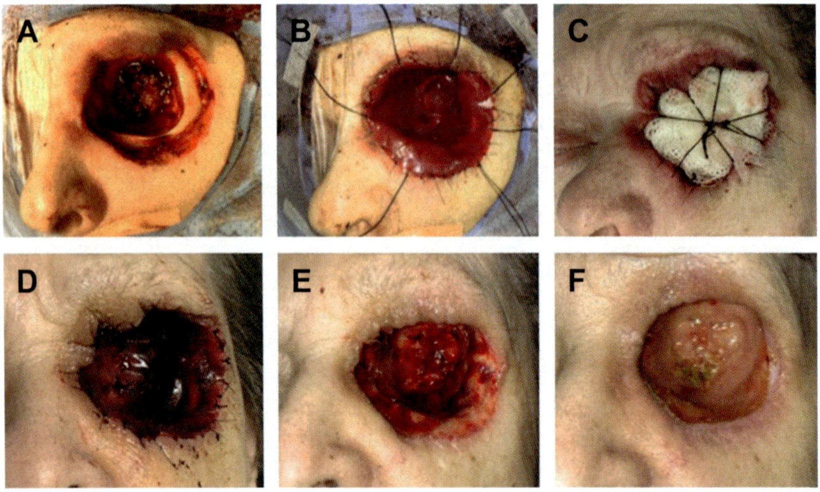

Fig. 3. Exenterated socket reconstructed with Integra. (*A–C*) Day of surgery. (A) Exenterated socket due to invasive squamous cell carcinoma, ready for reconstruction. (B) The Integra graft is placed within the socket and sutured to the surrounding soft tissue. (C) The long sutures are used for packing the socket. (*D*) One week postoperative. Image prior to the placement of a new Jelonet packing (Smith & Nephew, London. UK). Integra remains tightly adherent to the orbit. (*E*) Four weeks postoperative. The silicone layer was removed, exposing fully vascularized dermal layer. (*F*) Eight weeks postoperative. Epithelialization is complete. (*Courtesy of* Dr. Kalin-Hajdu, Université de Montréal, Montreal, Quebec, Canada)

AlloDerm was used for correction of various periocular volume defects. When used as interpositional graft, AlloDerm can be rolled or stacked without regard to its polarity [16]. Rubin and colleagues [3] used AlloDerm for 8 cases of upper sulcus defects; Shorr and colleagues [16] used AlloDerm for 5 other periocular deficits. Both presented good results with a recommendation for overcorrection. Good, sustainable results were also obtained by Kridel and Sturm-O'Brien [47], when the same material was applied to correct the tear trough deformity in 9 patients, and by Bee and colleagues [24] when it was used in 27 cases of periocular volume deformities and scar release. No complications were seen in any of the studies.

Canthoplasty

In cases of previous trauma or surgeries, reconstruction of the lateral canthus may be challenging due to atrophic scarring and tissue deficiency. In some instances, ADM materials have been used for reinforcement and anchoring.

In a retrospective study reviewing various implementation of Enduragen for oculoplastics procedures, 0.5-mm thickness grafts were used to reinforce and support the lateral canthus [27]. The grafts were either linear for lower lids or Y-shaped grafts for both upper and lower eyelids in 17 cases. Transient chemosis resolved within 2 weeks and most cases delivered good results.

DISCUSSION

ADMs provide an abundant, accessible, and easy to handle graft material. They address the surgeon's search for constant evolution in providing improved surgical outcome while reducing operating time and minimizing patient discomfort, both derive from avoiding a secondary donor site. They also comply with the human nature for exploration, innovation, and creativity. Nevertheless, these would not suffice unless encouraging, enhanced outcomes were obtained, as evident by the multiple studies published and the increasing number of available ADMs.

Created first as novel commodities for burn victims and full-thickness skin defects, ADMs have been gradually applied to a range of oculoplastics reconstructive procedures. Providing biocompatible, nontoxic, nonallergenic graft material that is easy to shape and fit to host tissue, these materials seem to incorporate well with minimal inflammatory response and to deliver satisfactory results.

The initial enthusiasm that accompanied the ADMs, however, gave way to accusations of contraction and instability, invariably compromising the reliability and predictability of the surgical outcomes. Furthermore, the infectious potential seemed hazardous enough to discourage their use. Nonetheless, at this point there are means and sufficient clinical experience to retrospectively observe these allegations and evaluate them.

Efficacy seems to be inconsistent and fluctuates between the different ADMs and the varied indications. ADMs applied in lower lid eyelid retraction, for example, delivered excellent results in numerous studies and with varied graft materials: AlloDerm [3,16,20,23–25], DermaMatrix [26], BellaDerm [6], tarSys [10], and Enduragen [21,28]. In the few available comparative studies, AlloDerm was found equivalent to hard palate graft [2,7,8,22], whereas both Enduragen and SurgiMend were equivalent to ear cartilage while causing less inflammation [9]. Good results also were seen with ADMs used as spacer grafts for thyroid-related upper lid retraction repair: AlloDerm [3,16], Enduragen [28], and bovine acellular collagen graft [29]; and for cicatricial ectropion with ReDerm [30]. AlloDerm [32,33], SureDerm [31], and ReDerm [5,34] all were used as tarsal substitute for reconstruction of full-thickness eyelid defects, with outcomes varying between indications and surgical techniques. Clinically, when the grafts were used as a spacer, aligned with conjunctiva, they were noted to incorporate into the host tissue and became indistinguishable from their surrounding within 2 months, and epithelial lining was complete in 2 weeks to 6 weeks [3,22,24,32,34]. In cases of graft contraction, apparent in some of the studies [10,16] and a measured average of 55% in 1 study [8], it was noted to not correlate to surgical failure.

Full-thickness periocular skin defects were better handled with Integra [35,36] than with AlloDerm [37], with the latter associated with less favorable outcome related to scarring. AlloDerm also failed to deliver reliable results when used for reconstruction of contracted socket [8], whereas Permacol was shown inferior to buccal mucosa for this indication due to contraction [40]. Contraction also seemed to damage the effect of volume augmentation using AlloDerm [3,16], although some reports presented stable results without resorption [24,47]. As for patch grafting for primary or secondary orbital implant, efficacy seems related to coverage of the graft. When the graft was covered completely by conjunctiva, good results were obtained with both AlloDerm [3,38] and Enduragen [39], while leaving exposed graft for secondary epithelialization delivered inconsistent outcomes when using AlloDerm [3,42,44] and failure when a Permacol patch graft was used [45]. Excellent results were noted when Integra was used for lining of exenterated socket [4,18,46], and encouraging outcomes were seen when Enduragen was used to enhance and support lateral canthus reconstruction [28].

Various factors that affect success rate can be identified. Graft contraction and resorption are some of the main disadvantages attributed to ADMs. In most indications, contraction did not seem to affect outcome. In most studies, however, the grafts were oversized to compensate for potential shrinkage.

The interface with a healthy vascularized bed is crucial because it provides ample inflammatory factors that facilitate invasion and population with host cells, whereas any compromise of the host tissue bed may delay integration of the graft [15]. This can contribute to the contraction and resorption seen when AlloDerm was used for full-thickness periocular skin defects, when the graft was rolled and placed for tissue augmentation, and when exposed orbital implants were covered by patch grafts while not covered by conjunctiva. Rubin and colleagues [3] postulated that in the latter, factors, such as desiccation of the exposed graft, mobilization of the implant, and low-grade infection, also could contribute to failure. Other factors that were found associated with worse outcome were previous flaps or grafts in the surgical area, smoking- either was stopped before or after the procedure, and congenital anomalies reconstruction [24].

Inherent differences in the components and biophysical characteristics between the various ADMs, attributed both to tissue source and processing, also may affect success rate. Enduragen was reported to be more rigid and provide more predictable and sustainable results then AlloDerm [27]. This may be supported by animal studies, where it was demonstrated to maintain its original shape while developing cartilaginous firmness, in contrast to AlloDerm, which evolved into a soft, poorly defined spherical shape [14]. Nonetheless, no study exists to compare the 2 substances in clinical setting.

Integra is exceptional in this matter, with a bilayer structure different from other ADMs: the outer silicone layer seems to guard the dermal layer from desiccation and contraction until fully vascularized. This makes Integra more suitable for coverage of large areas, such as in exenterated socket.

Complication rate is relatively low and ranges between 0% and 20% in most studies. In the larger studies, encompassing multiple procedures using Enduragen [21,28] or AlloDerm [16], the complication rate was even lower- 10% to 12% and 0.2%, respectively. A majority of the complications were mild and easy to manage and included transient chemosis or inflammation, pyogenic granuloma or cyst formation, and implant exposure. Only 1 study encountered infections [28], 1 study described rejection [21], and corneal abrasion was apparent only in 2 [9,28]. Unsurprisingly, complications can be related to both substance and surgical technique. Enduragen, for example, is more rigid than other ADMs; therefore, the graft was recommended to be devoid of right angles and placed away from the conjunctiva [28].

The risk of disease transmission is still theoretic. No case of graft-related disease transmission was noted in any of the studies included in this review. This finding complies with the vast experience with ADMs in other disciplines that has yet to establish any link between possible residual bacteria in the graft substance and pathogenesis in ADM-related surgery [17].

The cost of ADMs may still be an obstacle. This may be balanced with measurable parameters, such as reduced operating time, as well as other factors, such as low complication rate and patient comfort. The significance of graft price may fluctuate between private and public surgical settings and between procedure type and graft material. It would not be irrational to assume that the cost is prone to change with the increased popularity of ADMs and invention of new materials.

It is up to a surgeon's discretion to choose the right substance for reconstruction. Care should be taken to match the right ADM to procedure and to bring into account ADMs' drawbacks. Consideration should be given to patients who may be reluctant to have a human or animal-source graft in their body and to the cost-effectiveness of the ADM used for specific procedure. With so little evidence comparing the different ADMs in clinical practice, it is the surgeon's responsibility to determine the one that will bring about the best outcome and at the same time fits the clinical setting and patient preference.

SUMMARY

This study aims to review the main ADMs in oculoplastics practice and to assess their compatibility, efficacy, and safety as reflected in various publications.

ADMs have proved safe and effective in various oculoplastic reconstructive procedures. As with the traditional graft materials, ADMs are not flawless; however, they comprise an excellent alternative graft material while avoiding disadvantages related to both allografts and synthetic materials. The data collected may aid in future evaluation and decision making by the oculoplastics surgeon when planning a reconstruction that necessitates using graft. With additional, prospective comparative studies, better appropriate selection of an ADM may be enhanced.

References

[1] Park E, Lewis K, Alghoul MS. Comparison of efficacy and complications among various spacer grafts in the treatment of lower eyelid retraction: a systematic review. Aesthet Surg J 2017;37(7):743–54.
[2] Taban M, Douglas R, Li T, et al. Efficacy of "thick" acellular human dermis (AlloDerm) for lower eyelid reconstruction: comparison with hard palate and thin AlloDerm grafts. Arch Facial Plast Surg 2005;7(1):38–44.
[3] Rubin PA, Fay AM, Remulla HD, et al. Ophthalmic plastic applications of acellular dermal allografts. Ophthalmology 1999;106(11):2091–7.
[4] Rafailov L, Turbin RE, Langer PD. Use of bilayer matrix wound dressing in the exenterated socket. Orbit 2017;36(6):397–400.
[5] Gu J, Zhai J, Chen J. The use of acellular human dermis composite graft for upper eyelid reconstruction in ocular injury. J Trauma Acute Care Surg 2012;72(1):288–92.
[6] Scruggs JT, McGwin G Jr, Morgenstern KE. Use of noncadaveric human acellular dermal tissue (BellaDerm) in lower eyelid retraction repair. Ophthalmic Plast Reconstr Surg 2015;31(5):379–84.
[7] Li TG, Shorr N, Goldberg RA. Comparison of the efficacy of hard palate grafts with acellular human dermis grafts in lower eyelid surgery. Plast Reconstr Surg 2005;116(3):873–8 [discussion: 879–80].
[8] Sullivan SA, Dailey RA. Graft contraction: a comparison of acellular dermis versus hard palate mucosa in lower eyelid surgery. Ophthalmic Plast Reconstr Surg 2003;19(1):14–24.
[9] Barmettler A, Heo M. A prospective, randomized comparison of lower eyelid retraction repair with autologousauricular cartilage, bovine acellular dermal matrix (Surgimend), and porcine acellular dermal matrix (Enduragen) spacer grafts. Ophthalmic Plast Reconstr Surg 2018;34(3):266–73.
[10] Liao SL, Wei YH. Correction of lower lid retraction using tarSys bioengineered grafts for graves ophthalmopathy. Am J Ophthalmol 2013;156(2):387–92.e1.
[11] Tan J, Olver J, Wright M, et al. The use of porous polyethylene (Medpor) lower eyelid spacers in lid heightening and stabilisation. Br J Ophthalmol 2004;88(9):1197–200.
[12] Karesh JW, Fabrega MA, Rodrigues MM. Interpositional polytetrafluoroethylene grafts. Conjunctival biocompatibility. Ophthalmic Plast Reconstr Surg 1991;7(4):278–83.

[13] Cole PD, Stal D, Sharabi SE, et al. A comparative, long-term assessment of four soft tissue substitutes. Aesthet Surg J 2011;31(6):674–81.

[14] Gordley K, Cole P, Hicks J, et al. A comparative, long term assessment of soft tissue substitutes: AlloDerm, Enduragen, and Dermamatrix. J Plast Reconstr Aesthet Surg 2009;62(6): 849–50.

[15] Sclafani AP, McCormick SA, Cocker R. Biophysical and microscopic analysis of homologous dermal and fascial materials for facial aesthetic and reconstructive uses. Arch Facial Plast Surg 2002;4(3):164–71.

[16] Shorr N, Perry JD, Goldberg RA, et al. The safety and applications of acellular human dermal allograft in ophthalmic plastic and reconstructive surgery: a preliminary report. Ophthalmic Plast Reconstr Surg 2000;16(3):223–30.

[17] Mendenhall SD, Schmucker RW, Daugherty THF, et al. A microbiological and ultrastructural comparison of aseptic versus sterile acellular dermal matrix as a reconstructive material and a scaffold for stem cell ingrowth. Plast Reconstr Surg 2017;140(1):97–108.

[18] Ozgonul C, Diniz Grisolia AB, Demirci H. The use of integra® dermal regeneration template for the orbital exenteration socket: a novel technique. Ophthalmic Plast Reconstr Surg 2018;34(1):64–7.

[19] Patipa M. The evaluation and management of lower eyelid retraction following cosmetic surgery. Plast Reconstr Surg 2000;106(2):438–53 [discussion: 454–9].

[20] Kim KH, Baek JS, Lee S, et al. Causes and surgical outcomes of lower eyelid retraction. Korean J Ophthalmol 2017;31(4):290–8.

[21] Dailey RA, Marx DP, Ahn ES. Porcine dermal collagen in lower eyelid retraction repair. Ophthalmic Plast Reconstr Surg 2015;31(3):233–41.

[22] Chang HS, Lee D, Taban M, et al. "En-glove" lysis of lower eyelid retractors with AlloDerm and dermis-fat grafts in lower eyelidretraction surgery. Ophthalmic Plast Reconstr Surg 2011;27(2):137–41.

[23] Chang M, Ahn SE, Baek S. The effect and applications of acellular dermal allograft (AlloDerm) in ophthalmic plastic surgery. J Craniomaxillofac Surg 2014;42(5):695–9.

[24] Bee YS, Alonzo B, Ng JD. Review of AlloDerm acellular human dermis regenerative tissue matrix in multiple types of oculofacial plastic and reconstructive surgery. Ophthalmic Plast Reconstr Surg 2015;31(5):348–51.

[25] Kim KY, Woo YJ, Jang SY, et al. Correction of lower eyelid retraction using acellular human dermis during orbital decompression. Ophthalmic Plast Reconstr Surg 2017;33(3): 168–72.

[26] Lee EW, Berbos Z, Zaldivar RA, et al. Use of DermaMatrix graft in oculoplastic surgery. Ophthalmic Plast Reconstr Surg 2010;26(3):153–4.

[27] Symbas J, McCord C, Nahai F. Acellular dermal matrix in eyelid surgery. Aesthet Surg J 2011;31(7 Suppl):101S–7S.

[28] McCord C, Nahai FR, Codner MA, et al. Use of porcine acellular dermal matrix (Enduragen) grafts in eyelids: a review of 69 patients and 129 eyelids. Plast Reconstr Surg 2008;122(4):1206–13.

[29] Sun J, Liu X, Zhang Y, et al. Bovine acellular dermal matrix for levator lengthening in thyroid-related upper-eyelid retraction. Med Sci Monit 2018;24:2728–34.

[30] Gu J, Wang Z, Sun M, et al. Posterior lamellar eyelid reconstruction with acellular dermis allograft in severe cicatricial entropion. Ann Plast Surg 2009;62(3):268–74.

[31] Vahdani K, Siapno DL, Lee JH, et al. Long-term outcomes of acellular dermal allograft as a tarsal substitute in the reconstruction of extensive eyelid defects. J Craniofac Surg 2018;29(5):1327–31.

[32] Pushpoth S, Tambe K, Sandramouli S. The use of AlloDerm in the reconstruction of full-thickness eyelid defects. Orbit 2008;27(5):337–40.

[33] Hayek B, Hatef E, Nguyen M, et al. Acellular dermal graft (AlloDerm) for upper eyelid reconstruction after cancer removal. Ophthalmic Plast Reconstr Surg 2009;25(6):426–9.

[34] Jiaqi C, Zheng W, Jianjun G. Eyelid reconstruction with acellular human dermal allograft after chemical and thermal burns. Burns 2006;32(2):208–11.
[35] Chen TA, Ayala-Haedo JA, Blessing NW, et al. Bioengineered dermal substitutes for the management of traumatic periocular tissue loss. Orbit 2018;37(2):115–20.
[36] Thinda S, Wright HV, Mawn LA. Integra bilayer matrix wound dressing closure of large periorbital traumatic wound. Arch Ophthalmol 2012;130(2):217–9.
[37] Levin F, Turbin RE, Langer PD. Acellular human dermal matrix as a skin substitute for reconstruction of large periocular cutaneous defects. Ophthalmic Plast Reconstr Surg 2011;27(1):44–7.
[38] Kadyan A, Sandramouli S. Porous polyethylene (Medpor) orbital implants with primary acellular dermis patch grafts. Orbit 2008;27(1):19–23.
[39] Wu AY, Vagefi MR, Georgescu D, et al. Enduragen patch grafts for exposed orbital implants. Orbit 2011;30(2):92–5.
[40] Teo L, Woo YJ, Kim DK, et al. Surgical outcomes of porcine acellular dermis graft in anophthalmic socket: comparison with oral mucosa graft. Korean J Ophthalmol 2017;31(1): 9–15.
[41] Custer PL, Trinkaus KM. Porous implant exposure: incidence, management, and morbidity. Ophthalmic Plast Reconstr Surg 2007;23(1):1–7.
[42] Jung SK, Paik JS, Sonn UH, et al. Surgical outcomes of acellular human dermal grafts for large conjunctiva defects in orbital implant insertion. Graefes Arch Clin Exp Ophthalmol 2013;251(7):1849–54.
[43] Thakker MM, Fay AM, Pieroth L, et al. Fibrovascular ingrowth into hydroxyapatite and porous polyethylene orbital implants wrapped with acellular dermis. Ophthalmic Plast Reconstr Surg 2004;20(5):368–73.
[44] Park SJ, Kim Y, Jang SY. The application of an acellular dermal allograft (AlloDerm) for patients with insufficient conjunctiva during evisceration and implantation surgery. Eye (Lond) 2018;32(1):136–41.
[45] Alwitry A, Burns SJ, Abercrombie LC. Orbital implant exposure treatment with porcine dermal collagen patching. Orbit 2006;25(3):253–6.
[46] Patel SY, Tamboli DA, Mancini R. Two-stage rapid exenteration reconstruction to allow early radiation therapy for an aggressive orbital cancer. Int Ophthalmol 2018;38(2):833–6.
[47] Kridel RW, Sturm-O'Brien AK. Acellular dermal grafts for tear trough deformity in revision lower blepharoplasty. JAMA Facial Plast Surg 2013;15(3):232–4.

Advances in Ophthalmology and Optometry 4 (2019) 305–312

ADVANCES IN OPHTHALMOLOGY AND OPTOMETRY

Emerging Uses of Ultrasonic Instrumentation in Orbital Surgery

Edward J. Wladis, MD

Department of Ophthalmology, Ophthalmic Plastic Surgery, Lions Eye Institute, Albany Medical College, Albany, NY, USA

Keywords

• CUSA • Sonopet • Piezoelectric • Orbit • Orbital surgery • Orbitotomy

Key points

- While ultrasonic instrumentation has been used in other surgical arenas for years, this technology is currently being integrated into oculoplastic and orbital procedures.
- In light of its relatively specific frequencies, ultrasonic instruments theoretically may resect bone or specific tumors and may spare the surrounding soft tissue and vasculature.
- An emerging body of evidence indicates improved safety with these techniques, as they relatively spare delicate orbital structures and blood vessels.
- Ultrasonic instruments are quite similar to existing devices with which ophthalmologists feel quite comfortable. As a result, they may be rapidly integrated into existing surgical practices with smooth learning curves.

INTRODUCTION

Orbital surgery requires a delicate balance between the goals of the procedure and the avoidance of complications. Even in well-trained hands, these interventions carry serious risks, including vision loss, diplopia, and damage to sensitive, unforgiving orbital and intracranial structures [1–3]. These serious, vision- and potentially life-threatening complications may be avoided through

The author has nothing to disclose.
Disclosure: The author has no financial conflicts of interest to disclose.

E-mail address: wladise@amc.edu

https://doi.org/10.1016/j.yaoo.2019.04.012

the introduction of technologies that increase the margin of safety of these procedures.

Ultrasonic instruments have been successfully used in a variety of other surgical settings for several years. Thanks to cross-pollination efforts, these modalities have recently entered the oculoplastic and orbital surgical arenas.

Regardless of their indications, these instruments oscillate at frequencies that range from 20 to 30 kHz. Consequently, ultrasonic tools selectively cut through tissue with high mineralized content (ie, bone) or tissue with high water content (ie, tumor), but relatively spare adjacent soft tissue and blood vessels [4–6]. Although they were initially designed for dental work, these devices are routinely successfully used in several other fields, including craniofacial surgery, neurosurgery, hand, otology, and facial reconstructive surgery [7]. The heads of these instruments may be modified from saws for bone removal and tips for tissue aspiration to achieve particular intraoperative goals.

Within orbital surgery, 3 varieties of ultrasonic devices have been used. Specifically, piezoelectric saws, the cavitron ultrasonic surgical aspirator (CUSA), and the Sonopet aspirator and bone curette have track records in this field. In light of their properties, these technologies facilitate smooth osteotomies and precise surgical resections with decreased morbidity to the underlying soft tissue, decreased hemorrhages, and improved safety. Classically, this emerging class of instruments has been used in lateral and transcranial orbitotomies (for both osteotomies and tumor resection), dacryocystorhinostomies, and orbital decompressions. Given that its use in oculoplastic and orbital procedures reflects an adaptation of their roles in other surgical fields, ultrasonic equipment carries a safe and well-established track record. This report is designed to review the existing literature regarding the use of these instruments in orbital surgery, with the intent of highlighting their utility.

SIGNIFICANCE

Piezoelectric saws

Piezoelectric saws (Fig. 1) were initially developed as adjunctive equipment for dental implantology and maxillofacial surgery [4–6]. As with other ultrasonic technologies, these saws oscillate at a frequency that is specific for mineralized tissue, and relatively spares the underlying soft tissue, making their use ideal for lateral orbitotomies, in which the osteotomy permits access to the orbital soft tissue structures. In particular, this increased margin of safety facilitates orbital approaches in which trainees are involved, as the risk of damage to the unforgiving orbital parenchyma is diminished.

These saws carry certain other advantages that facilitate smoother surgical interventions. Specifically, the handpieces are illuminated, thereby improving the intraoperative visualization of the surgical field. Saline solution is continuously irrigated through the device tip, and the saw is thus constantly cooled. This feature decreases local tissue damage from thermal injury and serves to irrigate the field [7].

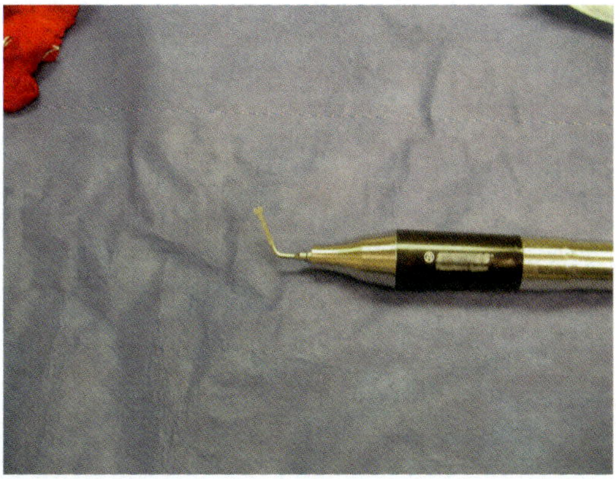

Fig. 1. Piezoelectric saw.

Histopathologic studies from other surgical fields strongly support the use of the piezoelectric saw in osteotomies. In both maxillofacial and orthopedic surgery, piezoelectric devices are associated with decreased thermal damage to adjacent structures than conventional drills and saws [8–10]. Furthermore, histologic evaluation of bone-related vessels in a rat model of piezoelectric-facilitated osteotomies demonstrated the absence of thromboses and occlusion [10]. After intervention with these devices, new bone seems to form much earlier than seen with conventional devices [11]. Together, these benefits should facilitate smoother bone healing and reduce postoperative complications.

The emerging body of literature regarding these devices strongly supports these theoretic implications. De Castro and colleagues [7] described their experience with the use of piezoelectric saws in 18 orbits of 16 patients. The devices were used as part of orbital decompression (n = 8), lateral orbitotomy (n = 5), transcranial orbitotomy (n = 4), and dacryocystorhinostomy (n = 1). The investigators specifically reported that the saw facilitated a very precise intraoperative dissection, and no patient in that series developed a complication that was related to the saw or within the soft tissue. Furthermore, although this study did not identify a control group for purposes of comparison, the patients who received treatment in this group had uncomplicated postoperative courses without evidence of bony defects.

Emerging data from studies that have explored the role of these saws exclusively in orbital decompression strongly suggest their efficacy. Kalwerisky and colleagues [12] reported the use of piezoelectric devices in decompression of the lateral wall of the orbit and described this instrument as "a useful adjunct." Spalthoff and colleagues [13] combined the use of these saws and computer-assisted planning in lateral decompressions in 2 patients with excellent results.

Expanding these qualitative results, Naik and colleagues [14] attempted to quantify the impact of piezoelectric saws on orbital decompression. The investigators compared a group of 13 patients who underwent 3-wall decompression with these devices with a cohort of 11 patients who received surgery with conventional devices and assessed infraorbital hypoesthesia with a scale that ranged from 0 ("normal") to 3 ("total loss"). Neither group experienced complications, and the surgical times were not statistically significantly different between the 2 groups. However, the group that underwent piezoelectric-assisted decompression experienced a dramatic reduction in hypoesthesia; this finding is consistent with the purported tissue-preserving benefits of this device.

In light of these advantages, studies that have documented the impact of these saws on orbital approaches have also demonstrated favorable results. Iacongeli and colleagues [15] discussed 20 patients who underwent supraorbital approaches and lateral orbitotomy with the use of piezoelectric devices to create the appropriate osteotomies. Piezoelectric-assisted lateral orbitotomies took "a few minutes longer" than those performed with conventional devices (ie, 7–12 minutes vs 5–7 minutes, respectively). Nonetheless, these saws were associated with "more precise" bone cuts with improved apposition, enhanced flap ossification, and better reconstruction, and they served to minimize blood loss and decrease postoperative pain. Furthermore, this group felt increased confidence, given the decreased risk of damage to the dura.

CAVITRON ULTRASONIC SURGICAL ASPIRATOR

The CUSA has a long track record in the management of intracranial lesions [16,17]. This modality (Fig. 2) oscillates at a frequency that is specific for tissue with high water and low collagen contents and therefore resects tumors without damaging the surrounding vasculature. As a result, intraoperative interventions are essentially hemostatic. In addition, the tip provides constant irrigation, aspiration, and dissection, meaning that the surgical field is quite clean and the surgeon has a free hand for tissue retraction and manipulation.

The CUSA has a similar appearance and function to standard phacoemulsification equipment. In addition, the foot piece is similar to that used in cataract surgery. As a result, oculoplastic surgeons have utility with this device, and it can be easily integrated into an armamentarium of surgical techniques.

Wladis and Kenning [18] documented their experience with the CUSA in the management of 4 orbitocranial tumors that were approached through a frontoethmoidal craniotomy. These investigators noted that the blood loss was minimal in these surgeries, and they did not detect any complications. In all cases, the CUSA facilitated excellent achievement of the preoperative goals.

ULTRASONIC BONE CURETTES AND ASPIRATORS

The Sonopet system functions similarly to the aforementioned devices. In essence, this technology oscillates at roughly 25 kHz and provides constant irrigation and aspiration, thereby improving visibility of the surgical field.

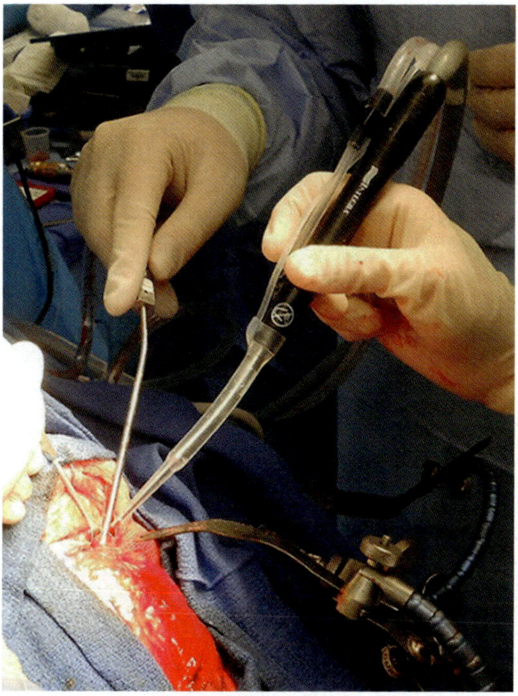

Fig. 2. Cavitron ultrasonic surgical aspirator.

As compared with standard drilling equipment, these ultrasonic aspirators generate less heat and spare the surrounding soft tissue.

The Sonopet system has been used in orbital and adnexal surgery with tremendous efficacy and safety. In an initial report, Sivak-Callcott and colleagues [19] discussed the use of this modality in orbital decompression (n = 13) and dacryocystorhinostomy (n = 6). The investigators concluded that this ultrasonic bone aspirator provided improved visualization and ease of use, and they noted that the tissue handling was safer. Consequently, they were able to perform these interventions in a more rapid fashion.

Similarly, Vrcek and colleagues [20] used the ultrasonic bone curette in the management of 3 cases of orbital lesions. The Sonopet was used to sculpt these lesions for debulking. They reported less soft tissue damage and thought that the constant irrigation and aspiration facilitated smoother, more precise tissue resection. In addition, they noted the ease of use of this modality, given the foot pedal that mimics the one used in standard phacoemulsification.

Although these investigations have explored the benefits of the Sonopet system in a qualitative manner, Cho and colleagues [21] directly compared ultrasonic bone removal (n = 18) with standard, conventional burring devices (n = 18) in lateral orbital decompression. These investigators reported that the 2 groups were not statistically significantly different, in terms of proptosis reduction, lagophthalmos, keratopathy, postoperative complications, and visual acuity. Nonetheless, the Sonopet resulted in a shorter operative time. Furthermore, subjectively, the investigators found that the ultrasonic device was easier to use, had decreased intraoperative "jerking," and fit well into tight surgical spaces.

Finally, Chappell and colleagues [22] evaluated the learning curve inherent to this relatively new modality. These investigators measured the surgical time of Sonopet-assisted endoscopic dacryocystorhinostomy in 20 patients, and they found that the duration of unilateral and bilateral procedures decreased by 36.4% and 33.9%, respectively, over the course of their series, underscoring the ease of integrating this technology to an existing surgical practice.

DISCUSSION

Optimal orbital and adnexal surgical interventions require delicate, precise intraoperative manipulation to ensure excellent postoperative outcomes and to avoid serious complications [1–3,23]. Thanks to cross-pollination with other surgical subspecialties, newer modalities that facilitate these goals and enhance margins of safety have rapidly revolutionized the nature of these surgeries. Fortunately, many of these technologies have been rigorously assessed, and their utilities may be thoroughly evaluated in meaningful manners.

Ultrasonic surgical devices have recently emerged from other fields, and, fortunately, their use in oculoplastic surgery is predicated on the long-standing record of safety and efficacy in other areas of surgery. These devices carry long histories of safe usage in maxillofacial and neurosurgical interventions and are therefore primed for integration into orbital surgery.

These instruments oscillate at frequencies that are specific for either mineralized tissue or tissue with properties that differentiate it from the surrounding orbital parenchyma, meaning that they may be safely used to achieve particular surgical goals (the creation of an osteotomy, resection of a tumor) without compromising the avoidance of complications (cerebrospinal fluid leaks, significant bleeding, etc). Furthermore, they cut precisely, generate less local heat, and leave the vasculature unperturbed, thus facilitating more rapid, smoother healing, and better apposition of bone. In addition, these modalities offer constant irrigation, aspiration, and dissection, meaning that surgeons have a clear view of the surgical field and a liberated hand for tissue handling and retraction.

As with any new device, integration into surgical practice necessitates a learning curve. However, the studies documented in this report indicate that the use of these tools is associated with a very rapid reduction in surgical time, suggesting a very rapid, easy learning process. Furthermore, several of these studies have demonstrated that ultrasonic devices decrease surgical time, as compared with standard equipment. This phenomenon may be due to the increased safety and improved hemostasis; given that surgeons do not have to interrupt the surgical process to stop bleeding and may proceed without constant concerns about the underlying soft tissue, they may be able to operate in a more efficient, rapid fashion.

These instruments are generally comparable to standard phacoemulsification equipment. The foot pieces for all of these devices and the CUSA and Sonopet hand pieces are quite similar to the devices used for cataract surgery. As a result, oculoplastic surgeons likely have some facility with these modalities, and the instruments may be rapidly integrated into surgical practice.

References

[1] Ting DJS, Lopez Perez M, Chew NJ, et al. A ten-year review of orbital biopsy: the Newcastle Eye Centre Study. Eye 2015;29:1162–6.

[2] Jacobs SM, McInnis CP, Kapeles M, et al. Incidence, risk factors, and management of blindness after orbital surgery. Ophthalmology 2018;125:1100–8.

[3] Massoud VA, Fay A, Yoon MK. Cerebrospinal fluid leak as a complication of oculoplastic surgery. Semin Ophthalmol 2014;29:440–9.

[4] Vercellotti T, DePaoli S, Nevins M. The piezoelectric bony window osteotomy and sinus membrane elevation: introduction of a new technique for simplification of the sinus augmentation procedure. Int J Periodontics Restorative Dent 2001;21:561–7.

[5] Vercellotti T. Piezoelectric surgery in implantology: a case report – a new piezoelectric ridge expansion technique. Int J Periodontics Restorative Dent 2000;20:358–65.

[6] Robiony M, Polini F, Costa F, et al. Piezoelectric bone cutting in multipiece maxillary osteotomies. J Oral Maxillofac Surg 2004;62:759–61.

[7] De Castro DK, Fay A, Wladis EJ, et al. Self-irrigating piezoelectric device in orbital surgery. Ophthal Plast Reconstr Surg 2013;29:118–22.

[8] Vercellotti T, Nevins ML, Kim DM, et al. Osseous response following resective therapy with piezosurgery. Int J Periodontics Restorative Dent 2005;25:543–9.

[9] Vercellotti T, Crovace A, Palermo A, et al. The piezoelectric osteotomy in orthopedics: clinical and histological evaluations (pilot study in animals). Mediterranean J Surg Med 2001;9:89–95.

[10] Von See G, Gellrich NC, Rucker MM, et al. Investigation of perfusion in osseous vessels in close vicinity to piezo-electric bone cutting. Br J Oral Maxillofac Surg 2012;50:251–5.

[11] Vercellotti T. Technological characteristics and clinical indications of piezoelectric bone surgery. Minerva Stomatol 2004;53:207–14.

[12] Kalwerisky K, Hill R, Czyz C, et al. Piezoelectric-assisted removal of the lateral orbital rim in lateral orbital rim advancement. Orbit 2012;31:63.

[13] Spalthoff S, Jehn P, Zimmerer R, et al. Modified lateral orbital wall decompression in Graves' orbitopathy using computer assisted planning. Int J Oral Maxillofac Surg 2018;47: 167–74.

[14] Naik MN, Nema A, Ali MH, et al. Piezoelectric surgery versus mechanical drilling for orbital floor decompression: effect on infraorbital hypoaesthesia. Orbit 2018;18:1–3.

[15] Iacongeli M, DiRienzo A, Nocchi N, et al. Piezosurgery as a further technical adjunct in minimally invasive supraorbital keyhole approach and lateral orbitotomy. J Neurol Surg A Cent Eur Neurosurg 2015;76:112–8.

[16] Jallo GI. CUSA Excel ultrasonic aspiration system. Neurosurgery 2001;47:695–7.

[17] Sears WR, Francis IC. Use of ophthalmic phacoemulsification instrument for tumors of the spinal cord. J Spinal Disord Tech 2004;17:41–3.

[18] Wladis EJ, Kenning TJ. Cavitron ultrasonic surgical aspirator-assisted resection of combined orbital and intracranial tumors. Orbit 2014;33:234–5.

[19] Sivak-Callcott JA, Linberg JB, Patel S. Ultrasonic bone removal with the Sonopet Omni: a new instrument for orbital and lacrimal urgery. Arch Ophthalmol 2005;123:1595–7.

[20] Vrcek I, Starks V, Mancini R, et al. Use of an ultrasonic bone curette (Sonopet) in orbital and oculoplastic surgery. Proc (Bayl Univ Med Cent) 2015;28:91–3.

[21] Cho RI, Choe CH, Elner VM. Ultrasonic bone removal versus high-speed burring for lateral orbital decompression: comparison of surgical outcomes for the treatment of thyroid eye disease. Ophthal Plast Reconstr Surg 2010;26:83–7.
[22] Chappell MC, Moe KS, Chang S-H. Learning curve for use of the Sonopet ultrasonic aspirator in endoscopic dacryocystorhinostomy. Orbit 2013;33:270–5.
[23] Margalit N, Ezer H, Fliss DM, et al. Orbital tumors treated using transcranial approaches: surgical technique and neuroophthalmological results in 41 patients. J Neurosurg 2007;23:e11.

Section X: Uveitis

Advances in Ophthalmology and Optometry 4 (2019) 313–323

ADVANCES IN OPHTHALMOLOGY AND OPTOMETRY

Ocular Inflammatory Disease in the Elderly Demographic

Irfan Khan, MD[a,*], Ashvini Reddy, MD[b]

[a]Department of Ophthalmology, University of Virginia, 1300 Jefferson Park Avenue, Charlottesville, VA 22903, USA; [b]Retina Division, Dean McGee Eye Institute, 608 Stanton L. Young Boulevard, Office 517, Oklahoma City, OK 73014, USA

Keywords

• Ophthalmic disorders • Elderly patients • Masquerade syndromes • Uveitis

Key points

- Ocular inflammatory diseases are a group of ophthalmic disorders that are relatively rare but associated with a disproportionate amount of visual disability throughout the world.
- The elderly represent a demographic in which ocular inflammation may actually occur at a greater frequency, and the evaluation of individuals presenting with such diseases warrants consideration of infectious disease and malignant inflammatory masquerades.
- The elderly may be at greater risk for adverse reactions to therapies used to treat ocular inflammation which necessitates careful observation.

INTRODUCTION

Ocular inflammatory disease encompasses a group of disorders that are characterized by inflammation of the uveal tract, sclera, optic nerve, and/or orbital tissues. Although some causes of ocular inflammation have been well characterized (namely drug reactions and ocular infectious diseases), most are undifferentiated, without any specific causative factors elucidated. Individuals of any age group can be affected with ocular inflammation, but the elderly demographic is of special consideration because of the unique diagnostic considerations and the increased risk of inflammatory "masquerade" syndromes mimicking primary immune-mediated ocular inflammation.

The authors have nothing to disclose.

*Corresponding author. *E-mail address:* ikhan@virginia.edu

https://doi.org/10.1016/j.yaoo.2019.04.013
2452-1760/19/Published by Elsevier Inc.

EPIDEMIOLOGY OF OCULAR INFLAMMATION IN THE ELDERLY

In most epidemiologic studies of ocular inflammatory diseases (most data are available for uveitis and its subtypes), the reported incidence data suggest that they are relatively uncommon diseases (range of 17–52 people for every 100,000 inhabitants) in all age groups, especially in comparison with other ophthalmic diseases such as primary open-angle glaucoma and cataract [1]. Despite this relatively low incidence, ocular inflammatory disease is responsible for a disproportionate amount of visual disability [1,2].

Although data are limited, some epidemiologic studies of ocular inflammation have specifically examined the incidence of uveitis presenting in older individuals (older than 60 or 65 years). Older data suggested that new-onset uveitis in the elderly was a relatively rare phenomenon. A 1962 review suggested that the incidence rate of new-onset uveitis in the 24- to 44-year-old age group was almost twice that of the greater than 65-year-old group (30 vs 14 per 100,000) [3].

Perhaps secondary to shifting demographics (increase in the number of elderly individuals) and better diagnostic tools and recognition of ocular inflammatory disease, more recent studies suggest that new-onset ocular inflammation in the elderly is not an uncommon clinical scenario. Although it is prudent to consider infection or malignancy masquerading as autoimmune inflammation in this age group, most diseases seen in these age groups seem to represent a primary, undifferentiated inflammatory reaction [4].

Chatzistefanou and colleagues [5] reviewed cases of uveitis in 138 elderly patients, noting that uveitis continues to occur de novo at a significant rate, with neoplasia occurring at a relatively low frequency overall, and idiopathic uveitis being the most common type of inflammation encountered. They also noted that, in terms of anatomic distribution of uveitis, anterior uveitis was the most common, followed by panuveitis (25.4%), posterior uveitis (16.7%), and, unlike younger individuals, the prevalence of intermediate uveitis was very low (1.4%).

Barton and colleagues [6] reviewed 71 cases of new-onset uveitis occurring after age 60 years, noting a median age of incidence of 69 years (range 60–93 years). In this cohort, 42.2% had acute anterior uveitis, 19.7% had chronic anterior uveitis, and 38% had posterior involvement. Again, most cases were undifferentiated, with some episodes occurring in the setting of other autoimmune diseases such as sarcoidosis and inflammatory bowel disease.

In a review by Favre and colleagues [7], of 435 patients with new-onset ocular inflammation, 21.8% were older than 60 years. Common forms of ocular inflammation encountered in these older individuals included granulomatous anterior uveitis, panuveitis, scleritis, sarcoidosis, and varicella zoster virus-associated uveitis. Entities such as HLA-B27-associated anterior uveitis, intermediate uveitis, Behçet's uveitis, Vogt-Koyanagi-Harada disease, and toxoplasmosis were not identified in this age group.

Interestingly, and perhaps even more reflective of the changing demographics in the United States population, the Northern California

Epidemiology of Uveitis study demonstrated that new-onset uveitis in the elderly was not a rare occurrence, but an increased incidence was found with advancing age, with the highest rates being seen in the population aged greater than 65 years, peaking at 102.7 per 100,000. Similar increased prevalence findings were noted, peaking at 234.6 per 100,000 in those aged greater than 65 years [8].

These findings were replicated by Reeves and colleagues [9] in their review of Medicare data, with a reported average annual incidence of uveitis of 340.9 per 100,000 in patients aged greater than 65 years. During the 9-year period in which data were collected, the prevalence of uveitis in this cohort doubled. Additional data characterizing the anatomic location of uveitis revealed that anterior uveitis was the most common subtype, with a mean incidence of 243.6 per 100,000, followed by posterior uveitis (76.6 per 100,000), and then panuveitis (41.7 per 100,000). Intermediate uveitis was very rarely encountered.

Studies of the immune systems and aging have described a variety of complex remodeling/restructuring events of both innate and the adaptive immunity with age. This process is called "immunosenescence," "immunopause," or "immune dysregulation." The 3 primary events in this process are a reduction in immune response, an increase in the inflammatory, and oxidation background and a production and release of autoantibodies [10].

Changes such as a reduction in immune response are implicated in the increased risk of malignancies such as lymphoma, and the increased release of autoantibodies could potentially explain some of the data described above that demonstrate a higher incidence of uveitis in the elderly population. It is important to note that not all autoimmune diseases occur more frequently in the elderly population, and the factors that curtail the development of certain diseases in the presence of the increase in autoantibodies are yet to be fully characterized. For example, the incidence of some diseases, such as giant cell arteritis, are almost always encountered in the elderly, whereas other diseases, such as systemic lupus erythematosus and Behçet's disease, are rarely encountered in this group.

In summary, ocular inflammatory diseases represent a relatively rare group of ophthalmic disorders in all age groups. Traditional views suggested that these diseases are even more rare in the elderly population, and that most presentations represent an infectious disease or a malignant masquerade. Review of more recent epidemiologic literature suggests that ocular inflammation is not uncommon in older individuals and some data even suggest a peak in incidence at older ages. In addition, although consideration of a masquerade is necessary in the assessment of any patient with ocular inflammation, most elderly people with uveitis or scleritis have an undifferentiated, primary immune-mediated process.

INFECTIOUS DISEASES

The assessment of an elderly patient with new-onset ocular inflammation must include a comprehensive examination and serologic and/or ocular fluid testing to exclude an infectious disease manifesting in the eye. The primary infectious diseases to consider in most populations are syphilis, tuberculosis (TB), and the herpesviruses.

Syphilis, caused by the spirochete bacterium, *Treponema pallidum*, has been observed to cause essentially all types of ocular inflammation. In many countries, including the United States and the United Kingdom, the incidence of syphilis has been increasing, contrasting the mistaken notion that this is a disease of the past that has largely been eradicated [11]. A recent case series analyzed a total of 50 eyes of 34 patients who had intraocular inflammation due to syphilis. Of these, 94% were men, and 75% were men who had sex with men. 29% were HIV-positive. The mean age at presentation was 41 years (range 20–75 years). Diverse presentations included anterior uveitis, intermediate uveitis, panuveitis (Fig. 1), retinitis, placoid chorioretinitis, and papillitis. Concurrent skin rash and/or headache were seen in 41% [11].

Although little data are available regarding trends in the incidence of ocular syphilis in the United States, specifically in the elderly, it is well recognized that syphilis can occur in any age group, as the infection may remain latent for decades before manifesting as ocular inflammation. Both treponemal (FTA ABS, syphilis IgG), and nontreponemal tests (RPR, VDRL) are obtained to confirm a diagnosis of ocular syphilis. Prompt treatment with intravenous penicillin G may reverse vision loss. In addition, because of the high prevalence of HIV co-infection, testing strongly should be considered in the elderly as well.

The herpesviruses, including varicella zoster virus (VZV), herpes simplex virus (HSV), and cytomegalovirus (CMV), are important causes of uveitis, scleritis, and retinitis in the elderly population. Some data suggest that

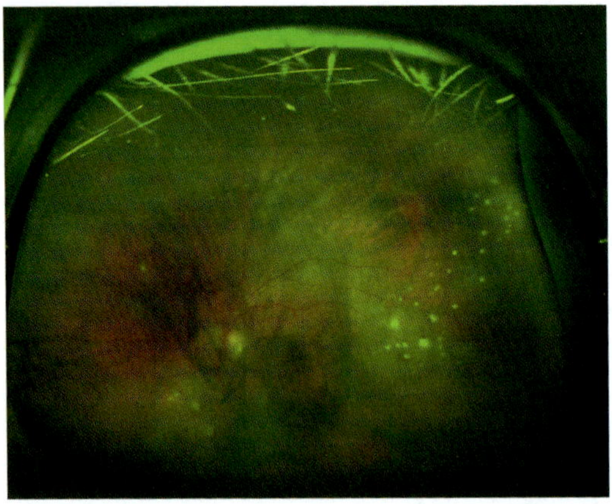

Fig. 1. A color fundus photograph obtained in a 73-year-old man diagnosed with syphilitic panuveitis. Note the vitreous opacities and multiple, circular chorioretinal lesions in the temporal retinal periphery. Vision loss at presentation was profound with rapid recovery after institution of antimicrobial therapy and systemic corticosteroids.

viral-mediated inflammatory diseases, particularly VZV uveitis and retinal necrosis, tend to occur in older adults [12,13].

Features that typify anterior uveitis caused by a herpesviral infection include intraocular pressure elevation, unilaterality, iris atrophy, and/or irregularity in the pupillary aperture, and corneal stromal inflammation, although the absence of one or more of these features does not exclude such infectious uveitis.

Retinal necrosis caused by herpesviral infections (usually VZV and HSV) is characterized by rapidly progressive peripheral retinitis and arterial occlusion in the presence of significant vitreous inflammation. The disease can result in permanent blindness and retinal detachment in a very short period of time. Consideration of herpesviral retinal necrosis is essential in any individual with posterior uveitis given the rapidity of progression and need for immediate antiviral therapy. Viral polymerase chain reaction (PCR) from either aqueous or vitreous fluid often is helpful in confirming the diagnosis.

Retinitis caused by CMV typically is encountered in individuals with AIDS or who are iatrogenically immunosuppressed, including patients with autoimmune disease, malignancy, or status postorgan transplant. Multiple reports of CMV show retinitis occurring, albeit rarely, in patients who do not have AIDS and are otherwise immunocompetent. Gupta and colleagues [14] presented 9 such patients in their review, noting that 7 of the 9 patients were greater than 60 years old. Other series and case reports reflect an older age at the time of diagnosis and may have additional risk factors such as diabetes mellitus, which in itself confers some degree of immunosuppression. Other cases have been associated with administration of intravitreal corticosteroid for macular edema, which results in local ophthalmic immunosuppression [14].

TB has been implicated as a cause of most forms of ocular inflammation. A long period of latency can occur between initial exposure and active ophthalmic disease, so this infection should be considered in the elderly who have risk factors such as close contacts with TB, incarceration, or time spent in endemic countries. Of note, most individuals with ocular inflammation caused by TB do not have any evidence of pulmonary TB or active TB affecting extraocular sites [15].

An additional infectious process that can cause fulminant ocular inflammation is endogenous endophthalmitis, which occurs when microorganisms in the blood stream cross the blood-retinal barrier. A recent review by Bjerrum and La Cour of 59 eyes with endogenous endophthalmitis noted an age range of 28 to 90 years, but a median of 66 years, indicating the skew toward older patients. Positive cultures were obtained in 51% of the cases from the blood and in 43% from the vitreous. *Streptococcus* species, and in particular *Staphylococcus aureus*, were the most commonly identified bacteria. Interestingly, despite investigation such as urine and blood cultures, a clear source was not identified in 36% of patients [16].

Many important infections should be considered in the elderly population that can cause severe inflammatory disease in the eye and result in significant morbidity, with some infections such as VZV and endogenous endophthalmitis occurring at greater frequency in this cohort.

MASQUERADES: ONCOLOGIC

Although we recognize that most elderly patients with new-onset ocular inflammation do not have a malignant masquerade (a malignant process that mimics ocular inflammation), it still is important to consider this diagnosis through careful examination, diagnostic testing, and a careful medical history and systems review, as the incidence is higher than in younger individuals with ocular inflammation. In addition, some masquerades such as intraocular lymphoma are notoriously difficult to diagnose, requiring clinicians to maintain a high index of suspicion, particularly when the pattern of inflammation evolves or does not persistently respond to treatments as anticipated.

In the previously mentioned reviews of older individuals with new-onset ocular inflammation, 3.4% of patients were noted to have intraocular lymphoma by Chatzistefanou and colleagues [5].

A primary central nervous system (CNS) lymphoma that involves the eye is known as a primary intraocular lymphoma. The incidence of primary CNS lymphoma is 4 to 5 per 1000 person-years among patients with AIDS and 0.3% per 100,000 person-years in the immunocompetent population [17]. Approximately 15% to 25% of patients with primary CNS lymphoma will have ocular involvement at the time of diagnosis [17].

Primary intraocular lymphoma usually affects the elderly, with the median age of onset being the sixth and seventh decades of life. Ocular involvement usually manifests as intermediate or posterior uveitis that is bilateral in 80% of cases (Fig. 2). Presenting symptoms often include the presence of new floaters or decreased vision. Pain, redness, and photophobia are rare but do

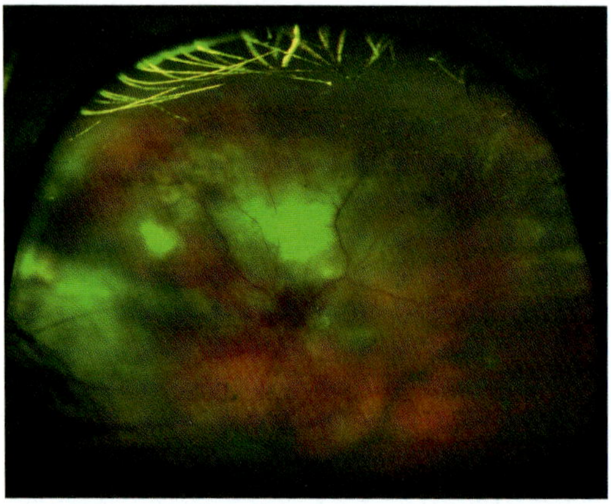

Fig. 2. A color fundus photograph of a 76-year-old woman treated for panuveitis who failed to respond to local and oral corticosteroids. Pictured are broad subretinal infiltrates and optic disc hemorrhage. Vitreous biopsy confirmed a diagnosis of primary vitreoretinal lymphoma.

not preclude a diagnosis of primary intraocular lymphoma. Initially, a variable response to corticosteroid occurs, given that the malignant cell is a lymphocyte, but over time the response may become limited with advancing ocular disease, or new symptoms that lead to the diagnosis of a definitive CNS lesion.

When lymphoma is suspected, diagnostic testing includes neuroimaging, lumbar puncture, and diagnostic vitrectomy (particularly if the imaging is unrevealing). The yield of diagnostic vitrectomy for this disease is variable, and repeat vitreous sampling, or sampling of subretinal lesions by chorioretinal biopsy, may be necessary to confirm a diagnosis. Newer analyses such as the interleukin 10 to 6 ratio (increased in lymphoma) and PCR for specific gene rearrangements can be performed on vitreous samples to aid in diagnosis [17].

In addition to primary intraocular lymphoma, other neoplasms may metastasize to the eye, masquerading as intraocular inflammation. Iris metastases can resemble anterior segment granulomas. Choroidal metastatic disease can resemble choroiditis, and associated ocular ischemia can cause inflammation. In the elderly population, paraneoplastic ocular inflammatory disease should be considered, because reports of inflammation and retinopathies in the setting of systemic malignancy exist. Lastly, given the increased incidence of malignancy in the elderly population, and with the advent and more widespread use of immune activators as treatments for various cancers, resultant drug-induced inflammatory reactions in the eye need to be considered in patients with new-onset uveitis and scleritis.

MASQUERADES: CHRONIC SURGICAL INFECTIONS AND SURGICAL STRUCTURAL COMPLICATIONS

Advancing age is associated with an increased incidence of ophthalmic disease such as cataract and glaucoma. Surgical interventions for these conditions pose risks for associated infections and complications that may manifest as ocular inflammation.

Infectious diseases causing variable amounts of intraocular inflammation may occur after cataract extraction either early in the postoperative course, or even years afterward as a more indolent process, as is seen in individuals infected with *Propionibacterium acnes*. Similarly, individuals may develop infections related to implantations of glaucoma drainage implants and scleral buckles that can manifest with cellular reaction in the anterior chamber and vitreous and/or scleritis. In these cases treatment often included the use of intraocular antimicrobial therapy, and can even necessitate removal of the implanted materials.

In addition, intraocular lens (IOL) placement can cause iris chafing (typically in the setting of a single-piece lens not within the capsule or zonular weakness and movement of IOL-capsule complex) that results in inflammation, pigment dispersion, and hemorrhage (anterior chamber/vitreous). These findings constitute the uveitis-glaucoma-hyphema syndrome, which can require surgical fixation of the IOL and/or explantation of the IOL to treat the inflammation and glaucoma [18].

AUTOIMMUNE DISORDERS AND PRESENTATIONS IN THE ELDERLY POPULATION

Most elderly patients with new-onset uveitis seem to have a primary autoimmune syndrome. Some important diagnoses in this category that are more common in the elderly demographic include sarcoid uveitis, Birdshot chorioretinopathy, and mucous membrane pemphigoid with ocular involvement.

Sarcoidosis is a multisystem inflammatory disorder of undetermined cause that manifests as noncaseating granulomatous inflammation. Chronic inflammation can lead to end-organ damage with resultant increase in morbidity and mortality. The eye is a commonly afflicted organ, and sarcoidosis can have diverse presentations, including conjunctivitis, scleritis, all subtypes of uveitis, optic nerve inflammation, and orbital inflammation.

The incidence of sarcoidosis has a bimodal distribution, peaking at age 20 to 30 years and age 50 to 60 years [19]. With regard to presentations in specific demographics, posterior uveitis is the most common type of inflammation in white patients (65%–83%), and this presentation also seems to be more common in elderly female patients (Fig. 3). Sarcoid posterior uveitis can present as choroidal granulomas, either solitary or multifocal. Lesions may be temporally distinct, with punched-out scars indicating previous active inflammation. Vascular sheathing (often of venules) with readily visible cuffs of heavier exudation are described as "candle-wax drippings" [19].

Birdshot chorioretinopathy is an inflammatory disorder of the retina and choroid of undetermined cause that is characterized by multiple hypopigmented choroidal lesions scattered throughout the posterior pole, vitritis,

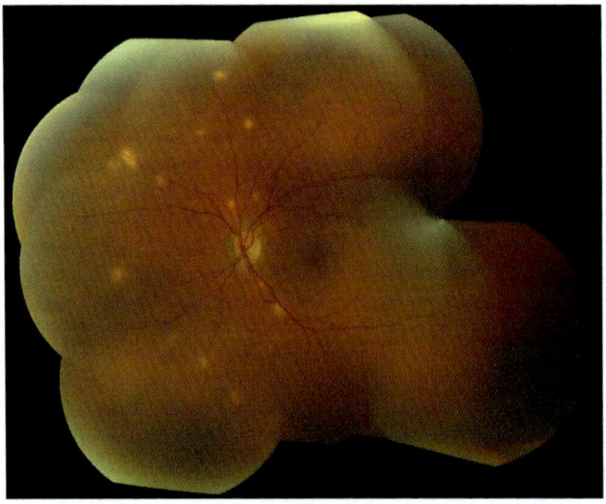

Fig. 3. A montage color fundus photograph of a 69-year-old white woman demonstrating multifocal chorioretinal inflammation. Investigation lead to the discovery of pulmonary hilar adenopathy consistent with sarcoidosis.

sectoral phlebitis, and progressive retinal dysfunction, which can lead to permanent vision loss. The average age at diagnosis tends to occur later in life: mean age at presentation is 53 years with a range of 15 to 79 years, and a slight female predominance [20]; almost 96% of reported patients are HLA-A29-positive. Given the chronicity of disease, patients often are treated with immunosuppressive therapy for years [20].

Within the umbrella of ocular inflammation lies cicatrizing conjunctivitis, which in elderly individuals can often be pathologically classified as mucous membrane pemphigoid (MMP) with ocular involvement. Chronic inflammation of the conjunctiva can result in progressing scarring, symblepharon formation, trichiasis, limbal stem cell deficiency, and corneal blindness. MMP tends to occur at older ages with the mean age at diagnosis typically in the seventh and eighth decades of life [21].

TREATMENT CONSIDERATIONS

For noninfectious ocular inflammatory disease, corticosteroid therapy (local or systemic) often is used initially to rapidly quell inflammation.

The need for therapy beyond corticosteroids is based on response to therapy and the establishment of chronic disease, for which steroid monotherapy may not be effective or the side effects/potential long-term complications may not be acceptable. Many of the steroid-sparing immunosuppressant therapies used for ocular inflammation can be used in the elderly population, but attention needs to be paid to potential interactions with the patients' concurrent medications (polypharmacy is common in the elderly) and careful and more intensive monitoring for side effects of immunosuppression may be necessary as older patients may be more sensitive to a given dose.

For example, corticosteroids have numerous potential side effects, including hyperglycemia. The systemic treatment for eye diseases study group investigated risk factors for hyperglycemia requiring medical therapy for control in individuals with uveitis treated with steroids. The relative risk of requiring antihyperglycemic therapy was greater in association with higher initial doses of steroid and older age (relative risk [per each additional 10 years], 1.46; 95% CI, 1.15–1.85; $P = .002$) [22].

When prescribing for ocular inflammation, adherence to treatment recommendations can be challenging in the elderly demographic for a multitude of reasons, including the increased risk of side effects and barriers that are cognitive in nature or related to decreased vision and/or hearing, which is more common in this age group. Efforts to aid patients in overcoming these barriers and actively engaging them in their treatment plans can help improve adherence and help select the most appropriate therapies as there are often multiple options [23].

SUMMARY

Timely diagnosis, appropriate testing and instituting proper treatment is challenging in many cases of ocular inflammation, and these challenges can be magnified in the elderly demographic. Epidemiologic data have established that ocular inflammation is not uncommon in the elderly. In addition to primary autoimmune disease, there are some diagnoses such as malignant and infectious masquerades that can occur at greater frequency in this population. Lastly, there are unique considerations in the treatment of elderly patients given greater sensitivities to therapeutics and challenges with adherence.

References

[1] Suttorp-Schulten MS, Rothova A. The possible impact of uveitis in blindness: a literature survey. Br J Ophthalmol 1996;80:844–8.

[2] Chang J, Wakefield D. Uveitis: a global perspective. Ocul Immunol Inflamm 2002;10: 263–79.

[3] Darreil RW, Wagener HP, Kurland LT. Epidemiology of uveitis: incidence and prevalence in a small urban community. Arch Ophthalmol 1962;68:502–14.

[4] Miserocchi E, Fogliato G, Modorati G, et al. Review on the worldwide epidemiology of uveitis. Eur J Ophthalmol 2013;23(5):705–17.

[5] Chatzistefanou K, Markomichelakis NN, Christen W, et al. Characteristics of uveitis presenting for the first time in the elderly. Ophthalmology 1998;105:347–52.

[6] Barton K, Pavesio CE, Towler HM, et al. Uveitis presenting de novo in the elderly. Eye 1994;8(3):288–91.

[7] Favre C, Tran VT, Herbort CP. Uveitis in the elderly. Klin Monatsbl Augenheilkd 1994;204(5):319–22.

[8] Gritz DC, Wong IG. Incidence and prevalence of uveitis in Northern California: the Northern California Epidemiology of Uveitis Study. Ophthalmology 2004;111(3): 491–500.

[9] Reeves SW, Sloan FA, Lee PP, et al. Uveitis in the elderly: epidemiological data from the National Long-term Care Survey Medicare Cohort. Ophthalmology 2006;113(2):307.

[10] Watad A, Bragazzi N L, Adawi M, et al. Autoimmunity in the elderly: insights from basic science and clinics – a mini-review. Gerontology 2017;63:515–23.

[11] Wells J, Wood C, Sukthankar A, et al. Ocular syphilis: the re-establishment of an old disease. Eye 2018;32:99–103.

[12] Lau CH, Missotten T, Salzmann J, et al. Acute retinal necrosis: features, management, and outcomes. Ophthalmology 2007;114(4):756–62.

[13] Takase H, Kubono R, Terada Y, et al. Comparison of the ocular characteristics of anterior uveitis causes by herpes simplex virus, varicella-zoster virus, and cytomegalovirus. Jpn J Ophthalmol 2014;58(6):1613–2246.

[14] Gupta S, Vemulakonda GA, Suhler EB, et al. Cytomegalovirus retinitis in the absence of AIDS. Can J Ophthalmol 2013;48(2):126–9.

[15] Agrawal R, Gunasekeran DV, Grant R, et al. Clinical features and outcomes of patients with tubercular uveitis treated with antitubercular therapy in the collaborative ocular tuberculosis study (COTS)–1. JAMA Ophthalmol 2017;135(12):1318–27.

[16] Bjerrum SS, la Cour M. 59 eyes with endogenous endophthalmitis – causes, outcomes and mortality in a Danish population between 2000 and 2016. Graefes Arch Clin Exp Ophthalmol 2017;10:255, 2023.

[17] Levy-Clarke GA, Chan CC, Nussenblatt RB. Diagnosis and management of primary intraocular lymphoma. Hematol Oncol Clin North Am 2005;19(4):739–49.

[18] Goodman DF, Stark WJ, Gottsch JD. Complications of cataract extraction with intraocular lens implantation. Ophthalmic Surg 1989;20(2):132–40.

[19] Rothova A. Ocular involvement in sarcoidosis. Br J Ophthalmol 2000;84(1):110–6.

[20] Shah KH, Levinson RD, Yu F, et al. Birdshot chorioretinopathy. Surv Ophthalmol 2005;50(6):519–41.

[21] Goldich Y, Ziai S, Artornsombudh P, et al. Characteristics of patients with ocular cicatricial pemphigoid referred to major tertiary hospital. Can J Ophthalmol 2015;50(2):137–42.
[22] Udoetuk JD, Dai Y, Ying G, et al. Risk of corticosteroid-induced hyperglycemia requiring medical therapy among patients with inflammatory eye diseases. Ophthalmology 2012;119(8):1569–74.
[23] Akinsoji E, Goldhardt R, Galor A. A glimpse into uveitis in the aging eye: pathophysiology, clinical presentation and treatment considerations. Drugs Aging 2018;35(5):399–408.

Advances in Ophthalmology and Optometry 4 (2019) 325–339

ADVANCES IN OPHTHALMOLOGY AND OPTOMETRY

Perioperative Management of Uveitic Cataracts

Judy L. Chen, MD, Pooja Bhat, MD, Ann-Marie Lobo-Chan, MD*

Department of Ophthalmology, Illinois Eye and Ear Infirmary, University of Illinois at Chicago, 1855 West Taylor Street, Chicago, IL 60612, USA

Keywords

• Uveitic cataracts • Pseudophakic macular edema • Uveitic macular edema

Key points

- Control of inflammation should be prioritized to promote successful cataract extraction, maximize visual outcomes, and minimize postoperative complications for patients with uveitis.
- No clear algorithm exists for the prophylaxis against or management of refractory pseudophakic cystoid macular edema in this susceptible population.
- Further studies are needed to establish the efficacy and role of steroid-sparing agents, including intravitreal anti–vascular endothelial growth factor and methotrexate, oral acetazolamide, and subcutaneous interferon alfa and somatostatin, for refractory postoperative cystoid macular edema.

INTRODUCTION

Cataracts commonly develop in patients with uveitis as a result of chronic inflammation and long-term steroid use. Although postoperative prognosis is significantly improved in these patients with the development of more potent antiinflammatory drugs and advances in microsurgical techniques, patients with uveitis remain at increased risk for postoperative complications, including persistent postoperative inflammation and cystoid macular edema. No standardized guidelines remain regarding prophylaxis against, and management of, cystoid macular edema following phacoemulsification in these patients.

Disclosure: The authors have no financial disclosures.

*Corresponding author. 1855 West Taylor Street, Suite 3.138, Chicago, IL 60612 *E-mail address:* alobo2@uic.edu

https://doi.org/10.1016/j.yaoo.2019.04.014

This article describes evidence from the literature regarding cataract surgery and lens implantation in patients with uveitis, with special emphasis on the evidence surrounding prevention and management of refractory cystoid macular edema.

SIGNIFICANCE

Preoperative optimization

Thorough patient evaluation is paramount to selecting appropriate candidates for surgery, counseling patients of potential outcomes, and anticipating operative challenges. Characteristics of patients and their uveitis can predict surgical and visual outcomes; individuals prone to more inflammation, such as younger patients and those with disease entities that affect the posterior segment, tend to do poorer. Overall, eyes affected by acute as opposed to chronic uveitis do better, and eyes with anterior uveitis have the best outcomes [1]. Patients with Fuchs heterochromic iridocyclitis have been found to have better prognosis than those with juvenile idiopathic arthritis and other types of anterior uveitis, although they also are at increased risk of intraocular pressure (IOP) increase following cataract surgery [1]. Among those with posterior or panuveitis, patients with Behçet disease, Vogt-Koyanagi-Harada syndrome, and sympathetic ophthalmia tend to have inferior visual outcomes because of preexisting ocular disorders, including optic atrophy and retinal ischemia, atrophy, and scarring [2,3]. Of note, this does not necessarily preclude these patients from visual improvement after cataract surgery. The Multicenter Uveitis Steroid Treatment (MUST) trial found that patients with noninfectious intermediate, posterior, and panuveitis who underwent cataract surgery experienced improvement in visual acuity of about 23 letters that was sustained over 9 months of follow-up [4]. However, these patients still remain more likely to develop postoperative inflammation and cystoid macular edema (CME), the major vision-limiting complication following cataract surgery in patients with uveitis. The UK Pseudophakic Macular Edema Study Group reported that a greater proportion of uveitic patients have small pupils, require additional surgical procedures, experience more intraoperative complications, and have poorer postoperative visual outcomes, often caused by their increased risk of CME [5,6]. Patients with preexisting, sight-limiting disorders should be advised of the reduced prognosis for visual improvement, with a detailed discussion of the risks, benefits, and expectations for surgery. In addition, once the decision has been made to proceed with surgery, identifying comorbidities is of utmost importance for planning the surgical approach. Many preexisting uveitic sequelae, including band keratopathy, miotic pupils, iris atrophy, posterior synechiae, and pupillary membranes, can complicate cataract extraction in these patients, and, therefore, it is crucial to perform a careful preoperative examination at the slit lamp to detect and prepare for these anatomic challenges.

Control of inflammation is vital to improving surgical and visual outcomes (Fig. 1). At this time, the standard recommendation is to maintain at least 3 months of quiescence before cataract surgery, which may necessitate the

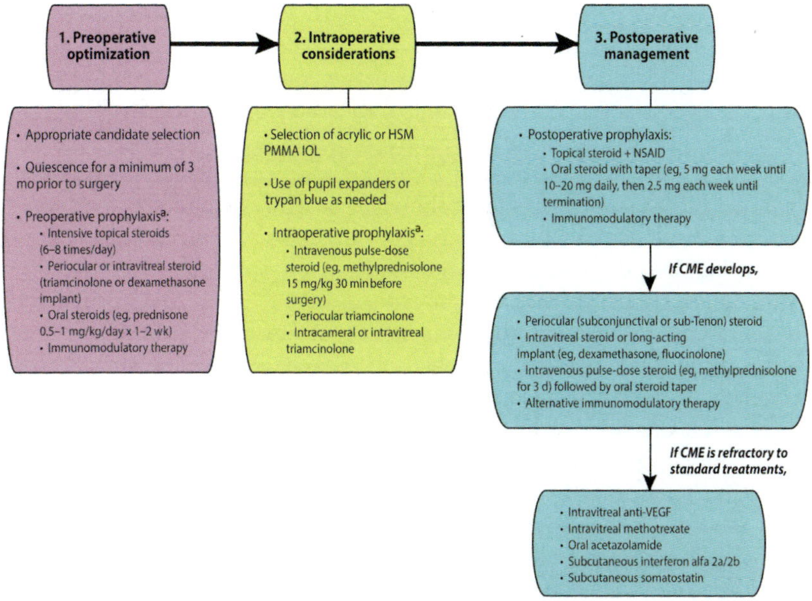

Fig. 1. Perioperative management considerations for uveitic cataracts. [a]Consider preoperative intraoperative prophylaxis for particularly high-risk patients, including those who are younger or have chronic inflammation, disease affecting the posterior segment, or a history of recurrent CME. HSM, heparin surface–modified; IOL, intraocular lens; NSAID, nonsteroidal antiinflammatory drug; PMMA, polymethyl methacrylate; VEGF, vascular endothelial growth factor.

use of immunomodulatory therapy for control of inflammation. Several studies have shown that patients who are quiescent for at least 3 months have comparable outcomes with the standard population undergoing phacoemulsification, whereas those with active inflammation within 3 months of surgery have greater risk of intraoperative and postoperative complications, as well as development of postoperative CME [7]. Current prophylactic inflammation control measures have overall been successful in preventing recurrence. In a longitudinal study out of Moorfields, 309 eyes with uveitis that underwent the prophylactic inflammation control measures (perioperative systemic prednisolone or intravitreal triamcinolone) had no significant increase in relapse of uveitis or change in topical or systemic steroid dosing following surgery compared with the presurgery period [8]. Uveitic eyes treated with perioperative oral corticosteroids have been found to have a 7-fold reduction in postoperative CME [7]. For the uveitic population, it is common to consider preoperative inflammation prophylaxis with oral steroids dosed at 1 mg/kg/d for up to 1 week before surgery. Periocular or intraocular steroids in the form of triamcinolone or dexamethasone implants have been used for prevention of inflammation. Intensive topical steroids (6 to 8 times per day) or intravenous methylprednisolone may serve as an adjunct or alternative to oral steroids. Mora and colleagues [9] performed a comparison of frequent topical steroids versus the same topical regimen combined with oral steroids for perioperative prophylaxis in patients with noninfectious uveitis, finding comparable outcomes in terms of improvement in visual acuity, intraocular pressure variation, central macular thickness, and uveitis relapse. A single dose of 15 mg/kg intravenous methylprednisolone 30 minutes before surgery has been shown to be equivalent to a 2-week course of oral prednisolone 0.5 mg/kg in terms of visual acuity outcomes and rates of CME at 7 and 90 days after surgery [10].

Although this article focuses on the management of noninfectious uveitides, it is important to mention that, for infectious uveitides, clinicians should consider prophylaxis with antimicrobials to prevent reactivation after surgery. For herpetic uveitis, clinicians should consider antiviral prophylaxis with oral acyclovir 400 mg twice daily or valacyclovir 0.5 g daily preoperatively and for 2 to 3 weeks postoperatively. Topical nonsteroidal antiinflammatory drugs (NSAIDs) are associated with less risk for herpetic corneal recurrence than topical steroids, and thus may be used concurrently to reduce the dose of topical steroid required in the postoperative period [11].

Intraoperative considerations

Intraocular lens placement and material selection

Traditionally, intraocular lens (IOL) placement at the time of cataract extraction has been deferred for patients at high risk for postoperative inflammation, such as those with intermediate uveitis and juvenile idiopathic arthritis, with secondary IOL implantation considered in the future if inflammation is well controlled. However, a recent meta-analysis of 89 articles revealed that more eyes that received IOL implantation at the time of surgery achieved vision of 20/40 or better than those that were left aphakic (71% vs 52%) [2]. However, this finding may be confounded by the general trend toward deferring IOL implantation in patients with poorly controlled disease, who are at more risk for underlying vision-limiting disorders.

As with standard cases, IOL placement in the capsular bag is ideal, but, if unable to be done safely, the IOL may also be placed in the sulcus or fixated to the sclera [11]. Given the increased risk of inducing inflammation, anterior chamber IOLs should be avoided in uveitic patients. Among the available lenses, implantation of acrylic and heparin surface–modified (HSM) polymethyl methacrylate (PMMA) IOLs is associated with better visual outcomes and less recurrent inflammation than non-HSM PMMA and silicone IOLs [2,3]. A Cochrane Review in 2014 reported the results of 4 randomized controlled trials, in which fewer eyes with hydrophobic acrylic IOLs developed posterior synechiae than eyes with silicone IOLs, but there were no significant differences found in risk of posterior capsule opacification (PCO), corneal edema, CME, or IOL decentration [12]. Silicone IOLs should generally be avoided because uveitic patients are at risk for posterior complications requiring future vitreoretinal procedures, including silicone oil placement.

Surgical planning

Several special techniques may be needed to successfully accomplish cataract extraction in uveitic patients. Often, clinicians perform synechiolysis for posterior synechiae and retract the iris using ophthalmic viscoelastic devices, iris hooks, and pupil expanders for miotic pupils [11]. Trypan blue can aid visualization during capsulorrhexis in white cataracts. In terms of surgical approach to lens removal, phacoemulsification and nuclear expression cataract extraction have been found to achieve similar visual outcomes [2]. For patients with chronic uveitis with posterior segment disorders, such as CME, vitreous opacities, or retinal or choroidal neovascularization, clinicians may consider combined cataract extraction with vitrectomy, which has been associated with more rapid visual recovery, although the data on the outcomes of this approach generally remain limited [13,14].

The addition of intraoperative steroids to the preoperative regimen has become instrumental for quelling excess inflammation after surgery in this population. Patients on chronic steroids should receive a stress dose on the day of surgery, either in the form of a 500-mg to 1000-mg bolus of intravenous methylprednisolone at the time of surgery or intravenous dexamethasone [14,15]. Injection of intracameral or intravitreal triamcinolone or surgical implantation of a fluocinolone acetonide implant can further decrease postoperative inflammation and fibrin formation in the anterior chamber, although these carry a significant risk of intraocular pressure increase [14].

Postoperative complications and management

Cystoid macular edema

One of the most common sight-limiting complications of cataract extraction is CME. Patients with uveitis are known to possess an increased susceptibility to developing pseudophakic CME, with the greatest risk in those affected by intermediate, posterior, or panuveitis; those who have had recurrent CME during flares; and those who have recurrent uveitis within 3 months of surgery [3,6]. The underlying mechanism is thought to be related to breakdown of the blood-ocular barrier secondary to surgical manipulation and postoperative inflammation, after which transudate accumulates within the retina with subsequent clinically significant edema [16].

Typically, patients are placed on a postoperative regimen of topical NSAIDs and steroids to attenuate postoperative inflammation and risk of CME (Fig. 2). A meta-analysis examining 16 randomized controlled trials with a total of 2898 eyes undergoing prophylaxis with topical NSAIDs or steroids revealed a decreased incidence of angiographic and clinically relevant CME, as well as improvement in vision versus controls [17]. The addition of topical NSAIDs to steroids has been shown to significantly reduce central foveal thickness and pseudophakic macular edema in high-risk eyes, including those with uveitis [18].

Should there be CME refractory to topical agents, clinicians typically escalate to local subconjunctival, posterior sub-Tenon, or intravitreal steroid

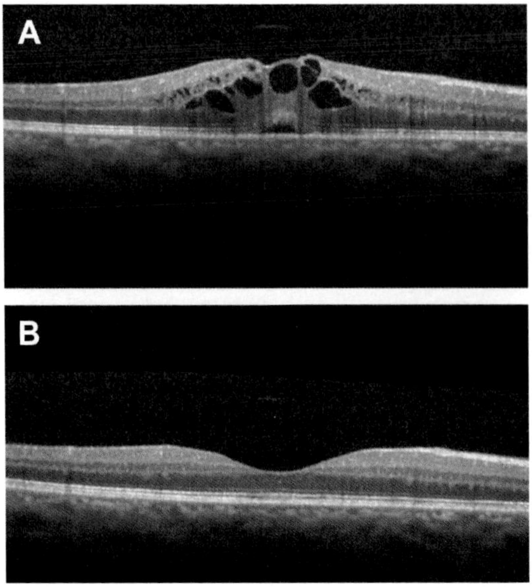

Fig. 2. (*A*) Pseudophakic CME and recurrent uveitis following cataract surgery in a patient with history of sarcoidosis. (*B*) Resolution of CME with topical corticosteroids (difluprednate) and NSAID (ketorolac) therapy.

injections, which are more potent than topical therapy and avoid the adverse effects of systemic steroids, such as hyperglycemia and hypertension. A comparative study among subconjunctival, sub-Tenon, and intravitreal steroids found that there were no significant differences in visual acuity improvement, central macular thickness, or tolerability among the treatments [19]. However, another study suggested that intravitreal delivery of triamcinolone is superior to orbital floor injections for macular edema, inflammation, and visual outcome after cataract surgery in patients with uveitis [20]. Intravitreal triamcinolone (IVTA) has consistently shown efficacy in uveitic macular edema, as well as in patients with posterior uveitis who experience pseudophakic CME [21–23]. In a study out of Moorfields, 19 eyes with posterior uveitis that did not undergo systemic corticosteroid prophylaxis before cataract surgery because of underlying conditions that were at risk for exacerbation (diabetes and hypertension) were given IVTA at the time of surgery [21]. No patients experienced a decrease in visual acuity, with 17 out of 19 achieving visual acuity of 20/40 or better; the remaining 2 were limited by optic atrophy and macular edema. Also no development of macular edema occurred within 4 months of surgery. Increased IOP occurred in 3 out of 19 patients, but was controlled medically and resolved after 3 months. This finding suggests that IVTA could be a good alternative to systemic steroids for prophylaxis against postoperative CME, although the study sample is small and only provides data for short-term follow-up.

Longer-acting steroid implants, including the intravitreal, sustained-release dexamethasone implant (Ozurdex) and surgically implanted fluocinolone acetonide implant (Retisert), also are used for refractory uveitic and pseudophakic macular edema, and have shown efficacy as a preventive measure against the occurrence of macular edema and recurrence of uveitis in the perioperative setting [24–26]. Williams and colleagues [27] reported results of a randomized controlled trial of 41 patients with persistent macular edema from uveitis or after cataract surgery who were randomized to 1 of 2 dosages of dexamethasone (350 or 700 μg) or observation; those who received the 700-μg dexamethasone implant had the most significant improvement in visual acuity and fluorescein leakage. Observed improvement in visual acuity and central retinal thickness seems to last for up to 12 months following implantation of dexamethasone, and these effects may be comparable with, or even superior to, those achieved by systemic immunosuppression [26]. These implants may be administered either before or at the time of cataract surgery, with benefits seen regardless of timing, although possibly to a greater degree when implanted closer to the time of surgery. Larochelle and colleagues [28] found a decrease in central macular thickness in patients who received the intravitreal dexamethasone implant and underwent phacoemulsification within 4 months of implantation. Those who underwent surgery within 4 weeks of dexamethasone implantation experienced a greater decrease in macular thickness versus those who had surgery greater than 4 weeks later. In terms of the fluocinolone acetonide implant, the MUST trial examined 148 eyes with uveitic macular edema randomized to Retisert or systemic immunosuppression; about two-thirds of both groups experienced improvement or resolution of macular edema, but the implant group was noted to have more quantitative improvement in retinal thickness [29]. Another study by Chieh and colleagues [30] evaluated 24 eyes with severe intermediate, posterior, or panuveitis requiring immunomodulatory therapy, periocular corticosteroid injections, or both who underwent phacoemulsification with IOL implantation and fluocinolone acetonide implant insertion during a single surgical session. These patients experienced improvements in visual acuity and central retinal thickness, as well as a decrease in uveitis recurrences and need for topical and periocular steroids and systemic immunosuppression. Although it seems that these implants have good efficacy for refractory disease and may improve outcomes following phacoemulsification, they also carry a significant risk of long-term intraocular pressure increase. Clinicians must take into account the status of the patient's optic nerve and presence of glaucoma before consideration of these implants, especially because further and persistent increase of intraocular pressure may necessitate eventual glaucoma filtering surgery [30].

Lower-dose intravitreal fluocinolone acetonide implants, including Iluvien and Yutiq, have recently been developed for use in noninfectious uveitis. Unlike Retisert, they can be administered in office, and incur less risk of cataract formation and glaucoma. A single case report in the literature from 2016 describes results of Iluvien implantation in a patient with intermediate versus panuveitis who experienced intractable inflammation and macular edema of the left eye despite aggressive topical difluprednate and a history of bilateral Retisert insertion [31]. Improvement in visual acuity and macular thickness occurred within 3 weeks of Iluvien implantation and was sustained through 8 months of follow-up, without increase in IOP or recurrence of active inflammation. Although further comparative studies are needed to elucidate these newer implants' relative impact on macular edema, they represent potential alternatives to Retisert with advantages of ease of administration and fewer adverse effects.

In addition, systemic therapy with oral and intravenous steroids has been shown to decrease the incidence of perioperative CME, and generally is recommended before surgery for patients with a history of severe inflammation, as well as monocular patients who lost their fellow eye to inflammation. A typical regimen of oral prednisone consists of 0.5 mg/kg starting 3 days before surgery, with a taper of 5 mg each week until a dose of 10 to 20 mg daily is reached, after which a more gradual taper of 2.5 mg each week is followed until patients reach presurgery dosing or the lowest required maintenance dose. Eyes treated with perioperative oral steroids have shown a 7-fold reduction in postoperative CME at 1 and 3 months after surgery [7]. It remains unclear whether local or systemic therapy is superior for CME. In a head-to-head study of 40 patients who received either intraoperative IVTA or postoperative oral steroids, postoperative CME was seen in 3 out of 20 patients in the steroid group as opposed to 1 out of 20 patients in the IVTA group, with lower central foveal thickness and more resolution of angiographic CME in the triamcinolone group [32]. In contrast, a comparison between intravitreal dexamethasone implant and postoperative oral steroids in 20 patients with uveitis who underwent phacoemulsification with IOL implantation found no significant difference in central macular thickness or IOP [33]. For patients who do not respond to oral steroids, a short course of intravenous pulse methylprednisolone may be indicated. Small studies of refractory pseudophakic and uveitic CME have shown improvement or resolution of disease within 3 days of IV methylprednisolone followed by a rapid oral taper, without a significant increase in IOP [34,35].

Posterior capsule opacification

PCO remains the most common late complication of cataract surgery among patients with or without uveitis. Strategies discussed here in relation to preoperative optimization, including deferring surgery until inflammation is controlled for at least 3 months, and implantation of acrylic IOLs may decrease the risk of PCO, although overall the rates remain high at about 18% at 10 years despite these measures [3,6,36]. In general, it is recommended to should wait until inflammation is controlled before attempting neodymium:yttrium-aluminum-garnet capsulotomy.

Intraocular pressure

Patients with uveitis are vulnerable to fluctuations in intraocular pressure. Hypotony may result from persistent inflammation and require increasing topical and systemic antiinflammatory therapy, particularly steroids that additionally serve to maintain intraocular pressure. In contrast, persistent increase of intraocular pressure may occur secondary to steroid response, in which case topical steroids may need to be tapered and oral and/or systemic immunosuppression for persistent inflammation increased. Of note, patients with Fuchs heterochromic iridocyclitis may specifically be at increased risk of IOP increase following cataract surgery [1].

Disease recurrence

Because of disruption of the blood-ocular barrier and promotion of inflammation during surgery, patients are at risk of disease recurrence following cataract surgery. Some cases may require increasing immunosuppression to regain adequate control. However, current prophylactic measures have overall been successful in preventing recurrence of inflammation. A recent longitudinal study by Sharief and colleagues [8] examined outcomes of 309 eyes of uveitic patients who underwent phacoemulsification with IVTA or postoperative oral prednisolone, compared with a control group that remained phakic. At 5-year follow-up, pseudophakic eyes had no significant increase in uveitis relapse or change in dosing of topical or systemic steroids compared with the presurgery period or control eyes.

PRESENT RELEVANCE AND FUTURE AVENUES TO INVESTIGATE

A suprachoroidal formulation of triamcinolone has been developed in the search for a treatment modality that limits the undesirable side effects of steroids, but still provides adequate drug concentrations to the posterior segment. In 2018, Yeh and colleagues [37] summarized findings of a randomized controlled study that followed 17 patients with macular edema caused by noninfectious uveitis who received a single suprachoroidal injection of 4.0 mg of triamcinolone. Importantly, patients who had a history of steroid-refractory disease were excluded from this study. Compared with the control group who received a dosage of 0.8 mg, the treatment group experienced both statistically and clinically significant decreases in retinal thickness, improvement of visual acuity, and reduction of anterior chamber and vitreous inflammation over a 2-month follow-up period. Adverse events were uncommon and largely injection related, including eye pain at the time of injection and conjunctival hemorrhage, but no serious ocular effects were noted in follow-up, including increase of intraocular pressure. This finding suggests that suprachoroidal drug delivery may be a viable future alternative for uveitic macular edema, although comparative trials with greater enrollment and longer follow-up are needed to determine whether reinjection is necessary, to explore the relative safety and efficacy of suprachoroidal injections to existing periocular and intravitreal options, and to elucidate whether IOP increase and glaucoma may still develop in the long term.

Several steroid-sparing agents are being studied to provide alternative options for preventing and managing refractory CME. Intravitreal anti–

vascular endothelial growth factor (anti-VEGF) is currently being investigated with some success reported for patients with refractory pseudophakic CME, for whom it is thought a need exists to stabilize the blood-retinal barrier by multiple mechanisms [38]. Most studies report results with bevacizumab, which has been associated with decreased mean macular thickness in patients with CME unresponsive to conventional treatment, including intensive topical steroids and NSAIDs, and periocular and intravitreal steroids [38–44]. One study has reported the use of bevacizumab as an effective primary treatment of pseudophakic CME [45]. For some patients, effect was dramatic and rapid, with resolution of chronic CME occurring within 2 weeks following 1 injection of anti-VEGF, and sustained in follow-up up to 12 months [40,43]. Other studies report response only after repeated injections [38,43]. No significant adverse events have been reported with intravitreal anti-VEGF injections in these patients. However, there seems to be significant variability in improvement of visual acuity, although this may be a function of the chronicity of underlying disorders. Ranibizumab has been studied in a large randomized controlled study of 156 patients with macular edema of uncommon causes; variable effects were seen among subgroups, with greater than 1-line improvement in visual acuity observed in patients with inflammatory conditions and after cataract surgery [46]. Overall, the evidence remains scant, and further studies are needed to establish the role of anti-VEGF agents for refractory pseudophakic CME [47]. It has not yet been determined whether intravitreal anti-VEGF may play a role in preoperative or intraoperative prophylaxis.

A few reports of intraocular methotrexate suggest some efficacy for inflammation and uveitic macular edema. In a study by Hardwig and colleagues [48], 8 out of 9 patients with uveitis treated with intravitreal methotrexate showed improvement in visual acuity, and 3 out of 4 patients with preexisting CME achieved visual acuity of 20/20. Another study, by Taylor and colleagues [49], of 15 eyes with exacerbation of noninfectious intermediate, posterior, or panuveitis and/or CME reported improvement in visual acuity and ocular inflammation after intravitreal methotrexate, with a decrease in dose of systemic immunosuppression. Relapse after 4 months was noted in some patients, but reinjection of methotrexate had similar efficacy. No adverse events have yet been reported with these injections, and intraocular methotrexate thus may represent an additional steroid-sparing option for patients with refractory uveitis and CME.

Systemic therapies for uveitic and pseudophakic CME currently being explored include acetazolamide, subcutaneous interferon, and subcutaneous somatostatin. Oral acetazolamide has historically been attempted with variable success in small cohorts; studies of patients with uveitic or pseudophakic macular edema have found a decrease in CME that may or may not ultimately affect visual acuity [50,51]. Subcutaneous interferon alfa-2a and alfa-2b injections have shown efficacy in small case series of patients with pseudophakic or uveitic macular edema refractory to topical NSAIDs, intravitreal anti-VEGF, acetazolamide, intravitreal triamcinolone, systemic steroids, and immunosuppression [52,53]. The studied regimens for these interferon injections often consist of a treatment dosage of 3 million or 6 million IU once or twice weekly for 4 weeks with a slow taper over months. Resolution of CME is noted within days and maintained up to 6 months after treatment in patients whose disease is refractory to 1 or more immunosuppressive agents [54–56]. The recent Evaluation of Birdshot Retine Choroidopathy Treatment by Either Steroid or Interferon-alpha2a (BIRDFERON) study evaluated 48 patients with chronic bilateral noninfectious uveitis complicated by macular edema who were randomized to treatment with subcutaneous interferon or systemic corticosteroids, or no treatment; comparable improvement in CME was observed in both treatment groups compared with controls [57]. Mild side effects, including fatigue, malaise, arthralgia, nausea, anorexia, and hair loss, have been reported with these injections, as well as serious adverse events, such as pancreatitis, necessitating discontinuation of therapy [56,57]. Of note, use of an eyedrop formulation of interferon alfa-2b was described in a 2018 case report of a patient with refractory pseudophakic CME; complete resolution of CME with 1 MIU/mL 4 times daily was reported after 12 weeks, with stability at 36-week follow-up [53]. In addition, subcutaneous octreotide, a somatostatin analogue, has also shown benefit for uveitic CME resistant to periocular and systemic therapies in case reports and small case series. Missotten and colleagues [58] conducted a study of 20 patients with refractory CME treated with long-acting octreotide injections, with reduction of CME reported in 70% of episodes within 2 to 4 months. Of note, recurrence of CME occurred in about 30% with discontinuation of treatment, suggesting patients may require repeat injections for sustained effect. However, among those who were successfully treated, nearly 40% maintained resolution of CME for more than 1 year.

To this day, cataract extraction in uveitic patients remains a unique challenge. Certain principles are clear in approaching these patients, including controlling inflammation for at least 3 months before surgery to optimize structural and functional outcomes following surgery. However, despite the well-known susceptibility of uveitic patients for postoperative CME, no clear algorithm exists for the prophylaxis of CME or treatment of refractory CME in this susceptible population, and this represents an avenue of research that could have significant bearing on these patients' postsurgical outcomes. This article has described the literature on established as well as alternative modalities for treating pseudophakic CME in patients with uveitis, but much of the data comprise small case series, case reports, and uncontrolled studies. Interpretation of data must therefore be performed with caution given the small number of subjects and heterogeneity of existing studies. Ultimately, this highlights the need for larger studies and, specifically, randomized clinical trials, which is particularly challenging because uveitic patients represent a small subset of the population undergoing cataract extraction. POINT (Periocular and Intravitreal Corticosteroids for Uveitic Macular Edema Trial, NCT02374060) was a recently completed trial that evaluated the relative efficacy of periocular triamcinolone, intravitreal triamcinolone, and the intravitreal dexamethasone implant in patients with macular edema secondary to uveitis; results are pending at the time of this publication. Some other ongoing clinical trials include SOAP (Study for Optimizing Anti-inflammatory prophylaxis, NCT03383328), which evaluates the timing of topical NSAIDs, as well as their efficacy compared with topical prednisolone and intraoperative sub-Tenon dexamethasone; ACME (Treatment of Macular Edema After Cataract Surgery with Subconjunctival Aflibercept, NCT03396861), which studies the utility of subconjunctival aflibercept for pseudophakic macular edema unresponsive to topical therapy; MEND (Macular Edema Nepafenac vs Difluprednate Uveitis Trial, NCT01939691), which compares the use of various individual and combinations of topical nepafenac, difluprednate, and prednisolone for uveitic macular edema; and MERIT (Macular Edema Ranibizumab vs. Intravitreal Anti-inflammatory Therapy Trial, NCT02623426), which compares the relative efficacy and safety of the dexamethasone implant, intravitreal methotrexate, and intravitreal ranibizumab for uveitic macular edema refractory to intravitreal steroids.

SUMMARY

Patients with uveitis represent a unique subset of the population undergoing cataract surgery and pose several challenges that require special consideration and strategy. Control of inflammation should be prioritized to promote successful cataract extraction, maximize visual outcomes, and minimize postoperative complications for patients with uveitis. Traditionally, this has been accomplished with intensive topical, oral, or intravenous steroids in the preoperative period, as well as intraoperative intracameral or intravitreal triamcinolone or longer-acting steroid implants, although the steroid burden subjects these patients to significant risk of intraocular pressure increase. With current prophylactic measures, structural and functional outcomes after surgery may be comparable with those for the nonuveitic population, but patients with a history of uveitis still remain at higher risk for postoperative CME, and no clear algorithm exists for the prophylaxis against or management of refractory pseudophakic CME. Intravitreal anti-VEGF and methotrexate, oral acetazolamide, and subcutaneous interferon alfa and somatostatin have all been reported to reduce and even resolve refractory cases of pseudophakic and uveitic macular edema, and may represent options for CME that does not respond to the standard topical, periocular, intravitreal, and systemic steroids. However, more studies are needed to establish the potential efficacy and role of these agents in the perioperative management of uveitic cataracts.

References

[1] Balta O, Sungur G, Acar MA, et al. Long-term results of cataract surgery in patients with anterior uveitis. Int Ophthalmol 2018;38:1399–407.

[2] Mehta S, Linton MM, Kempen JH. Outcomes of cataract surgery in patients with uveitis: a systematic review and meta-analysis. Am J Ophthalmol 2014;158:676–92.e7.

[3] Zhang Y, Zhu X, He W, et al. Efficacy of cataract surgery in patients with uveitis: a STROBE-compliant article. Medicine (Baltimore) 2017;96:e7353.
[4] Sen HN, Abreu FM, Louis TA, et al. Cataract surgery outcomes in uveitis: the multicenter uveitis steroid treatment trial. Ophthalmology 2016;123:183–90.
[5] Chu CJ, Dick AD, Johnston RL, et al. Cataract surgery in uveitis: a multicentre database study. Br J Ophthalmol 2017;101:1132–7.
[6] Chu CJ, Johnston RL, Buscombe C, et al. Risk factors and incidence of macular edema after cataract surgery: a database study of 81984 eyes. Ophthalmology 2016;123:316–23.
[7] Belair ML, Kim SJ, Thorne JE, et al. Incidence of cystoid macular edema after cataract surgery in patients with and without uveitis using optical coherence tomography. Am J Ophthalmol 2009;148:128–35.e2.
[8] Sharief L, Lightman S, Baltinas J, et al. Long-term effect of cataract phacoemulsification on the inflammation control and clinical outcome in uveitis patients. Clin Exp Ophthalmol 2018;46:1048–54.
[9] Mora P, Gonzales S, Ghirardini S, et al. Perioperative prophylaxis to prevent recurrence following cataract surgery in uveitic patients: a two-centre, prospective, randomized trial. Acta Ophthalmol 2016;94:e390–4.
[10] Meacock WR, Spalton DJ, Bender L, et al. Steroid prophylaxis in eyes with uveitis undergoing phacoemulsification. Br J Ophthalmol 2004;88:1122–4.
[11] Chan NS, Ti SE, Chee SP. Decision-making and management of uveitic cataract. Indian J Ophthalmol 2017;65:1329–39.
[12] Leung TG, Lindsley K, Kuo IC. Types of intraocular lenses for cataract surgery in eyes with uveitis. Cochrane Database Syst Rev 2014;(3):CD007284.
[13] Androudi S, Ahmed M, Fiore T, et al. Combined pars plana vitrectomy and phacoemulsification to restore visual acuity in patients with chronic uveitis. J Cataract Refract Surg 2005;31:472–8.
[14] Lobo AM, Papaliodis GN. Perioperative evaluation and management of cataract surgery in uveitis patients. Int Ophthalmol Clin 2010;50:129–37.
[15] Conway MD, Stern E, Enfield DB, et al. Management of cataract in uveitis patients. Curr Opin Ophthalmol 2018;29:69–74.
[16] Wielders LHP, Schouten J, Nuijts R. Prevention of macular edema after cataract surgery. Curr Opin Ophthalmol 2018;29:48–53.
[17] Rossetti L, Chaudhuri J, Dickersin K. Medical prophylaxis and treatment of cystoid macular edema after cataract surgery. The results of a meta-analysis. Ophthalmology 1998;105: 397–405.
[18] El Gharbawy SA, Darwish EA, Abu Eleinen KG, et al. Efficacy of addition of nepafenac 0.1% to steroid eye drops in prevention of post-phaco macular edema in high-risk eyes. Eur J Ophthalmol 2018; https://doi.org/10.1177/1120672118799626. [Epub ahead of print].
[19] Carbonniere C, Couret C, Bleriot A, et al. [Treatment of macular edema: Comparison of efficacy and tolerability of subconjunctival triamcinolone injections, sub-tenon's triamcinolone injections and intravitreal dexamethasone implant]. J Fr Ophtalmol 2017;40:177–86.
[20] Roesel M, Tappeiner C, Heinz C, et al. Comparison between intravitreal and orbital floor triamcinolone acetonide after phacoemulsification in patients with endogenous uveitis. Am J Ophthalmol 2009;147:406–12.
[21] Okhravi N, Morris A, Kok HS, et al. Intraoperative use of intravitreal triamcinolone in uveitic eyes having cataract surgery: pilot study. J Cataract Refract Surg 2007;33:1278–83.
[22] Sorensen TL, Haamann P, Villumsen J, et al. Intravitreal triamcinolone for macular oedema: efficacy in relation to aetiology. Acta Ophthalmol Scand 2005;83:67–70.
[23] Steeples LR, Anand N, Moraji J, et al. Clinical outcomes of intravitreal preservative-free triamcinolone preparation (Triesence(R)) for cystoid macular oedema and inflammation in patients with uveitis. Ocul Immunol Inflamm 2018;26:997–1004.
[24] de Oliveira Dias JR, Nunes RP, Goldhardt R. New drugs and new posterior delivery methods in CME. Curr Ophthalmol Rep 2017;5:160–8.

[25] Garcia JM, Isaac DL, Avila MP. Dexamethasone 0.7 mg implants in the management of pseudophakic cystoid macular edema. Arq Bras Oftalmol 2016;79:113–5.
[26] Khurana RN, Bansal AS, Chang LK, et al. Prospective evaluation of a sustained-release dexamethasone intravitreal implant for cystoid macular edema in quiescent uveitis. Retina 2017;37:1692–9.
[27] Williams GA, Haller JA, Kuppermann BD, et al. Dexamethasone posterior-segment drug delivery system in the treatment of macular edema resulting from uveitis or Irvine-Gass syndrome. Am J Ophthalmol 2009;147:1048–54, 1054.e1-2.
[28] Larochelle MB, Smith J, Dacey MS. Dexamethasone intravitreal implant in the treatment of uveitic macular edema in the perioperative cataract setting: a case series. Am J Ophthalmol 2016;166:149–53.
[29] Tomkins-Netzer O, Lightman S, Drye L, et al. Outcome of treatment of uveitic macular edema: the multicenter uveitis steroid treatment trial 2-year results. Ophthalmology 2015;122:2351–9.
[30] Chieh JJ, Carlson AN, Jaffe GJ. Combined fluocinolone acetonide intraocular delivery system insertion, phacoemulsification, and intraocular lens implantation for severe uveitis. Am J Ophthalmol 2008;146:589–94.
[31] Reddy AK, Burkholder BM, Khan IR, et al. Iluvien Implantation for Uveitis and Uveitic Macular Edema. Ocul Immunol Inflamm 2018;26:315–6.
[32] Dada T, Dhawan M, Garg S, et al. Safety and efficacy of intraoperative intravitreal injection of triamcinolone acetonide injection after phacoemulsification in cases of uveitic cataract. J Cataract Refract Surg 2007;33:1613–8.
[33] Gupta A, Ram J, Gupta A, et al. Intraoperative dexamethasone implant in uveitis patients with cataract undergoing phacoemulsification. Ocul Immunol Inflamm 2013;21:462–7.
[34] Abe T, Hayasaka S, Nagaki Y, et al. Pseudophakic cystoid macular edema treated with high-dose intravenous methylprednisolone. J Cataract Refract Surg 1999;25:1286–8.
[35] Kiew S, Forrester JV, Chee SP, et al. Intravenous 'pulse' methylprednisolone for the treatment of inflammatory cystoid macular oedema. Br J Ophthalmol 2012;96:1531–3.
[36] Chiu H, Dang H, Cheung C, et al. Ten-year retrospective review of outcomes following phacoemulsification with intraocular lens implantation in patients with pre-existing uveitis. Can J Ophthalmol 2017;52:175–80.
[37] Yeh S, Kurup SK, Wang RC, et al. Suprachoroidal injection OF triamcinolone acetonide, CLS-TA, for macular edema due to noninfectious uveitis: a randomized, phase 2 study (DOGWOOD). Retina 2018; https://doi.org/10.1097/IAE.0000000000002279. [Epub ahead of print].
[38] Rodriguez-Blanco M, Marticorena J, Gomez-Ulla F. Triamcinolone acetonide for refractory pseudophakic cystoid macular edema after intravitreal bevacizumab. Graefes Arch Clin Exp Ophthalmol 2009;247:427–8.
[39] Arevalo JF, Maia M, Garcia-Amaris RA, et al. Intravitreal bevacizumab for refractory pseudophakic cystoid macular edema: the Pan-American Collaborative Retina Study Group results. Ophthalmology 2009;116:1481–7, 1487.e1.
[40] Barone A, Prascina F, Russo V, et al. Successful treatment of pseudophakic cystoid macular edema with intravitreal bevacizumab. J Cataract Refract Surg 2008;34:1210–2.
[41] Barone A, Russo V, Prascina F, et al. Short-term safety and efficacy of intravitreal bevacizumab for pseudophakic cystoid macular edema. Retina 2009;29:33–7.
[42] Diaz-Llopis M, Amselem L, Cervera E, et al. [Intravitreal injection of bevacizumab for pseudophakic cystoid macular edema resistant to steroids]. Arch Soc Esp Oftalmol 2007;82: 447–50 [in Spanish].
[43] Mason JO 3rd, Albert MA Jr, Vail R. Intravitreal bevacizumab (Avastin) for refractory pseudophakic cystoid macular edema. Retina 2006;26:356–7.
[44] Spitzer MS, Ziemssen F, Yoeruek E, et al. Efficacy of intravitreal bevacizumab in treating postoperative pseudophakic cystoid macular edema. J Cataract Refract Surg 2008;34: 70–5.

[45] Arevalo JF, Garcia-Amaris RA, Roca JA, et al. Primary intravitreal bevacizumab for the management of pseudophakic cystoid macular edema: pilot study of the Pan-American Collaborative Retina Study Group. J Cataract Refract Surg 2007;33:2098–105.
[46] Staurenghi G, Lai TYY, Mitchell P, et al. Efficacy and safety of ranibizumab 0.5 mg for the treatment of macular edema resulting from uncommon causes: twelve-month findings from PROMETHEUS. Ophthalmology 2018;125:850–62.
[47] Ghasemi Falavarjani K, Parvaresh MM, Modarres M, et al. Intravitreal bevacizumab for pseudophakic cystoid macular edema; a systematic review. J Ophthalmic Vis Res 2012;7:235–9.
[48] Hardwig PW, Pulido JS, Erie JC, et al. Intraocular methotrexate in ocular diseases other than primary central nervous system lymphoma. Am J Ophthalmol 2006;142:883–5.
[49] Taylor SR, Habot-Wilner Z, Pacheco P, et al. Intraocular methotrexate in the treatment of uveitis and uveitic cystoid macular edema. Ophthalmology 2009;116:797–801.
[50] Pepple KL, Nguyen MH, Pakzad-Vaezi K, et al. Response of inflammatory cystoid macular edema to treatment using oral acetazolamide. Retina 2019;39(5):948–55.
[51] Whitcup SM, Csaky KG, Podgor MJ, et al. A randomized, masked, cross-over trial of acetazolamide for cystoid macular edema in patients with uveitis. Ophthalmology 1996;103: 1054–62 [discussion: 1062–3].
[52] Deuter CM, Gelisken F, Stubiger N, et al. Successful treatment of chronic pseudophakic macular edema (Irvine-Gass syndrome) with interferon alpha: a report of three cases. Ocul Immunol Inflamm 2011;19:216–8.
[53] Maleki A, Aghaei H, Lee S. Topical interferon alpha 2b in the treatment of refractory pseudophakic cystoid macular edema. Am J Ophthalmol Case Rep 2018;10:203–5.
[54] Butler NJ, Suhler EB, Rosenbaum JT. Interferon alpha 2b in the treatment of uveitic cystoid macular edema. Ocul Immunol Inflamm 2012;20:86–90.
[55] Deuter CM, Koetter I, Guenaydin I, et al. Interferon alfa-2a: a new treatment option for long lasting refractory cystoid macular edema in uveitis? A pilot study. Retina 2006;26:786–91.
[56] Plskova J, Greiner K, Forrester JV. Interferon-alpha as an effective treatment for noninfectious posterior uveitis and panuveitis. Am J Ophthalmol 2007;144:55–61.
[57] Fardeau C, Simon A, Rodde B, et al. Interferon-alpha2a and systemic corticosteroid in monotherapy in chronic uveitis: results of the randomized controlled BIRDFERON study. Am J Ophthalmol 2017;177:182–94.
[58] Missotten T, van Laar JA, van der Loos TL, et al. Octreotide long-acting repeatable for the treatment of chronic macular edema in uveitis. Am J Ophthalmol 2007;144:838–43.

Sheridan
Hanover, PA USA
September 6, 2019